D. M. Butler

D0131289

Helping Couples Change

THE GUILFORD FAMILY THERAPY SERIES
Alan S. Gurman, Editor

Helping Couples Change: *A Social Learning Approach to Marital Therapy*
RICHARD B. STUART

In Preparation
The Family Therapy of Drug Addiction
M. DUNCAN STANTON, THOMAS TODD, AND ASSOCIATES

Normal Family Processes
FROMA WALSH, EDITOR

The Process of Change
PEGGY PAPP

The Practice of Theory in Family Therapy
LARRY CONSTANTINE

Growth of a Therapist: Selected Works of Carl Whitaker
JOHN NEILL AND DAVID KNISKERN, EDITORS

Contemporary Marriage
HENRY FRIEDMAN, CAROL NADELSON, AND DEREK POLONSKY, EDITORS

Ethnicity and Family Therapy
MONICA MCGOLDRICK, JOE GIORDANO, AND JOHN PEARCE, EDITORS

Parent–Adolescent Conflict
ARTHUR ROBIN AND SHARON FOSTER

Depressed Families
DAVID RUBINSTEIN

Helping Couples Change

A Social Learning Approach to Marital Therapy

Richard B. Stuart
UNIVERSITY OF UTAH SCHOOL OF MEDICINE

FOREWORDS BY

Carlfred Broderick
UNIVERSITY OF SOUTHERN CALIFORNIA
AND

Alan S. Gurman
UNIVERSITY OF WISCONSIN

The Guilford Press
New York

© 1980 Richard B. Stuart
Published by The Guilford Press, New York
A Division of Guilford Publications, Inc.
200 Park Avenue South, New York, N.Y. 10003

Printed in the United States of America

Fourth Printing

LIBRARY OF CONGRESS CATALOGING IN PUBLICATION DATA

Stuart, Richard B.
  Helping couples change.

  (The Guilford family therapy series)
  Includes bibliographical references and indexes.
  1. Marital psychotherapy. I. Title. II. Series:
Guilford family therapy series. [DNLM:
1. Marital therapy. WM55 S932h]
RC488.5.S78   616.89'156   80-21949
ISBN 0-89862-604-8

A C K N O W L E D G M E N T S

Any work of this nature must be the product of the creative genius of many theoretitians, philosophers, researchers, and clinicians. I have attempted to acknowledge the specific contributions of the hundreds of seminal thinkers whose work is reflected in the techniques described herein. I would like to single out for special mention just a few of those whose impact upon my thinking has been especially profound. Mr. Jay Haley has been perhaps the most tireless and productive of those who foresaw the prominence of family relationships in the etiology, maintenance, and change of human behavior. Drs. John W. Thibaut and Harold H. Kelley developed a powerful language for analyzing the molecular components of social interaction in general, providing a means of free movement between understandings of dyads of all descriptions, from married to stranger pairs. Dr. Albert Bandura offered what amounts to a pragmatic philosophy of human behavior, one that truly recognizes the reciprocally determined centers of organization and control of human behavior. The late Dr. George Kelly presented a means of making order of human cognitions as they predict and guide behavior; while few specific references will be found to his work, his notion of "constructs" underlies many of the propositions to be found in this work. While the work of many researchers identified with behavior modification have played a role in shaping this effort, two have had a particular influence: Dr. Gerald R. Patterson offered a model of empirically derived practice that has provided guidance for me for many years; and Dr. Todd Risley has offered a comparable model for the creative use of quantified observation of the social world. Finally, many writer–therapists have helped to shape the logic presented here. These include such distinguished colleagues as Dr. Carlfred Broderick, Dr. David Olson, Dr. Don Jackson, Dr. Nathan Hurvitz, Dr. Clinton Phillips, and Dr. Paul Watzlawick.

Thanks are also due to a number of people on a more immediate level. All of the ideas presented in this volume were at least tested with if not derived from my interactions with over 1000 distressed couples seen over a 20-year period in sites as far apart as Manhasset, New York,

Ann Arbor, Michigan, Salt Lake City, Utah, and Vancouver, British Columbia. Without the input of these couples, this book could never have been written. Special thanks are also due to Dr. George Levinger, who carefully read and commented on the first draft, and Dr. Alan Gurman, who offered the same help with the penultimate draft. While the responsibility for all the flaws that remain in this volume rest with its author, many others were mercifully found in time to be corrected by these colleagues at the Universities of Massachusetts and Wisconsin. Mrs. Elaine Bennet offered encouragement and edited, typed, retyped, and retyped again the varied drafts of this manuscript. She did the work of editor, lexicographer, bibliographer, ally, and typist and deserves much of the credit for the actual production of a submissible final manuscript. Special thanks are also due to Mr. Seymour Weingarten, who as editor and publisher had the vision to cultivate the production of this effort and whose sure hand helped to make it a much more readable and potentially productive book.

My most important and heart-felt acknowledgment is rightfully addressed to my sons, Jesse, Toby, and Gregory. Without being asked, they were put in the position of giving up over a year of skiing, hiking, and other deserved and expected contacts with their father, who spent time, instead, closeted with his books and typewriter. I can never repay this lost time, but at the very least I would like to dedicate this book to them and offer my hope that in some way this work may help them to carve out new and productive options for their future years.

RBS
Salt Lake City, Utah

F O R E W O R D
by Carlfred Broderick

It has always seemed curious to me that while the neighboring fields of sex and family therapy have from the beginning been dominated by the contributions of a handful of strong, charismatic personalities, this has never been the case in the field of marriage counseling. Of course, there have been pioneers, such as Paul Popenoe, Emily Mudd, and Abraham Stone, but to my knowledge, none of these established an approach that has taken their name or inspired discipleship. Almost without exception, the handbooks and manuals in the field have been "eclectic" in the most dishwatery sense of that word, republishing articles from practitioners with minipassion on minisubjects. There have been some bright spots, of course. Don Jackson, in collaboration with William J. Lederer, published a marvelous little book on the dynamics of the marital dyad, *Mirages of Marriage,* but it was not aimed at the professional practitioner, and it never became the centerpiece of any particular therapeutic approach.

A number of books on the communication aspects of couple dynamics have attracted some disciples (for example, Bach & Wyden, *The Intimate Enemy,* 1969, or Miller *et al., Alive and Aware,* 1975). It has been generally acknowledged, however, that these approaches are too limited in scope and too rigidly formalized to serve as a general model for marital therapy. More promising is the recent work of Jacobson and Margolin (1979), which outlines a systematic behavioral approach to the treatment of marital problems.

But my nomination for the first entry in the charismatic-marriage-therapist sweepstakes is Richard Stuart. I am hopeful that this long-awaited publication of his philosophy and methods will attract followers and critics and make a general stir in the profession. It may be that the style of the book is not sufficiently self-proclaiming or fast-moving for that effect. Stuart is a philosopher and a scholar as well as a therapist, and it is clearly imperative to him to get into print his basic value premises and logical assumptions as well as his therapeutic approach.

He emerges as a committed behaviorist who is nevertheless in touch with the power of cognitive reframing, a theorist whose concepts are tempered by systematic research as well as by clinical experience, but most of all as a man rich in ideas. In my opinion no one since Jackson and Lederer has captured the realities of pair dynamics so well.

F O R E W O R D
by Alan S. Gurman

It was not very long ago that the field of psychotherapeutic practice once known as "marriage counseling" was described by many observers as "a technique in search of a theory." Actually, even that characterization was unduly optimistic since, as recently as the 1960s, there were few techniques that were specific to the treatment of couples. Then, what the field lacked in technical and theoretical substance was perhaps temporarily compensated for by the perseverance, if not the passion, of its advocates. Less than two decades ago, marital and family therapy could really offer therapists little more than a sort of broad philosophical "mind set" about the nature of suffering and growth in intimate relationships.

Marital and family therapists had enough problems to deal with in fighting for their place in the therapeutic sun, so that attention to getting their own houses in order was historically out of the question. At about the same time, the professional politics of psychotherapy at least as severely constrained the development of *behavioral* intervention with couples and families. Indeed, it was not until the decade of the 1970s that behavior therapy, generically speaking, became widely accepted among the major mental-health disciplines.

Moreover, the two most revolutionary (in the Kuhnian sense) movements in the mental health field since Freud's break with Victorian social thought were emerging quite independently. The odds of these two rebels forming a coalition against the prevailing forces of individual treatment and closed-system psychodynamicism must have appeared slight even early in the last decade: behavior therapy had emerged from academic psychology, and family therapy had, in large measure, been the product of creative maverick psychiatrists; these were not a pair of eligibles who were likely to consummate a lasting relationship.

But now the tides have shifted and the shoreline of psychotherapy will never look the same again. Increasingly, it is becoming accepted— and, in the fields of both family therapy and behavior therapy, championed—that what goes on between (and among) people is at least as important to consider for effective therapeutic planning as what goes on within them. Unfortunately, with rare exceptions, the convergence of the behavioral and family approaches has been fostered by few influential contributors to either field.

It is within this historical context that Richard Stuart's important book enters the scene. In these pages the reader is exposed to four Richard Stuarts! Stuart the social philosopher–theoretician, Stuart the empiricist–scholar, and Stuart the master clinician. Each of these Stuarts deserves to receive acclaim for "his" contribution. But the fourth Stuart is simply awesome: Stuart the integrator of years of clinical experience, clear-headed theorizing, and empirical evidence. Thus, this is a rare and landmark contribution to family therapy that will captivate and stimulate both the most vigorous of family scholars and the most pragmatic of family clinicians. And yet, there is an implicit humility in Stuart's contribution: his ideas are presented not with the evangelistic fervor that is often found in the *magnum opus* of one of the most creative minds in the field, but simply with an abiding confidence in the power of his therapeutic approach to produce change. Unlike many leaders in the field of psychotherapy, Stuart is able to put his case before the reader without ever succumbing to the ever-present temptation and opportunity to disparage alternative points of view.

More than any other contributor to the field of marital and family therapy, Stuart has both revealed explicitly the philosophical and value underpinnings of his treatment approach and presented a truly substantive linking of social psychological knowledge and clinical intervention. Even more concretely, Stuart offers an unusually clear model of the sequential stages of the therapeutic experience through which couples must progress if meaningful and durable clinical change is to occur. In addition to the obvious value of such a sequential approach for training purposes, this model should facilitate the research investigation of the essential components of the proposed treatment method to an extent matched by few other existing methods of psychotherapy, be they relationship-focused or individual-focused.

Finally, while I suspect that Stuart would not endorse the idea, I have found in my own practice that several of his specific techniques can be smoothly and effectively integrated into work with couples that is generally guided by a very different set of theoretical assumptions about marital relationships and marital change. For this reason as well as others, some of which I have mentioned, this book is certain to stimulate a great deal of attention and perhaps even controversy. It is a milestone in the continuing evolution of marital and family therapy.

PREFACE

It has taken over 20 years of practicing, studying, and teaching marriage therapy to gather the data and the temerity to write a text on this subject. Why now rather than 10 years hence? Because two commentators recently wrote, "Most therapists are about as poorly prepared for marital therapy as most spouses are for marriage" (Prochaska & Prochaska, 1978, p. 1), and I realize that, if true, this is not a condition that we need allow to continue. Indeed, I believe that the treatment philosophy, strategy, and tactics described in this book have matured to the point at which they can be cogently described and productively applied by clinicians with widely divergent ideologies and commitments.

I have endeavored to make this book different from most others in the vast clinical literature. Because I realize that there is far more myth than research underlying many therapists' clinical practice, I have attempted to explain the empirical basis for all the treatment recommendations that I can support. Where documentation is lacking, it is because I could find none, and readers with a research bent may wish to conduct studies in one or more of these areas. Because I realize that therapy is more productive when therapists thoroughly understand and are committed to the tools of their trade, I have provided detailed rationales for all of the major recommendations in this program, beginning with a justification of the very practice of marriage therapy and ending with the logic of an independently conceived program to maintain therapeutic gains. In addition, because I realize that therapists can successfully instigate changes in their clients' behavior only when their behavioral prescriptions are precise, I have taken pains to offer a step-by-step guide to the implementation of the therapeutic program found herein. I believe that these three objectives stand in rather sharp contrast to most of the books clinicians read—books that proffer their wares on the basis of faith rather than research, that assume but do not earn readers' commitment to the program, and that offer treatment techniques in hazardously global and nonspecific terms. It is my hope that the field is ready to receive a volume that is distinctive in these important ways.

Beyond these dissimilarities in form, readers will also find in this approach a number of points of difference with the content of conventional wisdom. Together with all of my contemporaries, for example, I was taught the nostrum that "Every individual is unique and this uniqueness must be understood if treatment is to succeed." Acceptance of this belief has meant that most clinical writers devote twice as many pages to the categorization of client distress than to its relief, with the result that fact gathering occupies much more of the traditional therapist's time than behavior-change efforts. I have come to realize that we are more alike than different, and that the process of relieving marital distress is generic, so that treatment can be offered as an action program, with significant change being accomplished in the very first session. I was also taught that I should "start where the client is." This led me, and many of my peers, to allow the client to direct the flow of therapy—in effect, putting the sickest person in the room in charge of the restorative process. During the intervening years I have learned that clients are the experts on the goals and content of their relationship, but they are miserable failures at developing a technique for achieving those goals. Accordingly, the treatment described herein is one in which the therapist plays a very active executive function and assumes proper responsibility for directing the ebb and flow of therapeutic events. As a third example, I was taught that every client gains more from the process of forming a therapeutic relationship with a caring professional than from any specific activities of the professional. I have since learned a countertruth, that "Love is not enough." Married couples enter therapy not in search of genuine change, but more often in search of a confederate who will help each learn to hold himself or herself blameless while pointing an accusing finger at the other. A benevolent, caring therapist is needed to help each person learn to accept responsibility for change in the interaction, but this major shift in perspective will come about only when the therapist bets more heavily on the deployment of technological skills than on being an accepting friend. These are just a few of the clichés that have been challenged in this book, some of which have been accepted, some of which have been rejected, and most of which have been qualified and refocused. As a result of these differences in form and content, I hope that readers will find here a somewhat innovative approach that will truly be a new learning experience.

I have tried to offer a "soup-to-nuts" package for marriage therapists, beginning with pretreatment assessment forms and presocialization audio tapes for clients' use, moving through an orderly series of behavior-change maneuvers to the development of materials intended to help clients maintain the gains achieved as a result of therapy. I am unaware of any other program that offers comparable supports, and I am pleased with these materials as a beginning-level effort. I am also painfully aware of the risks inherent in producing a program such as this. Some readers may spot flaws in the logic of this approach that were never obvious to me; others may find items presented as original (i.e., not documented) when earlier writers may have made the points both sooner and better. In addition, assumptions that I may have taken for granted and presented briefly may be very open to question for some readers and therefore may require much more detailed explication. Worst of all, however, is the risk that by the time the printer's ink has dried on these pages, I may have uncovered new beliefs or evidence that undermines some of the recommendations made in this book. I have had this experience more than once in the past: for example, when I became aware of the frivolity of *quid pro quo* contracts or the "direct" treatment of obesity upon learning that "this-for-that" exchanges are overly fragile and that the sources of the urge to overeat must be corrected before clients can be successfully taught eating-management techniques. For these reasons I hope that readers will approach this material with an open mind; that they will permit themselves to challenge some of the assumptions they have previously held dear; that they will give full consideration to the approach presented here; that they will incorporate into their own belief systems and practice those principles and practices they believe will be useful; and that they will stand as ready as I am to set these new beliefs aside when better ideas come along: they always do!

RBS
Salt Lake City, Utah

CONTENTS

Helping Couples Change

C H A P T E R 1

Why Treat Troubled Marriages?

COUPLES ENTERING THERAPY often present themselves as having major doubts not only about whether their own marriage is worthy of continuance, but also about whether the very institution of marriage is worthy of maintenance. In order to provide clients with the motivations needed to mobilize their efforts to improve the quality of their interaction, it is important for therapists to have a clear understanding of the current state of marriage. Therefore, this chapter reviews some of the facts that describe the rate of marriage formations and dissolutions. This review shows that we continue to marry at a fairly stable rate but that divorce rates are essentially on the rise. A number of explanations for the rising divorce rate are offered: explanations ranging from the fact that demographic factors create a large pool of available young women to the fact that society may now favor switching rather than fighting. The chapter then reviews some rather surprising statistics on the differential physical and psychological health status of the married and various currently unmarried populations. This review shows that on balance, both men and women who are married hold a clear edge in some very basic departments over those who have terminated their marriages, as well as a slight edge over the never-marrieds. While these parametric data do not permit individual predictions with confidence—that is, some who continue in marriages might fare worse than some who terminate—these data do point out some unexpected and sobering probabilities. With these facts available, therapists may be able to help client couples gain a perspective of both their own situation and the general trend in marital distress. The chapter then concludes with an overview of the intervention program that comprises the remainder of this volume.

Hardly a day passes without the media reminding us that marriage and family living as we know them today are in a state of rout. We are reminded that the divorce rate is rising beyond the top of the charts. Books describing alternative relationship forms are snapped up by the seeming hordes of despairing couples seeking "another way." The professional literature also extols the virtues of "single blessedness" (M. Adams, 1976; Stein, 1975), or voluntary childlessness (Veevers, 1975), or nonmonogamous (Knapp, 1975, 1976) and network marriages (Murstein, 1977; Ramey, 1975), and of communal living (Conover, 1975; Smith & Smith, 1974). Time and again storytellers offer sagas of couples bursting forth from troubled marriages, passing through brief transitional times of self-discovery, and then moving more or less happily ever after into fulsome new relationships or enlightened independence. News sources, nonfiction writers, professional researchers, and novelists alike all conspire to dampen our enthusiasm for marriage and weaken our faith in its very survival.

Marriage therapists working with clients experience yet another barrage of negative press about marriage. Our clients rarely enter therapy with a strong commitment to marriages that they hope to enrich. Much more often they ask for our help in resolving an intense ambivalence about staying together. They describe mixed feelings born of the realization that their relationships are habitually conflictual (the only sparks generated by dehumanizing thrusts and parries) or burned out (no sparks at all, although neither has given serious thought to leaving) or terminal (with both partners so much more involved in activities outside their relationship that their marriage is less important than virtually everything else in their lives). With these themes as counterpoints to the media blitz, it is small wonder that many therapists question the wisdom of applying their skills to the task of helping couples stay together.

The Facts

We live in a time of very rapid change. A recent issue of *Current Population Reports* (U.S. Department of Commerce, 1978) contains the following observations of the American population in 1977:

- The number of marriages (2.2 million) fell to only twice the number of divorces (1.1 million).
- Since 1970 the number of identified cohabitating adults rose 83%, to 1.9 million.
- For the first time the percent of 18- and 19-year-old women enrolled in college exceeded that of men (36% vs. 33%).

· Since 1970 the adjusted gross income of men has declined 4% on a constant dollar basis, while that of women has risen 9%.

These and other dramatic social changes that are not yet reflected in the statistician's broad brush strokes are clearly making a major impact upon the fabric of our society, and the survival of the hallowed institutions of marriage and the family is being questioned by professionals and lay people alike.

And yet, despite the adverse press concerning the slim chance that those marrying will find blissful relationships, and despite the fact that ever-increasing numbers of young and old alike are choosing to live together without marriage (Clatworthy, 1975; Cox, 1970), all but a very small percentage of those asked continue to express their avowed intention to marry sooner or later (Levinger & Moles, 1976; Rubin, 1973). For example, in a recent survey conducted by the Louis Harris organization and reported in the *New York Times* on January 23, 1979, it was found that fully 84% of a projectable national sample of men aged 18 to 49 considered family life "very important." In a hierarchy of values for daily life they ranked family life fourth behind health, love, and peace of mind, and ahead of work, friends, respect for others, education, sex, religion, and money, in that order.

Because marriage and family living continue to be highly valued, it should not be surprising that recent reports indicate the rate of marriage has been very stable for more than a century. In the year 1867, 9.6 adults per 1000 married (National Center for Health Statistics [NCHS], 1973b), while in the 12 months ending in January 1980, 10.6 adults per 1000 married (NCHS, 1980). It has been estimated that all but 3% or 4% of the adult population will marry during their lifetime (Carter & Glick, 1976; Glick & Norton, 1973; P. H. Jacobson, 1959), with almost all of us who can marry eventually doing so.

While the rate of marriage has essentially remained constant, divorce rates have plodded ahead, advancing by leaps and bounds in the last 15 years. Consider the following: In 1867 there were 0.3 divorces per 1000 adults. This figure touched 1.0 per 1000 in 1912; it reached 2.0 per 1000 in 1940; it passed 3.0 per 1000 in 1969; it hit 4.0 per 1000 in 1972; and it touched 5.3 per 1000 in 1979 (NCHS, 1973b, 1978b, 1979a). These statistics can be translated into more human terms when it is recognized that:

· While 70% of the 1969 marriages were "primary marriages" (i.e., those in which both bride and groom were marrying for the first time), the percentage fell to 59 by 1976 (NCHS, 1979b).
· Among those couples married in 1950, one-fourth were divorced by their 25th anniversary; one-fourth of the 1952 marriages were divorced by their 20th year; one-fourth of the 1958 sample parted

by their 15th year; and one-fourth of the 1965 sample withdrew their vows by the 10th year of their marriages (NCHS, 1979a).
· It has been estimated that while 20% of the ever-married women born between 1920 and 1924 will divorce, 38% of those born between 1945 and 1949 will do so (Glick & Norton, 1973).

While the rate of growth in divorces has slowed somewhat at the time of this writing (i.e., it has declined from an average annual growth rate of 11.5% between 1967 and 1973 to increases of 2%–4% in recent years [NCHS, 1979b]), in absolute numbers an ever-increasing number of men and women join the ranks of the formerly married. During the 12 months ending in January 1980, an estimated 1,169,000 divorces were granted, directly touching the lives of 2,338,000 adults (NCHS, 1980) and an estimated 1,194,000 children (NCHS, 1978b). Thus in one year alone enough adults were granted divorces to replace the entire population of cities the size of Baltimore, Boston, Cleveland, Dallas–Fort Worth, Houston, Minneapolis–Saint Paul, or Pittsburgh. Add the children, and only six metropolitan areas have populations greater than the number immediately affected by divorce in the single year of 1979.

Not only in the United States will roughly one-third of all adults (Glick & Norton, 1973) and children (Glick, 1975) experience marital or parental separation; similar although slower trends are found in virtually all Western nations (NCHS, 1970, 1978c). The forces that motivate couples to part are therefore clearly not unique to one country and may be endemic throughout the industrialized nations of the world.

The duration of marriage prior to divorce has fluctuated widely around a general average of 7.0 years (NCHS, 1973b), ranging from a low of 5.8 years in 1950, as hasty World War II marriages were dissolved, to a high of 8.3 years in 1900, perhaps reflecting the joys of the warmly regarded 1890s. Analysis of one cohort of divorcees showed that 23% divorced after less than 2 years of marriage; 16% divorced after 2–4 years of marriage; 24.6% divorced after 5–9 years of marriage; and 36.4% divorced after 10 or more years of marriage (NCHS, 1978c). Thus, roughly one-fourth of all couples who divorce believe that they discovered the awful truth almost before the sound of "Oh, Promise Me" has faded, while others learn that even a decade or more of sharing their daily bread is no guarantee that they will still be together during their graying years.

Those most likely to divorce are the young, the less well educated, and the poor (Carter & Glick, 1976; NCHS, 1973a, 1978b; U.S. Department of Commerce, 1973). The average age of divorcing men is 33.1 years, while their wives average 29.8 years of age (NCHS, 1978b). Some 32.3% of the divorcees in one cohort were childless, while 61.1% had at least one child under 18, and 6.6% had children, all of whom were 18 or older (NCHS, 1973a). Finally, the previously mentioned report (NCHS, 1978b) revealing that the average age of divorcing men was 33.1 years, and of divorcing women, 29.8 years, clearly shows that both have ample opportunity to try again.

Norton and Glick (1976) estimate that about 80% of those who divorce will make another try if their separation took place while they were young adults: the divorced are more likely to remarry than the widowed because the former tend to be younger than the latter; men are more likely than women to remarry; and those without children have better remarriage prospects than those who are parents (Thornton, 1977a). The U.S. Bureau of the Census (1976) projects the following time line for divorcing and remarrying Americans: they will stay in their first marriages for an average of seven years; they will enjoy their new-found singlehood for an average of only three years before remarrying; and they will remain in their second marriages for an average of five years, if it is destined to end in divorce. Rather than fleeing from marriage, divorcees born during the 1940s remarried after an average of only 1.9 years, while those born at the turn of the century waited an average of 6.3 years to make their second try (NCHS, 1973b).

While it is true that second marriages are twice as likely as first marriages to end in divorce (NCHS, 1978a), current evidence suggests that the two relationships tend not to differ markedly in the levels of marital satisfaction enjoyed by the partners (Glenn & Weaver, 1977). Rather, as Hunt and Hunt (1978) have suggested, remarried couples may be more likely to divorce simply because they tend to see divorce as the best response to the inevitable strains of married life. Messinger (1977) has suggested that with adequate preparation, second marriages can be helped to be very stable and satisfying encounters.

Some Interpretations

Many explanations have been offered for the rising divorce rate, whether in first, second, or even later marriages. For example, it has been suggested that modern marriages last longer than the marriages of yesterday. Carter and Glick (1976) speculated that death may have done to turn-of-the-century marriages what divorce does today. Discordant with this view, however, are the facts that marriages were ended long before death would have ended them, even in the days before sterilization, sewage, and penicillin, and that changes in longevity are more attributable to progress in controlling infant mortality than to success in extending life during the later years (NCHS, 1978b). Therefore, it cannot really be said that marriages today are more likely than marriages of the past to outlive their potential.

As another explanation, Glick (1975) believes that many people divorce simply because they failed to marry the right person rather than because of any defect in the institution. He wrote:

A certain amount of divorce undoubtedly grows out of the fact that the supply of acceptable marriage partners is very often quite limited and those who would be the most ideal partners never meet, or if they do, they may do so at the wrong time or become unavailable to each other at the optimum time for marriage. In other words, marriage partners are typically joined through a process of chance, often involving compromise, and if the compromise element is substantial, there should be no great surprise if the marriage is eventually dissolved by permanent separation or divorce. In view of the haphazard manner in which the important step of marriage is generally undertaken, and in view of the many frailties of human adults, the surprise may be that the proportion of marriages that last—to a happy (or bitter!) end—is as large as it is. (p. 22)

In addition to citing the less than ideal manner in which we generally decide to marry, Norton and Glick (1976) also ascribed some of the prevalence of divorce to the naive expectations that newlyweds have for the relationship they are entering. They note that modern-day couples expect to be each other's best friends as well as sharing the burdens of meeting the challenges of daily living, rearing children, and coping with the ravages of aging, while our forebears expressed little expectation of the first of these, using their energies to surmount the latter hurdles. Many writers call attention to the dangers of unrealistic marital expectations. For example, Cadwallader (1966) considers foolish the belief that men and women can love each other for life, while Arensburg (1960) considers utterly ill advised any attempt to concentrate so much procreative, emotional, and instrumental energy in a single relationship that as often as not is consummated under far less than ideal conditions. And Mead (1949) perhaps upstaged all of our contemporary cynics by writing 30 years ago that:

The American marriage ideal is one of the most conspicuous examples of our insistence on hitching our wagons to a star. It is one of the most difficult marriage forms that the human race has ever attempted, and the casualties are surprisingly few considering the complexities of the task. (p. 342)

Beyond the belief that it lasts too long and that it is inadequate to meet the burdens placed upon it, others have argued that marriage as an institution has suffered from the relaxation of the laws that bind partners together. However, the rates of divorce in "fault" and "no-fault" states are not markedly different (NCHS, 1973a; Wright & Stetson, 1978), although the change in laws most certainly reflects a shift in values from stigmatization of the divorced to viewing the one-time-married as a breed apart (Glick, 1975; Norton & Glick, 1976; Levinger & Moles, 1976).

Demographics can also reveal two "squeeze" phenomena that might force the divorce rate upward. The baby boom of World War II produced an unprecedented number of marriage-eligible women whose availability may have induced older men to leave their care-worn wives in favor of a fresher start (Norton & Glick, 1976). In addition, a sharp rise in out-of-wedlock pregnancies may have induced many to marry who would and perhaps should have gone their separate ways (Norton & Glick, 1976).

Finally, divorce may be a self-perpetuating phenomenon in several ways: An increase in divorces leads to the freeing of men and women to form new relationships, thereby inflating the opportunities for remarriage by the still-married group (Gunter & Johnson, 1978). Also, the probability is great that parents who divorce transmit to their children a view that divorce is a reasonable way to respond to marital crises, thereby increasing the chances that the children will divorce (Levinger & Moles, 1976; Pope & Mueller, 1976). The flood of divorced women entering or reentering the job market has made women a major pressure group for equal rights in employment. As they succeed in opening up opportunities for women to have more interesting and better-paying jobs, fewer women find it necessary to marry for economic reasons or to stay in their marriages to enjoy financial security (Glick, 1975; Norton & Glick, 1976).

What conclusions can we draw from this welter of observations? It is clear that most people still marry and that when their marriages fail they seek remarriage with increasing speed. Married is therefore what most American adults would like to be. It is also true that a combination of demographic and cultural forces strain the stability of modern marriages. While some of the forces that weaken marriage are intensifying (e.g., an increasing number of children living through their parents' divorce and likely also to divorce), others are changing. Among the positive changes is the fact that as the children of the post-World War II baby boom are being absorbed, the age of first marriage is increasing and the awareness of its limitations is becoming more realistic (e.g., Carter & Glick, 1976; NCHS, 1978b; Harris poll as reported in the *New York Times* and cited above). Therefore, on the basis of the cold, hard facts alone, it is clear that marriage as we know it is here to stay, for another generation or two at least, so therapists can and should work on enhancing and preserving marriages, as we have done for years.

The Impact of Divorce

The acid test of the wisdom of divorce can be found only in an assessment of its effects. In approaching this analysis, however, it is important to stress the fact that parametric or group data can point to general trends but cannot be used to predict the experience of any single individual in the group. Thus, while it will be shown below that divorce and separation have devastating effects on most of those who move apart, many individuals thrive in the new freedom of separated living. For example, divorce is believed to have diverse advantages for both men and women, including (1) a freedom from domestic routines; (2) an opportunity to rear children without the opposition of the other parent; (3) freedom from conflict with a troubled mate; (4) an opportunity to control one's own resources and life space; and (5) opportunities to make personally fulfilling choices without constraint through the need to consider the wishes of others (Brown *et al.*, 1976; Hetherington *et al.*, 1976). But divorce is very far from an unmixed blessing, as the following findings show.

Many reviewers have found that the health of divorced, separated, and widowed adults is inferior to the health of those whose marriages remain intact (e.g., Carter & Glick, 1976; Martin, 1976). Table 1 summarizes some of the findings of a major national survey undertaken by the National Center for Health Statistics (1976). It can be seen, controlling for age, that those who are married fare much better than those who are divorced, separated, or widowed on almost all categories. On some parameters singles do a little better than those who are married, but the researchers point out that their lower rate of pregnancy helps to reduce their rates of physician contact and short-stay hospital admissions.

Even more compelling data are presented in Table 2, which draws from several investigations. There it can be seen that married respondents have (1) lower mortality rates; (2) lower suicide rates; (3) lower rates of victimization through homicide; (4) lower rates of fatal auto accidents; and (5) decreased morbidity due to coronary diseases and cancer of the digestive organs, among others. Indeed, Kraus and Lillienfeld (1959) estimated that the ratio of age-adjusted mortality rates for the single, widowed, and divorced populations, relative to those still married, were 1.47, 1.46, and 1.84, respectively. These Johns Hopkins researchers concluded that divorced men pay a higher penalty for their action than do wives.

How can we explain the fact that, for example, each 1% increase in the divorce rate appears to be associated with a .54% increase in the suicide rate (Stack, 1980)? While some people clearly respond to divorce

Table 1. Age-adjusted rates of illness, disability, and use of medical services of adults age 17 and over by marital status for years 1971-1972[a]

Marital status	Incidence of acute conditions per 100 persons/yr		Restricted activity days/yr		Number of physician visits/yr		Number of days of hospitalization/yr	
	Male	Female	Male	Female	Male	Female	Male	Female
Married	157.8	188.8	16.2	18.9	4.4	6.6	12.9	8.0
Never married	149.5	176.4	17.0	17.2	3.8	5.3	11.9	8.3
Divorced	164.2	245.8	25.6	26.6	4.8	7.6		
Separated	—	247.1	27.3	33.3	5.3	7.4	11.9	8.3
Widowed	—	151.2	26.2	28.7	—	6.7		

[a]National Center for Health Statistics, *Differentials in health characteristics by marital status: United States, 1971-1972.* Bethesda, MD: Vital and Health Statistics, Series 10, No. 104, 1976.

Table 2. Age-adjusted rates of death from varied causes of adults aged 17 and over by marital status

Marital status	Mortality from selected causes (standardized rates for whites)[a]		Suicide (age-adjusted p/100,000)[b]		Victim of homicide (age-adjusted p/100,000)[c]		Death from auto accidents (standardized as % of rate of married persons)[d]		Death from coronary disease (p/100,000)[e]				Death from cancer: digestive organs (p/100,000)[e]			
									White		Nonwhite		White		Nonwhite	
	Male	Female	Male	Female	Male	Female	Male	Female	Male	Female	Male	Female	Male	Female	Male	Female
Married	100	100	18.0	5.5	8.6	3.0	100	100	176	44	142	83	27	20	42	25
Never married or single	134	130	33.2	7.7	16.3	3.2	155	103	237	51	231	112	38	24	62	33
Divorced or separated	221	144	69.4	18.4	39.2	10.6	371	328	362	62	298	113	48	23	88	35
Widowed	145	145	78.4	10.7	48.2	13.2	411	442	275	67	328	165	39	24	90	41

[a] National Center for Health Statistics, *Mortality from selected causes by marital status: United States, 1959–1961.* Bethesda, MD: Vital and Health Statistics, Series 20, No. 8, 1970.

[b] National Center for Health Statistics, *Suicide in the United States, 1950–1964.* Bethesda, MD: Vital and Health Statistics, Series 20, No. 5, 1967.

[c] National Center for Health Statistics, *Homicide in the United States, 1959–1961.* Bethesda, MD: Vital and Health Statistics, Series 20, No. 6, 1967.

[d] Unpublished data, National Center for Health Statistics. Cited in: H. Carter & P. C. Glick, *Marriage and divorce: A social and economic study.* Cambridge, MA: Harvard University Press, 1976.

[e] H. Carter & P. C. Glick, *Marriage and divorce: A social and economic study.* Cambridge, MA: Harvard University Press, 1976.

as a joyful liberation (Renne, 1970, 1971), others react to the experience of marital dissolution as though they had lost their only chance for happiness in this life. Lynch (1977) sees the loneliness that follows divorce as its major negative impact. Gilder (1974) considers the loss of future orientation suffered by divorcees as their major cross to bear, while Durkheim (1966) believes that in the loss of marital ties, divorcees lose their best defense against unrestrained self-interest, which leads ultimately to suicidal behavior. Still other writers (e.g., Gibbs, 1969; Maris, 1969) believe that the disorientation suffered by divorced persons may significantly undermine their life hold. Whatever the explanation, it is clear that devastatingly large numbers of divorced persons turn to suicide as what they may believe to be their only alternative to a lifetime of depression (Lester & Lester, 1972).

If they do not end their lives, divorced persons have a significantly higher rate of mental disorders than their married counterparts, as seen in some (Bachrach, 1975; Blumenthal, 1967; Briscoe & Smith, 1974), but by no means all (e.g., Porter, 1970), studies. Research reported in Table 3, however, shows clearly that when mental health differences do surface, they show the power of a tidal wave during a tropical typhoon, with risk rates of the formerly married exceeding those of the married by as much as 20-fold in certain categories.

Divorced men seem to suffer economically as well as emotionally and physically. The U.S. Bureau of the Census (1970) has shown that the average annual incomes of married men were significantly greater than those of men who were separated, divorced, widowed, or never married. The same study did find, however, that the annual incomes of divorced women were greater than the incomes of women who were still married, a finding at least partly attributable to the fact that more divorced than married women are employed full time. Overall, Morgan (1973) reported that family disruption resulted in an income loss on the order of 33% or more for men and some 16.5% for women. So great is the economic consequence of divorce that Gilder (1974) concluded his review of the statistics with the observation that divorce is a stronger correlate of poverty than is race.

In summary, it is clear that broad trends greatly favor the continued health and well-being of those who sustain their marriages. As suggested at the start of this section, divorce may be a liberating experience for two people who would have suffered emotionally, physically, economically, or otherwise had they remained together. But it can also signal the start of a gradual process of deterioration on these and other dimensions, with freedom bringing the potential for disaster much as it carries with it a hope for nirvana. Unfortunately, the marriage therapist cannot tell by looking at a couple whether either or both will prosper or

Table 3. Age-adjusted rates of admission to psychiatric outpatient clinics and to mental hospitals of adults 17 and over by marital status

| Marital status | Admissions to psychiatric outpatient clinics (p/100,000)[a] | | Admissions to state and county mental hospitals (p/100,000)[a] | | First admissions to mental hospital in Pueblo, Colorado—by disorder[b] | | | | | |
| | | | | | Functional psychosis | | Neurosis and psychosomatic | | Personality disorder | |
	Male	Female	Male	Female	Male	Female	Male	Female	Male	Female
Married	276.0	423.2	133	125	15.3	26.6	109.1	224.2	174.2	38.0
Never married	806.3	743.0	439	242	44.3	39.5	205.6	346.0	165.3	54.4
Divorced	1365.6	1621.7	2168	759	131.0	91.1	294.9	432.8	1408.9	227.8
Separated	310.9	286.3	2976	1066	0	59.7	81.1	99.5	365.0	39.8
Widowed	2653.8	2834.5	630	249	391.6	79.4	1436.0	111.1	3655.4	555.6

[a]R. W. Redick & C. Johnson, *Marital status, living arrangements and family characteristics of admissions to state and county mental hospitals and outpatient psychiatric clinics, United States, 1970.* Rockville, MD: National Institute of Mental Health, Statistical Note 100, 1974.

[b]B. L. Bloom, *Changing patterns of psychiatric care.* New York: Human Sciences Press, 1975.

die should they separate. Discussion of some of these sobering facts may, however, help the couple to consider more realistically the potential gains and losses that may be realized in the event they do decide to head in separate directions.

How Do the Children Fare?

Many couples still stay together for the "good of the children." Therefore, it is appropriate to ask whether the children gain or lose when parents remain together or go their separate ways.

Many studies have shown that when parents function poorly together, their children often pay the price through higher rates of deviance (e.g., Bugental & Love, 1975; Bugental et al., 1977; McPherson, 1970; Schuham, 1972). Haley (1969a) has speculated that when parents are in conflict, each is likely to bid for the support of one or more of the children in an effort to form a coalition against the other parent. This creates a climate in which the rules generated by each parent conflict with the expectations of the other, one in which rules are inconsistently enforced, and one in which the children often test the limits of the family system in upward-spiraling misbehavior. Therefore, intervention aimed at promoting consensus between the parents is a must, and the failure to promote parental agreement may be far more detrimental to the children's well-being than living in a single-parent home.

Bane (1976) has estimated that from 34% to 46% of the children of the 1970s will spend some portion of their first 18 years with single parents. She estimated that 2% of these children will be born out of wedlock; 20%–30% will experience their parents' divorce: 3%–5% will experience their parents' long-term separation; and 7%–9% will lose either or both parents through death. In this context, however, it should be noted that life with a single parent is only a brief transition for many of the children of divorce, because their parents either remarry or establish marriagelike relationships that reestablish a two-parent household.

As will be shown in Chapter 3, the presence of children appears to have an adverse effect upon the parents' satisfaction with their marriage (e.g., Glenn & Weaver, 1978; Hetherington et al., 1976, 1977). Other researchers have also shown that some children function better after divorce because many of the children's difficulties can be traced to their parents' distress (e.g., Hetherington, 1972; McDermott, 1970; Pemberton & Benady, 1973; Wallerstein & Kelly, 1976). These adjustment problems have been related to the financial hardship experienced by the custodial parent, to low rates of parent–child interaction as the custodial parent struggles to make ends meet and to construct a new social life (Shinn, 1978), and to the absence of parents of both sexes as models for the young (Olson, 1970). It has been noted, however, that many of these studies lack adequate controls, draw upon biased samples, and address the wrong questions (e.g., Herzog & Sudia, 1971; Brandwein *et al.*, 1974). For example, delinquency is more likely to be found among the children of broken homes (e.g., Monahan, 1957; Siegman, 1966; Silver & Derr, 1966), but so too is poverty, and it, rather than family dissolution, may best predict the children's delinquent acts. Moreover, many problems are found in children living in troubled yet intact homes. Therefore, those in single-parent families may hold a decided edge where certain problems are concerned (e.g., Johnson & Labitz, 1974; Nye, 1957; Oltmans *et al.*, 1977; Rice, 1975; Schneiders, 1965).

It can thus be said in conclusion that while parents seem to pay a high price for divorce, it is not clear that children do the same. With these findings in mind, marriage therapists should find encouragement for efforts to heal the hurts of conflicting parents, but they need not necessarily struggle to keep the warriors together in the interests of the young. While many a couple will stay together "to save the children," the therapist should be aware that the children of single parents are not necessarily worse off than the children of two parents, and they may, in fact, be even better off.

In light of these results, what should we as therapists do? We can work hard to help couples stay together, or we can use our talents to help them part with greater ease. Voices from the radical women's movement would have us free women from the ravages of "unholy matrimony" (e.g., Balogun, 1971; Bernard, 1972; DeBeauvoir, 1971; Tanner, 1971). And yet it has often been found that the psychological benefits of marriage are strong enough to outweigh its stressful consequences in the balance of positive and negative effects (Glenn, 1975), as many studies show that married women enjoy a sense of well-being often not equaled by the never-married or formerly married group. Moreover, there seems to be a phylogenetically determined drive to "pair-bond" (Ardrey, 1966) as we, in concert with other higher animals, choose a mate and defend our choice against all challengers. Even where communal living is encouraged, as in kibbutzim, women take the lead in forming family units (Tiger & Shepher, 1975). Therefore, the tide seems to flow in the direction of marriage and familism, and efforts to improve troubled marriages move *with and not against* this tide.

The existence of a stable marriage has many benefits (Purcell, 1976). It helps partners to carve out and to maintain a stable personal identity. It provides a foil for screening perceptions and motivations to improve their quality. It seems to enhance personal, professional, and social living and to reduce the pain of many physical and emotional stresses (Bloom *et al.*, 1978). It is also clearly very much the national choice, as shown by one national survey (Institute of Social Research, 1974) which concluded that "Marriage and family life are the most satisfying parts of most people's lives and being married is one of the most important determinants of being satisfied with life" (p. 4).

Clearly, marriage is not a bed of roses. There are weaknesses in the institution in both the general and the particular. Marriage therapists can use their expertise to try to remedy some of the flaws in the cultural conceptions of marriage just as we can use our skills to help individual couples to improve their marital experiences. By the same token, two-parent families are not necessarily better than single-parent families, and we can use our skills to try to help both family forms to reach their goals.

Our science falls far short of equipping us to look at troubled couples and determine which can and which cannot make major and dramatic changes. Indeed, we have all experienced the unexpected, with some "bright-prospect" couples never showing change, while other "impossible" combinations leave our office with very much improved marriages. Therefore, the best that we can do is to begin helping each couple plan and carry out changes in the way they treat each other, then to evaluate the personal meaning of these changes so that they can decide intelligently whether to stay together or to move apart. We can achieve these goals by guiding our clients' efforts to (1) assess their own contributions to their marriages, good and bad; (2) formulate plans for change; (3) develop the skills to reach these goals; and (4) learn how to harvest the data from these personal experiments as supports for future actions. Accordingly, the approach taken in this book makes the general assumption that marriages can be vital, alive, and productive; it also assumes that only the couple can tell whether their relationship can fulfill the hopes they shared when they spoke their vows; and it assumes that these judgments can be made wisely only when concerted efforts have been made to improve the quality of the couple's interaction.

Outline of the Approach That Follows

In Chapter 2 will be found an overarching rationale for marriage therapy. This chapter begins by prompting therapists to clarify their values. It then offers three philosophical pillars for the present technology: from philosophical humanism comes respect for the individual's freedom in the context of a predictable environment; from operationalism comes justification for limiting the language of the method to testable and verifiable terms; and from positivistic idealism comes a recognition that change in relationships is possible only if the individuals are willing to act *as if* their goals were within reach. This chapter then reviews the theoretical contributions of systems theory, social exchange theory, and interactional psychiatry. Systems theory lends an appreciation of the role of information flow in selecting and maintaining organizational direction. Social exchange theory affords a language of investments and returns for understanding reinforcement as the lifeblood of all encounters, and together with systems theory, it points up the threats to relationship stability inherent in the fact that each party always has the option of alternative encounters. Finally, interactional psychiatry contributes the conception of balance in relationships mediated by the intermeshing of rules that structure the ways in which each person can invest in and receive returns from an encounter, whether it is stable or changing. Taken together, these varied points of view help to formulate a philosophy of marriage and a rationale for its management when stresses are encountered.

Chapter 3 builds upon the theories presented in Chapter 2 and offers a strategy for relationship management. The theoretical approach adopted in this volume can best be described as one representing an expression of social learning theory. The essential elements of this theory are described, as are the three basic tactics of behavior change that it generates. The social-learning-theory approach is shown to be one that embraces nearly all aspects of operational theories of behavior, whether the data are expressed as thoughts and feelings or as overt behaviors, with each of these primary elements significantly impacting upon the other and all playing a role in every instance of human behavior. Techniques for changing expectations and relabeling experiences are offered as means of modifying thoughts and feelings, with both seen as fundamental to the techniques offered for changing behavior. In turn, suggestions are made for the modification of behavior by first changing small daily molecular behaviors and then changing the larger interaction patterns that are the molar units of human interaction.

Marital assessment is discussed in Chapter 4, where it is shown that the quality and rate of many different behaviors, in light of the context of their occurrence, affect the level of commitment to the relationship felt by both partners. A multitrait, multimethod approach is taken to the description of the partners' behaviors and reactions to their marriage, rather than simply relying upon diagnosis to classify their interaction patterns. Assessment in this sense is intended to provide data useful for planning and evaluating marriage therapy. To aid these processes, specific recommendations are made for instruments that measure the partners' level of affect, their goals and resources, their reactions to treatment, and the general impact of therapy upon their personal, parenting, and work performance.

In Chapter 5 is found a review of the essential characteristics of the approach taken here. These treatment methods depend upon an action-oriented, conjoint, ahistorical, time-limited strategy of goal attainment. To achieve these characteristics, the intervention must be highly structured. Specific recommendations are made to prepare clients and therapists alike to move easily into this structured exchange. The skeleton of the treatment structure is provided by the goals of therapy aimed at positive change through positive influence techniques. The therapist is cast in the roles of model, educator, and facilitator of change through a master contract, one form of which is presented. The other forms found in this chapter provide a systematic means for planning intervention techniques and for monitoring progress in cohorts of couples. The chapter concludes with recommendations for adapting these tools for use with special client groups.

The "caring-days" technique described in Chapter 6 is advocated as a method both of demonstrating to each spouse that change is possible and of giving them an opportunity to request and to offer changes that will help each to build more commitment to their relationship. When successful, caring days can generate significant changes in the details of the couple's daily interaction during the first seven days of therapy, a very firm foundation upon which to build subsequent suggestions for change.

Chapter 7 deals with what for many therapists is the *sine qua non* of relationship treatment: communication change. A somewhat novel approach is taken in this chapter, however, based upon a careful reading of the social science literature, which suggests that *planned rather than complete communication* is the lifeblood of human encounters. Therefore, the program suggested here calls for training the partners in listening skills, in the ability to make carefully planned self-statements, in the ability to make requests constructively, in the ability to give and receive feedback, and in the ability to clarify the messages that have been received in order to improve understanding.

Behavioral contracts are the subject of Chapter 8, for they are the means through which couples can be helped to achieve their major objectives. The contractual model presented here is "holistic," not the *quid pro quo* contract that has often been suggested. Accordingly, the partners are asked to exchange items from lists of desired behaviors, with each free to choose how and when he or she will opt to do things that please the other.

More generalized strategies for planning the core elements of the interaction are discussed in Chapter 9, which is aimed at building the partners' problem-solving skills. This chapter recognizes that the planning of concerted action requires each person to have a clear idea of the limits of his or her authority. Therefore, the "powergram" form is presented as a means of helping the spouses to identify the relative levels of authority that each has and would like to have for making decisions in major areas of their lives. Based upon these data, the couples can be helped to design a model for predicting who will have both the freedom and the responsibility to make decisions in each of the areas. Some decisions will be made mutually, others unilaterally upon consultation with the spouse, and still others will be made separately by one spouse or by the other. As is shown in the chapter, an equality of areas is less important than an equitable distribution of authority as seen by both partners. The chapter concludes with a realistic review of the steps that the couple can be helped to take in meeting the challenges they face.

With these various skills under their belts, the couple should have experienced a marked diminution in the level of their conflict. Chapter 10 is aimed at building their skills for coping with those conflicts that still persist. The chapter recognizes three degrees of conflict: first-degree conflicts are issue-specific; second-degree conflicts escalate to attacking the other person; while third-degree conflicts move further to attacking the core symbols of the relationship. On the assumption that a clear victory is a loss all ways, the chapter presents a rationale for a two-winner model of conflict resolution and then goes on to suggest a series of guidelines adapted to a stage concept of conflictual behavior.

Chapter 11, written by Drs. Freida Stuart and D. Corydon Hammond, codirectors of the Sex Therapy Unit in the University of Utah School of Medicine, presents a detailed description of techniques used for the management of sexual problems. It has been recognized for many years that distressed couples complain of problems in their sexual interaction almost as often as they complain about difficulties in their social exchanges with one another. "The other woman" was the most common complaint in a study of help-seeking marriage therapy clients in the 1950s (Turner, 1954), followed by "nagging." Levinger (1966) found "sexual incompatibility" ranked with in-law trouble in the sources of marital distress cited by male divorce applicants. DeBurger (1967) analyzed the content of letters sent to the American Association of Marriage and Family Counselors (now Therapists) in search of guidance. He found that an overwhelming 42.1% of those sent by men expressed concern with sex, while among women, 31.0% cited problems with affectionate relations and 20.6% noted sexual difficulties. Finally, in a study completed in the 1970s (Bentler & Newcomb, 1978), it was again found that sexual concerns placed high among the concerns of distressed couples. Therefore, marriage therapists should be able to understand and, ideally, to offer service to couples presenting complaints about their sexual interaction.

Clifford Sager (1976) has noted that "sex therapy and marital therapy deal with different aspects of the same entity and are almost always clinically interrelated" (p. 555). The bedroom is the arena in which many couples play out the drama of the joys and discord of their waking hours. Sex requires openness and therefore vulnerability. It is the essential expression through which many people test their masculinity and femininity. It is the powerful expression through which many partners test one another's love. For all of these reasons, sex is both the consequence and the cause of the full panoply of marital interactions (Meisel, 1977).

When couples entering either marriage therapy or sex therapy have been contrasted, it has been found that both groups seek changes in both the social and sexual aspects of their interaction. For example, Frank et al. (1976) found that "the overall frequency of sexual difficulties was quite similar in the two groups," while "the couples seeking sex therapy seemed to be experiencing considerable marital discord" (p. 560). They found, for example, that 75%–80% of the women seeking sex therapy complained of "difficulty in reaching orgasm," "inability to have orgasm," and "difficulty maintaining excitement." An average of 57% of the women requesting marriage therapy had the same complaints. Among men, "ejaculating too quickly" was the main complaint of both the sex therapy and the marriage therapy samples, followed by "difficulty in maintaining an erection" for the former and "disinterest" for the latter. In the social sphere, 52% of the sex therapy applicants and 69% of the marital therapy group expressed "difficulty discussing problems" as a principal concern. In the same vein, 46% of the sex therapy group and half of the marital therapy group expressed the feeling that "spouse does not fill emotional needs." It is therefore clear that the two populations present many of the same characteristics, the principal differences being that those seeking sex therapy:

> seemed to be more comfortable with one another, less conservative in their outlook, and more thoughtful in their approach to their life and their problems. In general, the sex therapy patients were happy with their spouse and involved in basically affectionate relationships, whereas the relationships of the marital therapy couples were characterized by antagonism. (Frank et al., 1976, p. 561)

Because of the greater risk-taking and therefore greater trust demanded by sex therapy, it is recommended here and elsewhere (e.g., Kaplan, 1974; Meisel, 1977; Sager, 1974, 1976) that sexual difficulties be addressed *after* relationship skills have been assessed and developed, if needed, to promote that level of trust in one another that is required for successful participation in sex therapy. The techniques that will then be described for sex therapy naturally derive from the pioneering work of Masters and Johnson (1970) and Kaplan (1974), but they include some very special adaptations that are the unique contributions of Hammond and Stuart, who produced these chapters.

It is hoped that clinicians will either develop sex therapy skills themselves through participation in any of a number of evolving training programs, or that they will at least become sufficiently knowledge-able about sex therapy to be able to prepare clients for referral to trained sex therapists.

Finally, in Chapter 12 readers will find a discussion of techniques that can be used to maintain the changes induced by the treatment. For this presentation a review of the major assumptions underlying the treatment techniques explained throughout the book is offered. Maintenance is still the stepchild of all intervention approaches, and the recommendations made in this chapter are tentative and in need of testing. They are presented here, however, in an effort to stimulate the therapist's attention to this critical problem as well as, hopefully, to offer some useful action recommendations.

The materials presented in this volume offer a detailed description of one carefully developed approach to marital treatment. With the assessment materials described in Chapters 4, 9, and 11, and the audio-cassette tapes described in Chapters 5 and 12, those wishing to use the basic social-learning-theory approach to marriage therapy will have all of the materials they need. No effort has been made in this volume to deal with such important issues as means of adapting the approach to those situations in which either or both spouses present severe behavior disorders or to the integration of marital therapy into efforts to manage the behavior disorders of children. These, and issues like them, are extremely important and require volumes exclusively allocated to each topic. Therefore, the basic approach is fully described here, but readers will have to turn elsewhere to find discussions of their adaptation to special situations.

As it is the responsibility of all professionals to remain sensitive to the data of their own experiences and those generated by others through the media of publications, workshops, and other training activities, it is hoped that readers who are influenced by this book to modify some aspects of their practice will do two things: they are strongly advised to monitor continuously the impact of their use of these techniques; and they are urged to open themselves to learning about still other alternative programs so that they can constantly compare this one with others, choosing those elements of all points of view that yield the most lasting positive therapeutic approaches. Our clients deserve no less than our highest level of thoughtfulness in selecting treatment approaches and our highest level of skill in delivering the techniques that we have chosen.

C H A P T E R 2

Values and Philosophy in Selecting Marital Therapy Goals and Methods

ALL HUMAN INTERACTIONS are guided by the values and philosophies of the parties concerned. Values and philosophies determine those aspects of our experience that we label as events, the meaning we ascribe to these events, the way in which we plan from our experience toward selecting and achieving our goals, and the manner in which we evaluate the success of our collective efforts. While generally the concern of ethicists and philosophers, none of us can act independently of our values and philosophies, even if they are not explicit. Unfortunately, despite the ethical and moral responsibilities of professionals to control personal biases in offering human services, these biases are rarely made explicit; therefore, this chapter begins with a framework for identifying values basic to the practice of marital therapy.

It is a given that every therapist operates from a value base. It is also a given that each professional must identify his or her value premises in order to protect clients from unwarranted value-based interventions. In this sense, values are regarded as essentially neutral. However, it is positive to become aware of value premises and to inform clients about the nature of value-governed interventions just as it is negative to inflict upon clients such values as the belief that divorce is bad (or good), that employment of wives and mothers is harmful (or helpful) to family stability, or that intimacies with other partners hinder (or help) marital stability.

After suggesting a means of discovering one's values, this chapter concludes with a detailed explanation of one of the philosophical traditions that is basic to the treatment approach found in this volume. Philosophy is to intervention theory what values are to the practitioner's actions: it provides shape and meaning to what otherwise might be a heterogeneous potpourri of treatment techniques. While such traditions as philosophical humanism lend to social learning theory its belief in the capacity of humans to be the arbiters of their own fates, and pragmatic philosophy lends its stress upon the role of experiential data in planning human behavior, it is the postulates of idealistic positivism that provide a unique rationale for efforts to change human behavior. This approach suggests that we all act on incomplete knowledge of the probable outcome of our acts; that is, we act "as if" we had the power to make safe and accurate predictions of the events that will follow from our actions. When clients formulate negative assumptions and act as if they were valid, they freeze themselves in the pain of their distress. Conversely, when they can be helped to make positive assumptions and change their actions accordingly, they are free to make great strides forward in their lives. This philosophy of "as if" therefore provides the basis for that optimism and trust that must precede any attempt to alter the course of human behavior.

The chapter then concludes with an exploration of three theoretical traditions that have helped to shape the current state of social learning theory. Systems theory provides a means of understanding the way in which information helps to shape, maintain, and change social interactions. From it is developed a strong rationale for heavy reliance upon communication patterns utilizing positive feedback. Social exchange theory provides for predicting constructive changes to occur as the result of therapeutic efforts to evoke a broader range of positive actions by each spouse. Because behavioral science has produced no better means of overcoming problematic behavior in open social settings than the generation of positive actions that are incompatible with the negatives, the facilitation of positives is viewed as the single most powerful tool available to the therapist. Finally, the interaction approach developed principally at the Mental Research Institute is cited as a useful basis for conceptualizing marriage therapy goals. This bellwether group has identified the cardinal significance of metacommunications inherent in all nonverbal and verbal actions as means of defining, adhering to, or changing the basic, implicit rules that guide all behavior of every couple. Rule identification and change, when necessary, stand as capstones in the hierarchy of the goals of marital therapy.

Value Bases of Therapeutic Practice

Whether we are private citizens or professionals, every action that we take originates from and is evaluated within the context of our values. Values may be institutional to the extent that they are conveyed through formal or informal teaching in family, school, work, community, and religious settings. They may also be idiographic to the extent that they are inferred from personal experience. We all tend to describe our own actions in lofty value terms that are sometimes close to and sometimes far from reality. Cynics often argue that values are readily sacrificed to the pragmatics of self-interest, but even such sacrifices are value-governed. Indeed, we cannot act independently of our values; values influence the way we label our experience at the hands of others and the way we plan our reciprocating acts; and our efforts to find meaning in the diverse experiences of our lives are mediated by our values.

Skinner (1953, 1971) believes that "shoulds" and "oughts" have no place in scientific discourse, and that the real meaning of these prescriptions and injunctions can be found only in the consequences of each set of actions. Others, however, believe that a theory of values is essential as a means of predicting and thereby potentially redirecting important classes of behavior. While Skinner (1953) has argued that science is and must be neutral, Einstein (1950) wrote that "Scientific statements of facts and relations, indeed, cannot produce ethical directives" (p. 127). He then argued that values must be brought to the scientific process, whether at the level of determining which problems to study, which methods to use in these investigations, or how, when, and where to apply the results of the process of discovery. Indeed, it was the readiness of scientists to set value considerations aside that led to the atrocities so painfully unveiled during the Nuremberg trials. Therefore, value considerations must be operative in every application of the methods of science and the knowledge so produced, and application of the principles of behavioral science in human service operations is no exception to this moral imperative.

THE NATURE OF VALUES

Rokeach (1973) has defined values as "an enduring belief that a specific mode of conduct or end-state of existence is personally or socially preferable to an opposite or converse mode of conduct or end-state of existence" (p. 286). Anthropologists (e.g., Kluckhohn & Strodtbeck, 1961) have noted the great similarity among the superordinating value orientations found in diverse cultures, perhaps expressing a universal dimenison in all of humanity's efforts to cope with the puzzles of life and death. These broadly accepted notions have a cognitive conception that addresses a belief in the desirable, an affective component that is elicited when values are accepted or challenged, and an action component that signals behaviors considered congruent or incongruent with the value.

We may have values that prescribe either the means or the ends of our actions (Hilliard, 1950; Kluckhohn & Strodtbeck, 1961). In either case, values guide us in efforts to make discriminations among alternative courses of actions as well as to differentiate ourselves from others. Values that prescribe means provide the basis for professional norms (Williams, 1968), while values prescribing ends contribute to attitudes toward all facets of society (Rokeach, 1968). Professional norms are hierarchically organized (Maslow, 1959) and relate to a series of beliefs about all phases of the therapeutic enterprise. For example, while we all treat our clients as though we have ready answers to fundamental questions about our values, we seldom take the trouble to state them. Below are just some of the scores of beliefs that stem from values in the daily activities of every marriage and family therapist. Each reader should complete the following statements and pause for a moment to investigate how influential each of them is to his or her practice:

1. I believe that a good marriage has the following characteristics . . .
2. I believe that the stress that weakens marriages can best be explained by . . .
3. I believe that marriage has the following functions in today's world . . .
4. I believe that when married people have inconsistent desires which tend to result in conflict, each should . . .
5. I believe that the best way to be of help to distressed couples is . . .
6. My beliefs about social and sexual contacts outside the marriage are . . .
7. My beliefs about the maintenance of marriages that may not offer the range of satisfactions desired by both spouses are . . .
8. My general beliefs about divorce are . . .
9. When real conflicts exist between spouses' personal desires and the demands of their relationship, I believe that the issue should be decided by . . .

Try to determine what contributions each of the following sources of values has made to your belief systems:

1. Your personal experience in the same or similar situations.
2. Your religious views.
3. Your sense of the times, of the social patterns in each of these areas.
4. Your recall of the behavioral science and of theoretical writings in support of each belief, taking care to identify specific sources to guard against replacing a professional data base with an amalgam of the first three sources.

In point of fact, virtually all of us would have extreme difficulty in both stating and supporting the beliefs that are fundamental to the daily practice of our profession.

In our defense, answers to questions like these require soul-searching inventories of our personal, religious, social, and professional values. Knapp (1975) has recently shown that marriage counselors do own up to holding strong values about such client behaviors as extramarital sex. She found, for example, that 28% of the counselors whom she surveyed personally approved of sexually open marriages, and that 43% would be supportive of this arrangement for their clients. In contrast, only 13% approved of and 23% would support recreational swinging. Interestingly, one of the best predictors of these counselors' reactions was their personal experience. Therefore, in the interest of protecting clients from any unwarranted intrusion of the therapist's values into their own deeply meaningful decisions, every client has the right to expect the therapist to state his or her own value judgments in the context of the questions that are asked (every question expresses a point of view) and the instigations offered. For example, the therapist might say, "I believe that sexual contacts outside of marriage potentially weaken commitment to the marriage. Now it is important for us to explore whether your experiences of this sort contribute to or detract from your willingness to be giving to one another in the most productive of ways." While value statements such as these offer no fail-safe protection for clients, they do put both the therapist and the clients on notice of the possible direction of value-governed influence attempts, and these help to limit any unwanted ill effects of clinical influence, for the client is then free to abort one therapeutic encounter in an effort to establish a potentially more productive (for him or her) therapeutic relationship with another clinician.

Basic Elements of a Treatment Philosophy

A general treatment philosophy influences every therapeutic decision, whether governing the selection of who will and will not be offered help, the goals of the service rendered, the techniques used to achieve the established goals, and the criteria by which therapeutically mediated changes are evaluated.

Many of the current therapies draw some of their philosophical bases from the assumptions of philosophical humanism, a branch of contemporary American philosophy that strongly recognizes the capacity of humans to change creatively (Lamont, 1949). The more operational philosophies, such as the operant approaches, also draw their respect for the value of data as the basis of human reason from pragmatism and operationalism (Burtt, 1946). The social-learning-theory approach draws some of its uniqueness from a third philosophical tradition, idealistic positivism, a "school" in name only, for it boasts but a single adherent, a German philosopher named Hans Vaihinger, whose chief activity took place during the first two decades of the 20th century. His outstanding achievement was a single volume, *The Philosophy of As-If*, written in 1877 but not published in German until 1911 and not in English until 1924. Reference to his work is rarely seen (exceptions are the writings of H. Ellis, 1923, Sahakian, 1968, and Wolf, 1951); and yet his beliefs are consistent with basic notions in the development of the philosophy of science and are at the core of this and other successful programs of therapeutic behavior change.

The work of Vaihinger can be traced to several sources. Bentham contributed the notion that certain words like "right" are fictional yet needed because discourse would be impossible without them. Stammler contributed the belief that nature can never be known directly, but instead can be apprehended only through the medium of ideas. Windelband conceived of philosophy as the science of values in logic, ethics, and aesthetics—opening to philosophers the full sweep of human experience. Schiller contributed a distaste for monistic philosophy that relied upon one-fact explanations and thereby opened to pragmatic philosophers the full sweep of the study of values and aesthetics. Finally, Vaihinger expressed positive values in opposition to Schopenhauer's fatalism. For Vaihinger, human beings had an unlimited potential for change, while, in sharp contrast, Schopenhauer had written: "Who can enjoy life who has seen into its depths!"

Vaihinger's contribution to this approach lies in his appreciation of the role of fiction in all productive human thought. A fiction is a belief that we treat *as if* it were true even though its validity may not yet have been established. He believed that without use of fictions, we could never move beyond present experience in formulating a vision of the future; indeed, that we could not ever change our experience in daily living. He also viewed the principle of *as if* as something basic to all social institutions. For example, he recognized that some crime is situationally induced, and he believed that other criminal acts are willful and capricious. He asserted that society had to treat all criminals *as if* their crimes were willful in the absence of a preponderance of evidence to the contrary. He thus extended his philosophy to applications beyond the province of the logician and the physical scientist. While not making specific reference to the role of conditional thinking in social situations, James (1948), at the turn of the century, offered the following parable:

A whole train of passengers (individually brave enough) will be looted by a few highwaymen, simply because the latter can count on one another, while each passenger fears that if he makes a movement of resistance, he will be shot before any one else backs him up. If we believed that the whole carful would rise at once with us, we should each severally rise, and train-robbing would never even be attempted. There are, then, cases where a fact cannot come at all unless a preliminary faith exists in its coming. (p. 105)

James thus believed that all cooperation requires all parties to act *as if* the others share their goals. A shared willingness to take the risks implied by such an assumption is at the core of all collective action.

Later, George Kelly (1955) recognized the psychological application of this principle, while not tracing its origin to Vaihinger. In his "fixed-role" therapy, Kelly asked his clients to act *as if* they did not have the problems that distressed them. For example, the shy college student was instructed to act *as if* he were self-assured when he approached girls on campus, and the depressed husband was asked to act toward others as though his depression were under control. This same instigation underlies all of the now-fashionable assertive therapies. Also, other approaches relying upon *in vivo* counterconditioning are premised on the therapist's success in reassuring the client to act *as if* the feared event would not follow his or her actions.

The same principle is fundamental to all attempts to promote change in marital and family behavior. Distressed family members often complain that their feelings of love for the others have died. They plaintively ask therapists to help restore those treasured feelings before they begin, anew, loving behaviors toward their mates. But feelings of love can grow only through interaction with the other; therefore, the key to relationship change is that the love-lost client must act toward the other *as if* loving feelings were alive and well, for only then will the other's loving actions be stimulated—actions that can truly support our client's love for his or her mate. Therapeutic behavior change of every sort is therefore seen to depend upon the therapist's skill in encouraging the client's willingness to reach beyond reality and to summon the willingness to act *as if* the world were a welcoming place, for it must remain the forbidding place it is believed to be until these new behaviors occur.

As another plank in this platform of therapeutic change, the principle of *as if* also offers a temporary resolution of the problem of determinism versus free will. "Determinism" is a belief that "claims that everything that happens happens necessarily and in accordance with some regular pattern of law" (W. T. Jones, 1975, p. 422); "free will" adopts the doctrine of contingency, which asserts that events do not occur in any necessary or predetermined chains. Philosophers have recognized that individuals sometimes do things that appear to be quite random (an attack upon determinism) and yet there is a clear orderliness to human behavior (an attack upon free will).

The therapist must come to terms with these opposing doctrines. If all behavior is determined, then treatment can hardly be expected to produce change, unless, perchance, its outcome were foretold as well.

But if all behavior were the result of free will alone, then the therapist could hardly be expected to have an impact upon the client's actions. If full weight were given to these opposing viewpoints and therapeutic action was delayed until the issue was resolved, such action would be a long time coming. Therefore, the principle of *as if* comes into play again.

Applying the principle without so naming it, James (1948) has advocated that we plan our actions *as if* we were free to make the necessary decisions, and *as if* our behavior were sufficiently determined to make our causal hypotheses and predictions of outcome plausible guesses. In this way the therapeutic enterprise can go forward before the final resolution of the determinism–free-will issue, which has been a concern since the dawn of our civilization.

SUMMARY

The philosophy underlying the treatment approach in this book can be traced to varied traditions. Philosophical humanism provides an appreciation for the potential for change in all areas of human striving. Pragmatism and operationalism provide their respect for the data base essential to all scientifically responsible therapeutic ventures. As perhaps the strongest and most unique tradition, however, idealistic positivism provides a rationale for the willingness to venture into the unknown through actions as if the journey will be rewarded. Every therapeutic approach draws upon philosophical assumptions such as these. It is only through making them explicit that the values which guide the approach can be formalized for the review that must be ongoing. Having stated the more fundamental philosophical assumptions in this approach, it is now time to turn to a review of some of its basic theoretical assumptions. These fall into two categories: theories of relationships and theories of behavior change.

Theory in the Practice of Marriage Therapy

Values and philosophy, as described at the start of this chapter, provide part of the context in which decisions are made about therapeutic theory and practice. With regard to the theory resulting from these considerations, viewpoints are polarized in some extreme and absurd ways. First, some have argued that there is no theory of marriage and family functioning (e.g., Feidman, 1976; Floyd, 1976) and that the field basically relies upon merchandising clichés and part theories rather than attending to the business of theory development and testing. On the other hand, others, like Wolberg (1965), have noted a trend toward theoretical orthodoxy that contains the potential of stultifying professional growth. He wrote, "What seems like the truth of today may be the exploded myth of tomorrow" (p. 356). Second, some well-known writers and researchers (e.g., Cashdan, 1973; Gomes-Schwartz, 1978; Rice *et al.*, 1974; Sundland & Barker, 1962; Wallach & Strupp, 1964) believe that theory is irrelevant to practice. For example, Stieper and Wiener (1965) contended that "there is little evidence that 'schools' of therapy or type of training have significant effects on the effectiveness of psychotherapy" (p. 63), while Strupp and others (Strupp *et al.*, 1969) repudiated the senior author's earlier position by finding that "There is substantial evidence that therapeutic changes occur in a broad front and that they are independent of the therapist's theoretical position and professional affiliation" (p. 135). In a third paradox, some writers, like M. Cox (1978) and Roth (1969), argue that it is irresponsible to be anything other than eclectic in approach because no currently available theoretical system can possibly be sufficiently broad to encompass all clinically relevant phenomena; but others have argued that eclecticism is an illustration of theoretical incompetence and a sign of the absence of theoretical rigor. As an example, Watzlawick *et al.* (1967) have pointed out the following situation, in which they feel that diverse theoretical approaches are utterly inconsistent:

> If the foot of a walking man hits a pebble, energy is transferred from the foot to the stone; the latter will be displaced and will eventually come to rest again in a position which is fully determined by such factors as the amount of energy transferred, the shape and weight of the pebble, and the nature of the surface on which it rolls. If, on the other hand, the man kicks a dog instead of a pebble, the dog may jump up and bite him. In this case the relation between the kick and the bite is of a very different order. It is obvious that the dog takes the energy for his reaction from his own metabolism and not from the kick. What is transferred, therefore, is no longer energy, but rather information. In other words, the kick is a piece of behavior that communicates something to the dog, and to this communication the dog reacts with another piece of communication-behavior. This is essentially the difference between Freudian psychodynamics and the theory of communication as explanatory principles of human behavior. As can be seen, they belong to different orders of complexity; the former cannot be expanded into the latter nor can the latter be derived from the former; they stand in a relation of conceptual discontinuity. (p. 29)

If theory exists and if it has the requisite blend of specificity and eclecticism, it is still not clear that its application has a significant impact upon therapeutic behavior and outcome. With some recent exceptions (e.g., Sloane *et al.*, 1975; Tuma *et al.*, 1978), traditionally cited studies reached the conclusion that experience has a stronger effect upon practice than theoretical orientation. For example, despite their theoretical orientations, Fiedler (1950, 1953) found that in contrast to inexperienced therapists, those with more years of practice formed closer alliances with their clients. Compared with the inexperienced, more practiced clinicians were also found to be more flexible and less given to extremes (Fey, 1958) and more active and willing to take responsibility for treatment control and outcome. Therefore, it is not clear whether book learning or the effects of many years in the therapist's chair has a greater effect upon clinical practice.

Wile (1976, 1977) has offered an interesting and valuable solution to these various dilemmas. He contended that therapists have both "official" and "unofficial" theories: the former derive from formal training, the latter from experience and general values and philosophies of living. Some therapists and clients subscribe to one or more of the theories of therapeutic change that Wile identified: he believes that change can be ascribed to the therapeutic relationship; to willpower; to catharsis, restitution, and/or revenge; to a bromide theory that minimizes the distress; or to destiny and/or providence. He believes that synchrony between the orientations of therapist and client leads to effective treatment outcomes, while dyssynchrony in these values is cited as the cause of premature terminations and/or poor therapeutic results.

The position taken here can be best stated as a response to each of these apparent paradoxes. First, as noted earlier, it is assumed that every maneuver in life, personal and professional, must be governed by an implicit set of values and an implicit theory of behavior. It is the responsibility of every therapist to explicate and appropriately control his or her biases. Second, it is the responsibility of the therapist to make certain that therapeutic actions are guided in large measure by formal theories as opposed to personal biases. Third, it must be recognized that theories differ in levels of abstaction, in the criteria used for determining the relevance of data, and in the rules of inference through which these data are fed into hypothesis formulation and testing. Therefore, diverse theories may be useful as guides in describing and explaining different aspects of clinically relevant behaviors; but any time two or more theories are used to explain the same phenomena, they must be matched for level of abstraction, data base, and rules of inference. Unfortunately, therapists are apt to slip from theory to theory without regard to these considerations, motivated by convenience and/or the preference of clients for one orientation as opposed to another.

As a further point, it is recognized that experience may guide therapists in learning the inadequacies of existing theories that fail to rise to the challenge of clinical practice. Experience may build their confidence in interacting with clients along the lines of some generally accepted principles of relationship management and behavior change, turning to theoretical language more as a rationale for decisions already made than as a guide in the making of those decisions. Therefore, it is incumbent upon therapists to formalize their master strategies for behavior change, to determine which elements are and which are not compatible with the currently available formal theories, and then to present their approaches to clients as a rationale for the service that is to be offered. The next section presents a language that can facilitate this articulation.

Endler and Magnusson (1976) have identified four broad classes of currently used behavioral theories: trait theory, psychodynamic theory, situationalism, and interactionalism. Trait theory originated in the work of Allport (1937) and Cattell (1950) and is concerned with observing individuals' overt behavior and their responses to pencil-and-paper tests, and using these data to predict future behavior. This is classified as a response–response (R-R) theory. These theories have definite heuristic appeal, but they falter when it is realized that behavior is more likely to vary across diverse situations than to occur consistently, irrespective of situational characteristics (Endler, 1973; see, too, Chapter 4, this book).

Psychodynamic theory is the second approach that is still in wide use. Endler and Magnusson (1976) classified it as a special case of R-R theories and feel that it suffers from the same weaknesses as the broader classificatory approaches: decades of research have failed to provide the support needed for the application of this theory to the task of helping to manage the lives of people in distress. For example, many of the theories in this approach are bidirectional and therefore irrefutable. Homosexual behavior, as one case in point, may be ascribed to overly indulgent or to overly rejecting mothering. In the same vein, savers may be termed "anal retentives," although they may be very free with money on certain occasions. Inference and labeling in the psychodynamic tradition may therefore be considered somewhat capricious, especially when employed by those who have not learned the cautions taught in formal training in the method.

"Situationalism" is the third class of theories identified by Endler and Magnusson (1976). It is illustrated by the work of Skinner (1953) and attributes much if not all of the variance in human behavior to the impact of environmental events that prompt and consequate responses. For example, researchers such as Risley (1977) and Stuart (1972) have explained what is commonly termed "self-control" in terms of delayed, differential social reinforcement for more constructive behaviors. For example, the alcohol-prone individual who passes up a drink so that he or she can later boast to a spouse about this major feat of self-management demonstrates not self-control but a choice between a lesser (alcohol) and a major (attention by a significant other) reinforcement.

These stimulus–response (S-R) theories have been criticized on many grounds. The most telling criticism is that of Kaplan and Anderson (1973), who asserted that social behavior is far more additive than is assumed by S-R theorists. For example, while Byrne and Nelson (1965) argued that the level of attraction between two people is a function of the value of the reinforcements that they mediate for each other, a more sophisticated analysis would show that the values they assign to their exchanges are complex in origin and profound in effect, greatly influencing the cue and reinforcement value in ways not encompassed by a simple functional analysis.

Endler and Magnusson (1976) consider "interactionism," as represented by the work of Bowers (1973), Endler (1973) and Mischel (1968, 1973), the approach to follow because it avoids the unsupported assumptions of R-R and psychodynamic theory and the incompleteness of S-R theory. Bandura's (1977, 1978) "reciprocal determinism," or his belief that all behavior is always reciprocally interactive with the social, physical, and personal environments in which it occurs, is perhaps the essence of this approach. In this S-R—R-S-R-S . . . model, consistencies in human behavior are ascribed to environmental regularities, and yet change in behavior is possible through the expansive use of the human potential for creativity.

The approach taken in this book falls into the broad "interactionalism" category just described. It traces its roots to systems theory, social exchange theory, and the interactional perspective of the Mental Research Institute group, with each of these frameworks being analyzed in the operational terms of the functional analysis of behavior. A brief overview of each of these schools of thought is now in order.

SYSTEMS THEORY

While the Mental Research Institute (MRI) group first called attention to the applicability of systems theory to family description change, the fact that its tenets are the irreducible dimensions of the other programs requires that it be described first.

General systems theory can be traced to the work of Von Bertalanffy (1950, 1968), Wiener (1954), and Ashby (1963), who synthesized the general principles; to Beer (1966), Buckley (1967), Klir (1969), Laszlo et al. (1974), and Ball (1978), who applied the principles to social organization; and to the MRI group and others (e.g., Bate-Boerop, 1975; Murray, 1975), who applied the principles to marriage and family therapy. Simply stated, a *system* is any set of interacting functional relationships that transform inputs into outputs. Every system can be characterized by a *state* or a measurable condition. The state of the system is affected to some degree by the *input and output vectors* and constraints that affect its processes. For a couple some controlled inputs are income, contacts with others, and sought-after activities; some uncontrolled inputs are acts of God, illnesses, and arbitrary changes in the jobs of either spouse.

The *constraints* under which they operate include the availability of other housing or employment, any physical limitations that they might have, or economic or other limitations on their freedom of activity. All of these forces combine to keep the family in a dynamic or ever-changing state as it fashions its outputs such as its size, income, level of health, and related consequences of the interaction.

Open systems are those engaged in a constant interaction with aspects of their environments. Often forces outside the system attempt to have an impact upon the intrasystem state, but this effect is neutralized by an *inertia* that produces a *time lag in response* which softens the response. For example, if all of the couple's friends begin to buy expensive new cars, they may feel some pressure to do so as well, despite their limited resources. During the process of deliberation, however, they may acquire the needed capital. These time lags differ from *time delays*, which are also inertial products. In this instance, however, the effect of the change is swift and dramatic. For example, when the last child leaves home for good and the couple are left with the need to work out a situation in which they must each provide the basic stimulation desired by the other, the changes that they must make are sudden and profound and, in the language of systems theory, are often *"destabilizing."*

The exchange between couples and their environment is accomplished through the process of feedback and feed forward. In *feedback* information about the effects of an action are fed back to the couple. These response-produced data can then be used to plan their next action—a *feed-forward* phenomenon. When negative data are processed as guides, the resulting action is to stabilize the system. On the model of the heat-activated thermostat that turns the furnace on when a negative state is detected (i.e., the temperature has fallen below a preset level), it is suggested that when one spouse tells the other to stop doing something annoying, the interaction can do no more than return to the state that existed before the objectional action took place. Conversely, *positive* data have a destabilizing effect in the sense that they stimulate system change. For example, when one spouse expresses appreciation for actions of the other, these actions can be expected to recur and to be expanded, changing the state of the interaction.

Inertia-produced *stability* can be adaptive to the extent that it allows the system to preserve its identity and inhibits its overreaction; but it can also paralyze the system's ability to adapt to change in the external environment. System functioning tends to be related within upper and lower *boundary limits* that establish the thresholds for change. For example, when the wife tells her husband that his last action was the straw that broke the camel's back, she has told him that his behavior has moved beyond the action-triggering level. Systems theorists have offered two models for predicting this level. Some contend that an *additive* model is useful; for example, a certain number of running days in which he left his dirty laundry on the bathroom floor will trigger action, according to this model. The *multiplicative* model, on the other hand, assumes that inputs have a cumulative effect; for example, the laundry on the bathroom floor becomes a problem only when the husband has been unpleasant at breakfast for a few days, buried himself in the evening newspaper rather than conversing with his wife, and criticized his wife for earning too little money.

Every system maintains some level of equilibrium over the long run, reflecting the operation of a somewhat planful feedback and control process; for example, the wife, angered by the laundry problem, may choose to do nothing lest she trigger an even more unpleasant countermove on her husband's part. To maintain state balance in families, input information must generally flow upward while output information must flow down. That is, the parents must receive information about the children's actions, their own incomes, and relationships with the community, etc., and they must send down constraints and performance demands. This is true because according to systems theory only the highest echelon can have all of the data necessary to make wise planning decisions. This explains—in part at least—the findings reported in Chapter 9 that unclear lines of authority characterize deviant families.

These, then, are the basic elements of systems theory as it applies to marriage and family interaction. The system is seen as a process that undergoes constant change as it adjusts to inputs and fashions outputs in light of the constraints under which it operates. The lifeblood of the system is information that feeds back from the outcomes of its actions so that it can be fed forward into plans for further action. The drama of the living system is its effort to preserve much of its current identity through negative feedback and inertia, while at the same time attempting to adapt successfully to a changing environment that requires it to use positive feedback as a basis for never-ending change.

SOCIAL EXCHANGE THEORY

The social psychological theory that is most compatible with systems theory is social exchange theory. As seen in reviews by Nord (1969) and Simpson (1972), the architects of this view of social relationships as a bargaining process are Thibaut and Kelley (1959), Homans (1961), and Blau (1964), with inputs from the full sweep of the behavioral sciences.

From economics comes the concept of a "*good*"—anything that is sufficiently scarce and valued to motivate one person to give up something else to get it (Homan *et al.*, 1961). Goods can be exchanged for some *generalized reinforcer* like money (Croome, 1956) on a demand curve

(L. J. Friedman, 1962) until an equilibrium point is reached balancing supply with demand. In social relationships the goods are the reinforcements that each person mediates for the other, and social approval (Blau, 1964; Homans, 1961) is chief among these rewards. Demand for these reinforcers is influenced by both their absolute value and their availability in other relationships.

From sociology social exchange theorists have derived the concept of *role:* both a set of expectations of how one should behave (Parsons, 1951) and a set of interactional behaviors (Sarbin, 1954). Applying economic terms to role behavior, Jackson (1957) has shown that one's adherence to role expectations can be plotted according to a "return potential model" in which an optimal behavioral level is determined by offering enough, but not too much, approval. As regards ego's behavior, there is thus a point of maximum potential return for all actions that he or she might take. As regards alter's behavior, however, there is a range of tolerable behaviors that ego might take (Sherif & Sherif, 1956). Together, the expectation of how ego will act, ego's expected level of return, and the span of alter's tolerance of ego's behavior all combine to form a *norm* of their particular interaction. The norm may be general in that it is accepted throughout their community, but whether or not it is general it will affect the interaction between ego and alter in very idiographic ways. For example, the environment in which the couple lives might generally disfavor employment by wives unless the family is in dire straits. But any particular husband and wife are free to define "dire straits" in terms of their own goals; and boredom and loneliness during the day may, for one couple, provide the justification that only extreme economic emergency would provide for another.

Social psychology has contributed two important notions to social exchange theory. The first is the general theory of social comparison (Kelley & Thibaut, 1978), which derives essentially from Helson's (1951, 1959, 1964) concept of adaptation. Consistent with this theory, it is assumed that people constantly scan the range of reinforcement available to them, choosing a path of action that they believe will lead to the greatest level of reinforcement. For example, Jane evaluates her interaction with husband Bob in light of her enjoyment of time with him relative to her enjoyment of time with other people in her life. She will decide to go skiing with Bob if she feels that her enjoyment of his company will be greater than the satisfaction that she forgoes by not skiing with other friends. In this sense, every relationship is fragile to some degree, potentially vulnerable to more apparently attractive encounters with others.

The second contribution of social psychology to social exchange theory is the concept to conformity (Allen, 1965; Hollander, 1960a, b), which is defined as the willingness of ego to yield to alter's pressure for a change in his or her behavior. Ego will make the shift in part because of the influence of group norms (Willis, 1965) and in part in order to ingratiate himself or herself to alter (E. E. Jones, 1964) so as to sustain the relationship. But ego may also "counterconform" (Crutchfield, 1963; Krech *et al.*, 1962), should this alternative seem to offer a greater payoff. For example, Jane is an aggressive skier and Bob tends to be more conservative. Jane may lead off in the run down the hill, with Bob struggling to control his worry in order to sustain her pace. At a certain point in his increasing rate of descent, Bob may decide that safety of life and limb is more important than earning Jane's respect, so he may start to do broader turns, allowing Jane to reach the lift line long before he does. Because of his counterconforming behavior, Jane is then faced with the choice on the next run of slowing her speed, which would mean conformity with his implied request, or continuing to ski fast, which is her counterconforming alternative.

Together these various concepts have fed into a theory of social relationships conceived of as bargaining experiences. Each person is believed to make a *bid* to *invest* certain *resources* in the hope of making a profit. For example, each time Bob tells Jane that he loves her, he is investing verbal commitment in the hope of influencing her behavior and/or feelings in some desirable way. Each such bid, however, also involves actual or potential *costs*. By investing in Jane, Bob forgoes the opportunity to invest in others; and in making any investment, Bob, of course, runs the risk of wasting a resource through its nonreinforcement by Jane. Bob must also face the problem of *diminished marginal utility*, as his resources may lose their reinforcing properties over time through satiation or the loss of their novelty.

A fall in the value of outcomes mediated by a relationship is reflected in the couple's constant measurement of their experience together. Jane has gone back to school and has been stimulated and excited by her work. Her enthusiasm is a dimension that Bob had not experienced before, and he is very pleased with it. Jane's behavior has therefore surpassed his expectations or, in the parlance of social exchange theory, his *"comparison level."* For Jane, on the other hand, home has become a dreary place compared with the excitement of the university. She is therefore registering unfavorable readings of her marriage on her *"comparison level for alternatives."* Had her evaluation of her experience with Bob merely fallen below her expected level of satisfaction (her comparison level) she would merely have been disappointed, but when it falls below her perceptions of the joys that can be had in other relationships the stability of her relationship with Bob is threatened. If her experience falls below her comparison level but is still above her comparison level for experience—that is, if she has less than she had hoped to get but more than she thinks she could have in any other relationship—she is regarded as *involuntarily* remaining in the present relationship. She would stay there *voluntarily* only if her experience matched her expectations and was beyond that which she believes she could enjoy elsewhere.

Social exchange theorists believe that relationships are stable when they can be characterized as being *reciprocal* or as showing *distributive justice.*

Lévi-Strauss (1957) believes that reciprocity is basic to all social order. For example, he believes that one man gives up sexual access to his sisters and daughters on the assumption that other men will do so as well. Gouldner (1960) considers the norm of reciprocity the basis of all social exchanges. Homans (1961) offered the following general principle:

> A man in an exchange relation with another will expect that the rewards of each man be proportional to his costs—the greater the rewards, the greater the costs—and that the net rewards, or profits of each man be proportional to his investments—the greater the investments, the greater the profit. (p. 75)

Blau (1964) viewed reciprocity as the "voluntary actions of individuals who are motivated by the returns that they expect, and typically do, in fact, bring from others" (p. 91). While reciprocity may be egoistically motivated, it is not necessarily a calculated and self-serving motive. Brittan (1973), for one, observed that:

> I give gratitude to those who have helped me, not because I believe it will stand me in good stead in the future, but because I have no other way of responding to the other's actions—in this sense the exchange is almost automatic. (pp. 141–142)

Even today, despite or perhaps because of the general turmoil surrounding values in human relationships, couples express a high degree of commitment to the ideal of reciprocal, egalitarian marriages (Douglas & Wind, 1978). However, it is important to bear in mind that reciprocity implies neither symmetry nor equality but relationships based upon equity. One team of researchers (Turner et al., 1971) identified six classes of social reinforcements: love, status, information, money, goods, and services. They observed a tendency to exchange each kind of reinforcer for one of the same, but this tendency was not absolute and could best be regarded as a "conditional probability." In the same vein, others (Raush et al., 1974) found that couples were likely to exchange in kind the same types of six communications: cognitive, resolving, reconciling, appealing, rejecting, and coercive. But they, too, found these exchanges to be probabilistic rather than absolute.

Given these observations, it is not surprising that Gottman *et al.* (1976b) found that immediate communication reciprocity did not differentiate clinic from nonclinic couples. Instead they found some support for a *"lag Markovian model"* of interaction in which reciprocation could be observed only through an expanded time frame. This tendency toward general reciprocation has been well documented (e.g., Robinson & Price, 1976; Wills *et al.*, 1974). Unfortunately, the expectation that one's spouse will *immediately* reciprocate can often lead to frustration and anger. While strangers may reciprocate immediately, spouses don't, and the expectation that they will do so may contribute to shattered illusions among many couples. Therefore, while reciprocity may be the norm that maintains all stable reactions, a mature expectation recognizes that relationship debts are more likely to be repaid next month or even next year as opposed to tomorrow. Therefore, *reciprocity should be viewed as an elastic norm of stable relationships.* Spouses often feel quite well compensated for their investments in their relationships when they expect and receive a just return, and they feel ill used when haunted by the belief that they have been and will continue giving substantially more than they are getting. The operation of this norm thus becomes a matter of subtlety, patience, and abiding trust or, in its absence, anguish.

From a social exchange theorist's point of view, human relationships can best be understood as encounters in which both parties bargain for the greatest possible personal and shared outcomes by making investments in light of their potential returns and costs. Stability is brought to relationships through the capacity of each person to increase his or her investments as a means of sustaining the other's interest. Instability stems from the fact that everything that transpires within the encounter will be evaluated by both parties in terms of the potential rewards from other relationships: strain often increases within relationships when outside attractions surpass those from within. This instability, however, may be one of the greatest strengths of any relationship. Because either party may, at any time, decide that another relationship may be more rewarding, effort must constantly be expended in the present relationship to sustain the other's interest.

THE INTERACTIONAL APPROACH

Those affiliated with the Mental Research Institute in Palo Alto—a program founded in 1958 and still running strong—characterize their efforts as "the interactional approach." This group has generated scores of journal articles, many of which have been collected in three volumes (Jackson, 1968a, b; Watzlawick & Weakland, 1977), and several books that should be basic reading for every marriage and family therapist (Haley, 1963b; Watzlawick *et al.*, 1967; Watzlawick *et al.*, 1974).

The interactional approach draws from systems theory a respect for the importance of information in regulating interaction, and it draws from social exchange theory a conception of interaction as a rule-governed relationship. Rather than generating basic theory, the cardinal contribution of the MRI group has been the clinical application of these core concepts in an effort to make the planning and execution of effective intervention more of a reality.

Jackson (1965a; see also, Greenberg, 1977) draws heavily upon the work of Shibutani (1961), who believed that "human nature and the social order are products of communication" (p. 21), and Wiener (1954), who believed that human adjustment depends upon the adequacy of the information available to the person. For Watzlawick et al. (1967), the study of human behavior equates to the study of "pragmatics" or the relationship of signs to their users. Following the lead of Bateson (1951), Jackson recognized that the information conveyed through communication is of two sorts: the "report" dimension contains the objective message, while the "command" instructs the message recipient as to how the message is to be taken—that is, it defines the relationship between the two individuals as mandated by the message sender.

Observing that redundant patterns develop in all relationships, Jackson (1965b) recognized that the command or "metacommunication" dimension of information exchanges contributes to the development of a set of relationship rules between the interactors. A rule is to a relationship what RNA is to cell growth: it provides the foundation for the morphogenesis of the way people will relate to one another. Rather than being a thing, however, Jackson cautioned that rules are metaphors, or, as Haley (1962) suggested, they are constructions imposed upon relationships by observers. Unique to each dyad in the family, the rules are rarely explicit; rather, they are generally understood: they are analogous to Garfinkel's (1964) conception of "constitutive rules" which penetrate our awareness only when they are broken. For example, we have rules for the distance between conversing strangers: we almost always obey these unspoken rules and become aware of them only when we feel the menacing proximity of a stranger who steps inside the invisible circle that we draw around ourselves.

Jackson (1965b) used the term "norm" interchangeably with "rule" in order to relate his use of the concept to that of Thibaut and Kelley (1959). He believed that rules set baseline expectancies for each member of the family. Using as an analogy Bernard's (1924) concept of "dynamic equilibrium" and Cannon's· (1929) notion of "homeostasis," Jackson believed that within dyads patterns of rules develop that perpetuate the interaction in the future along the lines that have developed in the past. The patterns that develop are essentially reciprocal in nature, governed by the dictum *quid pro quo* ("something for something"), in Jackson's view. Unfortunately, the something that one member of a pair "gains" as compensation for his or her investment may in fact be a significant psychological penalty.

Rather than viewing marital stress as the result of the pathology of the individual spouses, Jackson (1965b) believes that dysfunctional interactions produce stress. Specifically, he wrote:

> The individual differences which are unquestionably present in marriage are seen as results of the active process of working out this unique and difficult relationship, not as the primary cause of the relationship phenomena. (pp. 18–19)

Elsewhere, Jackson (1965a) illustrated one way in which interaction can be pathogenic. He offered the following vignette:

HUSBAND: Hey, I can't find any white shirts!

WIFE: I'm sorry, dear, they're not ironed yet.

HUSBAND: Send them to the laundry! I don't care what it costs!

WIFE: We spend so much on groceries and liquor, I felt I should try to save a few pennies here and there.

HUSBAND: Listen, for *!!&*, I need shirts!

WIFE: Yes, dear, we'll see about it.

Jackson noted that the wife has not specified whether she will or will not either iron the shirts or send them to the laundry. She has, therefore, neither accepted nor challenged her husband's authority; rather, she has, in the language of the interactional approach, "disqualified" both him and his message. Disqualification involves the sending of a message that is incongruent with the command dimension of the message that has been received (Sluzki et al., 1967). Disqualification may be accomplished through evasion, sleight of hand (such as taking the message too literally), withdrawal, and many other communicational subversions. When distortions of this sort persist, they are either challenged directly and resolved or, as is more often the case, accommodated into a persistent pathology-generating exchange. The husband in Jackson's illustration might accept the wife's effort to undermine his authority as his investment in their relationship; as a return on his investment, he might implicitly ask his wife to indulge his overuse of alcohol, as she implied in her message to him.

Ferreira (1977) believes that many of these covert bargains are struck at a behavioral level but then are fashioned cognitively into a series of family myths. These are shared beliefs that are *quid facti, quid juris*—questions of fact and belief at the same time. They are also beliefs that function as self-fulfilling prophesies (see below), for they control the eventual behavior that is taken to be the proof of their validity. For example, the husband and wife in Jackson's illustration might agree that the wife is "not mechanically minded." On the basis of this *folie à deux* she may refuse to learn to drive, forcing him to chauffeur her wherever she wishes to go. Haley (1967) has indicated that these myths and covert interactions feed into the formation of unholy coalitions that bisect families and are schizophrenogenic in effect. In a series of classic studies, workers at the MRI illustrated other patterns that develop through the stabilization of rules born of distorted communication. Rigid patterns of symmetry (both spouses opting for same actions) and complementarity (spouses playing interlocking roles) are one illustration of these destructive balances (Sluzki & Beavin, 1977); the problems of scapegoating (Watzlawick *et al.*, 1970) and overconstruction (Riskin & Faunce, 1970) are others. Together these observations contribute to Haley's (1967) clarion call for a therapeutic focus on the interactional context of pathology for virtually every clinical service. Tracing the dynamic growth of family therapy during the 1960s, Haley noted:

> Disturbed children were once treated as *the* problem; then the parents were given individual treatment in addition; and finally, parents and child were treated as a group. Recently it has been so taken for granted that the disturbed child is a "product" of marital problems of the parents that the child is excluded and only the parents treated. This shift toward assuming that the "cause" of an individual's behavior resides in the context in which he is living reflects the basic changes that have taken place in the orientation of psychiatry in less than a decade. (p. 26)

The interactional approach thus focuses on communication as the medium through which couples exchange overt information and the more important covert information about their relationship. While the social exchange theorists focus on the explicit exchange of reinforcements in the relationship, the interactional group moves "beneath the skin" of encounters to study the implications of the bargains that are overtly struck. They find in the data produced by such an analysis a fruitful way of describing social processes and, through this description, a way of redirecting their flow. Later chapters of this book draw heavily upon the therapeutic strategies generated by their approach, so they will not be summarized here.

None of these three approaches has reached the level of total predictive accuracy. In principle, it should be possible to assign weights to input and output data; it should be possible to identify for each individual the rules for combining bits of information of differing weight; and therefore, it should be possible to explain most of the variance in human behavior. In practice, however, our ability to quantify these processes falls far short of its goals. Therefore, each of the approaches that have been reviewed must be regarded as a model, the relevance of which must be tested anew in each application.

From *systems theory* the current approach gains several assumptions: the couple is seen as living in an ever-changing relationship; the change is prompted by environmental inputs and limited by environmental constraints and its own inertial force; the flow of information fed back from outside and fed forward in planning is the lifeblood of the couple's adjustment; positive feedback can promote system change, while negative feedback enhances system stability; and a multiplicative model of information effects probably best characterizes the way in which spouses process data utilizing their individual and collective output efforts. From *social exchange theory* the current approach draws these assumptions: relationships can be understood as bargaining encounters in which each person makes investments expected to yield an equitable return; each person evaluates the returns mediated by the relationship in light of a personal set of expectations of how much the relationship *should* yield and how much satisfaction could be derived from alternative relationships; the stability of the present relationship therefore depends upon its providing a return equal to the investments that each party makes, providing the relationship mediates more reinforcements for both parties than either believes they could have in other relationships. From the *interactional approach* comes recognition that the metacommunicational dimension of all verbal and nonverbal communications defines the interpersonal meaning of the message, and that the shared beliefs about the relationship that develops through this means become the rules of its process—rules that may generate either health or pathology.

While several recent commentators have focused on lacunae in the development of theories for marriage and family counseling (e.g., Floyd, 1976; Glisson, 1976; Paquin, 1977; Vincent, 1977), the range of alternatives available as guides for planning intervention is rich, and it is no longer either necessary or responsible for therapists to "fly by the seat of their pants." If we do not yet have perfect visibility we at least have some sound theoretical instruments to guide us. As Olson and Sprenkle (1976) have observed, "the field of marriage and family counseling is no longer in its infancy" (p. 317). We have reached the point at which it is reasonable to expect a very rapid and productive stage of sophisticated theory development, at least as far as intervention techniques are concerned, if not in the area of predicting and explaining the changing dynamics of marriage and family living.

In the next chapter several different constellations of intervention methods are discussed within the rubric of two master intervention theories. In turn, each of these general conceptions spawns the specific techniques of intervention that comprise the present approach.

Techniques of Therapy Based on Social Learning Theory

SOCIAL LEARNING THEORY represents the culmination of the philosophical and theoretical traditions reviewed in the last chapter. It resists definition beyond indicating that it assumes a dynamic interaction between what have been regarded as the three fundamentals in human behavior: a physical being with thoughts and feelings, a series of covert and overt behaviors, and a set of environmental factors that set the stage and provide the consequences for these behaviors. Recent developments within the social-learning-theory tradition have tended toward carelessness in their treatment of the cognitive and behavioral elements of this reciprocal interaction. An attempt is made here to analyze these elements in light of their relative contributions to various stages of the therapeutic process. Cognitive forces are seen to play a major role in prompting new behaviors and in integrating the effects of these actions as measured in the environmental response to them. The actual promotion of interaction change is, however, essentially a behavior-change process. To help clinicians differentiate these stages of treatment, techniques are suggested for relabeling experience in an effort to modify its emotional impact and to change expectations to make new behavior more likely. Techniques are then offered for changing the details of social interaction in order to bring the relationship to the point at which a second level of technique is possible, one aimed at promoting change in the way in which couples handle the larger issues in their relationship. These assumptions and techniques make up social learning theory as it is applied here, and together these elements form the basis for each successive stage of marriage therapy.

The preceding chapter laid out a framework for identifying the values of a marital treatment approach; it also offered a description of the philosophical and theoretical underpinnings of the techniques to be described here. As has been suggested, the philosophy can be traced to major developments in Western philosophy beginning during the latter half of the 19th century. The theoretical background is more contemporary, stemming from developments in social psychological theory and research spanning some four decades. All of these traditions flow together in what has been called "social learning theory," a term that reflects not a unitary system but a number of more-or-less related approaches. Miller and Dollard (1941) were perhaps the first to coin the term in their effort to synthesize the writings of behavior theorists like Hull, Pavlov, and Thorndike, cultural anthropologists like Ogburn, and psychoanalytic writers in the Freudian tradition. The approach was best expressed in their now classic *Personality and Psychotherapy* (1950). In this volume Dollard and Miller stressed their drive–response–cue–reward theory, in which some motivational force (drive) facilitated attending to a stimulus which was organized as either an inner (thought) or overt (behavior) response that generated an environmental consequence (reward). These pioneers in modern psychological theory thus called attention to the interaction between personal, behavioral, and environmental factors in understanding human behavior.

Rotter was next to use the "social learning" concept in the title of his seminal volume, *Social Learning and Clinical Psychology* (1954). He was mainly interested in applying the triadic model to matters of primary concern to clinical psychologists, and therefore he placed major emphasis upon internal forces as the major stuff of which overt behaviors are made. In that resect he may well be the essentially unacknowledged father of the contemporary "cognitive-behavior-therapy" tradition. Bandura's classic *Principles of Behavior Modification* (1969), as well as his later writings (e.g., Bandura, 1977, 1978), extended this tradition further and, in important respects, brought to it a truer balance between its three elements. In Bandura's (1978) words:

> Personal and environmental factors do not function as independent determinants; rather they determine each other. Nor can "persons" be considered causes independent of their behavior. It is largely through their actions that people produce the environmental conditions that affect their behavior in a reciprocal fashion. The experiences generated by behavior also partly determine what individuals think, expect, and can do, which in turn affect their subsequent behavior. (p. 345)

The individual is thus seen as both the partial cause and the partial result of an interaction between his or her covert and overt actions and the reactions that these behaviors elicit in others.

This dynamic interaction may be best illustrated in the "interdependence matrix" described by Kelley and Thibaut (1978) in the long-awaited update of their forceful earlier work (Thibaut & Kelley, 1959). They defined the matrix for any dyad as:

> the way in which the two persons control each other's outcomes in the course of their interaction. It is constituted by specifying the behaviors important to the relationship that each of them may enact and by assessing the consequences for both persons of all possible combinations of their respective behavior. Thus each cell in the matrix defines a possible interpersonal event. The flow of their relationship can be described in terms of the sequence through which it moves. (1978, p. 3)

The matrix thus describes both the options open to each party and the probable payoff that taking either option might yield. For example, a woman seated alone at a table in a coffee shop is joined by a man who occupies what appears to be the only vacant seat. She has the option of opening her book in a sign of obvious disinterest or of smiling and offering a casual greeting. He has the option of simply apologizing for intruding on her privacy or of making a bid to start a conversation. The chances that each person will choose one of the available options over the other is influenced by the "given matrix" that each person brings to the situation. The given matrix is the set of expectancies that each person has learned from experience in the environment in the past coupled with an assessment of the extent to which these factors bear upon the current situation. This is immediately transformed into the "effective matrix" of each person, which represents his or her active interpretation of the currently operative contingencies. The actions taken by each party are the result of the probabilities of success that each sees as the probable outcome of either action. Following the expression of either distancing or welcoming maneuvers by one, this datum is fed into the given matrix of the other insofar as it is a past experience, only to be transformed into an altered set of expectancies in a modified effective matrix. Hence, it is through the interaction of given and effective matrices that social learning theorists visualize the interplay of the personal, behavioral, and contextual factors that are believed to be intrinsic in all human behavior. This relationship has been symbolically represented by Bandura (1978), not as a unidirectional approach

$$B = f(P, E)$$

not in a partially bidirectional approach

$$B = f(P \leftarrow \rightarrow E)$$

but as a truly bidirectional approach

$$
\begin{array}{c}
B \\
\diagup \quad \diagdown \\
P \leftarrow\!\!\!\rightarrow E
\end{array}
$$

in which P refers to the constitutional, cognitive, and affective characteristics of the person, B refers to all of the person's covert and overt behaviors, and E refers to the environmental context in which the actions take place.

EVALUATING THE IMPACT OF CONSTITUTIONAL AND SITUATIONAL
FACTORS ON BEHAVIOR

Weighting the elements in a theory has the effects of establishing the relative importance and of suggesting an optimal sequence of interventions that emanate from that theory. Early thinkers in this general tradition had their own points of view concerning weights and sequences. For example, in attempting to understand the linkage between internal processes and external events, Thorndike (1898) speculated that stimuli elicited mediating processes (r-s) that in turn elicited responses by the actor. Tolman (1932) later gave a cognitive flavor to these mediational processes by characterizing them as expectancies and values, while Hull (1943) contributed a conception of response patterns as having habit strength and drive properties. Because of the persuasiveness of these giants of American psychology, the field waffled between cognitive orientation, as suggested by Tolman, and behavioral orientation as advocated by Hull (Bowers, 1973; Weiner, 1972).

An attempt has been made to overcome this schism by writers in the "cognitive-behavior-modification" tradition (e.g., Bandura, 1977; Meichenbaum, 1977; Mischel, 1973; Mahoney & Thoresen, 1974). This attempt at theoretical unification, however, may be made at the cost of some degree of therapeutic specificity and effectiveness. A look at some of the theoretical research of the past two decades may help to point out why this is the case.

The critical questions of this controversy for the marriage therapist are : (1) To what extent are thoughts the antecedents of behavior? (2) Is it reasonable to expect that a change in clients' thought patterns will have a great impact upon their actions? In response to the first question, writers like Bem (1967) have found that individuals often act and later try to provide a cognitive frame of reference for their actions, rather than thinking through issues carefully before taking action. Who among us, for example, has not often asked with justifiable annoyance, "Now why in heaven's name did I do that again when I knew it wouldn't work?" Therefore, while writers whose work is of great interest to clinicians (e.g., Ellis, 1962; Frank, 1961; Kelly, 1955) have suggested that thinking disorders are part and parcel of almost every form of psychological stress, evidence has yet to be adduced showing that thought disorders precede rather than result from stress. In response to the second question, Ledwidge (1978) noted that two decades of research by a distinguished group of behavioral scientists (e.g., Bem & McConnell, 1970; Festinger, 1964; J. G. Taylor, 1962) have shown not only that efforts to change clients' attitudes have met with sporadic success, but that the results of successful attitude-change programs often dissipate quickly unless environmental-change programs are made to support the newly introduced attitudes.

Researchers like Kaplan and Anderson (1973) have made valiant attempts to bridge the chasm between cognitive and behavioral biases in understanding and predicting human action. The weight of evidence, however, supports the notion that certain aspects of behavior may be under cognitive control, while others are more under environmental control; and it may very well be best to recognize the segmentation in these control systems. Analyzing this problem, Greenspoon and Lamal (1978) have observed that cognitive theories arose in idealistic and mentalistic traditions, while behavioral theories grew from positivistic and physicalistic traditions. As a result the two approaches have different definitional structures, with cognitive theories stressing connotative and implicit meanings in contrast to behavioral theories which stress denotative and ostensive meanings. When this discrepancy is coupled with the fact that even the internal operational terms of cognitive theory are inconsistent with the external operational terms of behavior therapy, it would seem as though the two theories are irreconcilable unless the core elements of both are compromised. These considerations lead to the conclusion that efforts to bridge the gap between the two approaches could profitably be abandoned (Greenspoon & Lamal, 1978). Instead, much might be gained through respecting the differences between these approaches and using each for the purpose to which it is best suited.

Both the necessity for and the advantages to be gained from treating cognitive and behavioral variables separately can be understood if we return to our analysis of behavior theories through a study of constitutional, behavioral, and environmental variables. In the first instance, let us imagine that things are going well in our lives. In this case we take full responsibility for the positive outcomes and feel that our personal characteristics explain most of the variance. However, when things go poorly for us, the self-ascribed importance of our own characteristics pales as we attribute the responsibility for the unhappy turn of events to what we conceive to be a hostile environment. This tendency to externalize the responsibility for negative events is supported by a fairly extensive body of clinical evidence showing that we all tend to punctuate descriptions of our less fortunate social experiences by bracketing each of our actions within two actions by others.(Watzlawick et al., 1967). For example, Bob might describe a negative exchange with Jane in the following terms:

JANE: Why are you home so late, Bob?

BOB: I was delayed at the supermarket.

JANE: That is incredible disregard for my feelings.

Bob appears the innocent in this description, which leaves out the fact that he went out for a few items an hour and a half before his return. By omitting his initial actions, Bob casts June in an undeservedly poor light, but one that is face-saving for himself.

Meanwhile, when others view an individual's behavior, they tend to attribute major importance to his or her personal disposition (Jones & Nisbett, 1971; Nisbett et al., 1973; Storms, 1973). For example, Jane is likely to explain the above exchange by observing that Bob "is always self-centered and unconcerned with the feelings of others." Unlike Bob, she sees him (i.e., his "personality") as the culprit and not his environment (e.g., her behavior). She, in fact, shares this orientation with traditional therapists, who take a "trait" orientation in their assessment of their clients' distress.

From the foregoing analysis it should be clear that clients would prefer to take responsibility for things when they go well and to project them onto others when things go sour. The protagonists in their lives tend to do the same, so the burden of responsibility is shifted from one to the other at times of stress. Trait-oriented therapists can reinforce self-perceived strengths at good times and are pitted against the client in a basic conflict during stressful times. This approach is sorely lacking, however, because it overlooks the pivotal importance of the interaction between the two people. He is no more wrong than she is wrong: they are wrong to the extent that their interaction does not yield the outcomes they both seek. Unfortunately, the therapist with a strong cognitive orientation joins clients in their faulty and incomplete assumptions to the extent that they lay excessive responsibility upon the individuals, agreeing with Bandura's (1978) assertion that "cognitive events are controlling, not controllable" (p. 347). In contrast, the social-learning-theory view is that one's ideas about an interaction are the consequence of preconceptions brought to that relationship tempered by interactive experiences, so that cognitions are believed to be both controlling and controlled by social interaction rather than one or the other.

When we use this formulation to explore the natural history of the rendering of therapeutic instigations (Kanfer & Phillips, 1969), we can find the proper places for cognitive as opposed to behavioral changes. (An instigation is an instruction given during treatment sessions calling for changes in behavior between sessions.)

Whether the instruction is to increase the rate of a behavior already in the client's repertoire, to apply this existing behavior in new situations, or to develop new behaviors for familiar or new situations, the instigation itself is a cognitive change, and it is reasonable to assume that it will be most readily accepted if the client is offered a rationale for the recommendation. The client must then accomplish the behavior change, and the results of the new action must be recognized, interpreted, and integrated into the client's constructs in order to play a role in the planning of subsequent behaviors. Accordingly, the following sequence of techniques seems relevant:

1. Cognitive change to potentiate new action.
2. Behavior change to potentiate new experience.
3. Cognitive change to potentiate the repeat of the desired actions by conceptualizing their effects.

Therefore, rather than the two approaches (behaviorism vs. cognitive theory) being treated as though they were compatible and applicable at the same time and with the same results, their differences should be recognized, and they should be applied sequentially in the service of the goals for which they are each uniquely adapted. This is the way in which reciprocal determinism can realize its vast clinical potential; treating differences as though they are alike can only sabotage the utility of this fertile approach.

In summary, then, the conception of social learning theory that is applied here recognizes the profound power of reciprocal determinism among the personal, behavioral, and situational forces that can be seen to shape every human interaction. No one of these factors is believed to be more powerful than any other, for a change in one clearly has a major impact upon the remaining two. It is believed that some level of understanding of each element is necessary if we are to achieve a reasonable level of awareness of the true dynamics of human relationships and if we are to be able to harness the potential of these relationships to accomplish directed change. But pursuant to a natural history in the operation of these elements, it is assumed that it is necessary to treat them unequally during varied stages of marital therapy. Some change in the personal characteristics of thoughts and feelings are believed necessary for promoting initial behavior change. Prompting further behavior change to promote enhanced social interaction is a second step. Finally, aid in the cognitive integration of the true meaning of these changes is considered the third interventive maneuver. The therapist who is oriented toward social learning theory thus needs two sets of basic skills if change is to be achieved: skills in modifying thought and feeling patterns and skills in translating these modified internal states into new and more effective overt behaviors. These are the subjects of the following two sections.

Changing Thoughts and Feelings

As suggested above, modified thought and feeling patterns are both the antecedents and the consequences of changed behaviors. Relabeling is a technique through which negatively charged beliefs can be toned down or even changed to positive events. Changing expectations is a means of modifying patterns of thinking. Both will be discussed in greater detail.

RELABELING

The first cognitive-change technique stems from the realization that all humans strive constantly to make sense of their experience (Carson, 1969), and that their success or failure in doing so hinges upon the language that they adopt for construing the inner and outer events of their lives (G. Kelly, 1955; Mowrer & Ullman, 1945). Depending upon the way that we label our experiences, we can bias our reactions negatively or positively, and we can facilitate or hamper our taking constructive action. As Chesterton (1960) has observed, "An adventure is only an inconvenience rightly considered. An inconvenience is only an adventure wrongly considered" (p. 315).

With regard to social experience, we all use selected categories for describing other people's traits, abilities, attitudes, and behaviors, and we have our own beliefs as to how these phenomena interrelate (Rosenberg & Jones, 1972). For some time (e.g., Bruner & Tagiuri, 1954; Rosenberg & Olshan, 1970; R. A. Jones, 1977) it has been suggested that we carry with us an "implicit theory of personality" or a "map of personality space" (Cronbach, 1958). Hays (1958) saw this set of trait labels as a "relatively stable scheme of expectations and anticipations about others, which is gradually built up through direct and vicarious experience" (p. 288). The traits that provide the major dimensions of these labels are, in Hays's view, the familiar good–bad, warm–cold, and dominant–submissive variables. Several writers (e.g., Brittan, 1973; Goffman, 1959; McCall & Simmons, 1966) have noted that these labels provide the basis for both the definition of others and the delineation of concepts of self as opposed to one's construction of others. For example, Josh, a Northerner, might have some very distinct views about southern women. He considers them feminine, frivolous, flighty, and socially irresponsible. His wife, Ellie, was born in Atlanta. He found her attractive enough to marry, but both of them are haunted by his unspoken ideas about the way southern women must behave. The fact that he buys her pink clothes, jokes about her overdrawing the checking account, encourages her to change her mind often, and baits her in discussions of social issues are all his means of engineering responses in her that confirm his beliefs.

With regard to marital interaction, Watzlawick (1976) offered the following example of a labeling problem:

> If, for instance, a husband defines his view of the nature of the marriage by stating, "I know that you despise me," and the wife tearfully retorts, "How

will I ever be able to convince you that I love you?", there is no way of establishing objectively who is right and who is wrong and what the nature of the relationship really is. (p. 120)

In this situation, both partners use what Watzlawick *et al.* (1974) have termed "first order labels"—gut reactions to the immediate events. They could, with help, learn to use "second order labels" instead, suggesting to the husband that the wife's withdrawal is not motivated by her dislike of him but by her effort to respect her privacy; and to the wife that the husband's doubts are a result of his genuine desire for closeness rather than an attack on her actions.

Weakland *et al.* (1974) suggested that clients can be helped to change their labeling behavior by treating some interactions *as if* they were not problems, and by correctly labeling others as challenges that should be met. If labels are distorted in a positive direction, they are likely to trigger positive emotions, which, in turn, help to create positive situations. Indeed, it has been shown that a little "Pollyannaism" can pay rich dividends in relationships among both single (Scott & Peterson, 1975) and married (Huesmann & Levinger, 1972; Levinger & Senn, 1967) dyads. Therefore, helping couples to arrive at the most positive labels they can find for one another's behavior can have a profound therapeutic effect. Even if the labels are totally incorrect when formed, they can often go far toward creating the quality of interaction that they describe.

Another approach is to train the spouses in taking the role of the other, a skill considered by G. H. Mead (1934, 1938) to be the foundation of all social organization. Stuart (1967) has illustrated the way in which the gradual acquisition of the ability to shift perspectives—to "decenter"—seems to lie at the base of children's gradual acquisition of objective notions about the physical world and subjective notions about social relationships. Feffer (1970) has demonstrated the manner in which this skill facilitates social interactions among adults, while Mehrabian (1970) has asserted his belief that building decentering skills is a major component in successful psychotherapy with adults, and Steinfeld (1978) recognized its facilitative effect upon change in marital interaction. In essence, the clients are taught to move away from a totally egocentric conception of their interaction and to grasp instead some notion of the other's goal and reactions. When successful, this change is one of those believed by many marriage therapy clients to be one of the major achievements of their therapeutic experience (Brown & Manela, 1977).

As labels can be inaccurate because of the tone attached to them and because they may stem from an overly narrow, personal perspective, they can also be troublesome if they focus upon the wrong aspect of the other's behavior. Hurvitz (1970) has attributed much of the variance in couples' distress to their overuse of terminal vocabulary and underuse of process vocabulary. Terminal language uses words that may or may not be accurate and that may or may not fit the situation but, even if accurate and fitting, offer no alternatives for action and often have rather destructive implications. Hurvitz offered nine types of terminal statements, including psychodynamic interpretations (e.g., "She has an oral fixation"), psychological name calling (e.g., "He's mentally ill"), and assertions about one's own or the other's desire and/or ability to change. Instrumental language, the alternative to terminal words, also may or may not be accurate and fitting, but these words have action implications and are the conceptual building blocks for change. The six subtypes of these terms offered by Hurvitz include recognition of discontinuities in communication, observations of habitual but changeable action patterns, and comments on potentially avoidable patterns of reaction.

The terminal language of which Hurvitz wrote is essentially aimed at classifying the person, while the instrumental language is aimed at describing modifiable events. For example, at the start of treatment the husband might say that his wife "is a depressive." This is a terminal statement because if the wife is a depressive there is nothing that he or the therapist can do to change her. It is the role of the therapist to help the husband (1) describe aspects of his wife's behavior that he would like to change; (2) describe ways in which his actions contribute to her behavior; (3) plan ways for changing his behavior so that her behavior can change; and (4) then follow through on these changes and evaluate their effect. The development of a more appropriate problem-solving language is thus followed by an expansion of the clients' conceptions of their stress, which is broadened from an "other-focused" to an "interaction-focused" approach.

CHANGING EXPECTATIONS

It is inevitable that we formulate expectations of how others will treat us based upon the way we label their behavior (Wegner & Vallacher, 1977). We then act toward them *as if* the labels were correct. Therefore, even if the labels were originally false, our subsequent actions make them true, and the label was, in effect, a "self-erasing error" (R. A. Jones, 1977; Mischel, 1968; Ross, 1977; Snyder *et al.*, 1977, p. 644). Many years ago, Thomas and Thomas (1928) observed that "If men define situations as real, they are real in their consequences" (p. 1104). Merton (1957) recognized the mechanisms through which prophecy becomes reality in the following terms: "In the beginning, a false definition of the situation evoke[s] a new behavior which makes the original false conception come true" (p. 423). Others (Jones *et al.*, 1962) have pointed to the fact that ego also pays the price for his or her negative self-fulfilling prophecies: when alter is induced to act negatively toward ego because of the latter's negative-label–inspired actions, then ego's self-appraisal pays the price.

These self-fulfilling prophecies have a certain positive function in that they do make the world a more predictable place to be (Rawlings, 1975). If by imposing our own construction on the events around us we can—in part at least—force these events to conform to our expectations, we can take strides toward making our worlds more predictable places and allow ourselves to relax to some degree and devote our energies to constructive purposes. Moreover, when two interacting parties share the same expectations, they tend to feel that their relationship exists on a higher plane, even though the shared outlooks may not be "true." Hence, it has been found that married (Chadwick et al., 1976; Hicks & Platt, 1970; Laws, 1971; Levinger & Breedlove, 1966; Meyer & Pepper, 1977) and unmarried (Hansen & Donoghue, 1977; Miller & Geller, 1972) dyads whose world views are similar tend to enjoy more stable relationships, in addition to—or perhaps because of— their greater ease of conflict resolution.

Harry (1976) found that expectations change over the life cycle of the marriage, and from his observations it is clear that effective adjustment in marriage depends upon a flexibility in expectations. For example, the courting couple may come to expect casual and relaxed evenings during their early childless years while both are employed and disposable income is high. Later, however, when overtime work cuts into their pleasures as both struggle to support a home large enough for their two young children, they will be quite unhappy if their expectations have not changed. In the same vein, he married her with the expectation that he would "bring home the bacon" while she would maintain their "home sweet home." That arrangement worked well until their youngest went off to school; then she felt the need for more fulfillment in her life, asked him to share the housework, and went off to find a full-time job. As long as her behavior is incongruent with his expectation, he is headed for considerable stress. Clearly, balance can be restored either by his changing his expectation or by her turning back into the home. Both the promotion of flexibility in expectations and the accommodation of expectation to reality can obviously do much to facilitate satisfaction with many aspects of marital interaction.

Expectations that are unrealistic can often pose a serious problem for the stability of the marriage, the success of therapy, and the well-being of both spouses. Arkowitz (1973) reported that while engaged women are more unrealistic in their expectations than those who are married, so, too, were women entering their second or later marriages. One can explain some of the variance in the high divorce rate during the first two years of marriage (see Chapter 1) in terms of the incompatibility of the lofty expectations of courting couples with their immediate postmarital experience. The high divorce rate of second and third marriages can also be at least partially explained by a comparable lack of realism, coupled with the fact that if divorce has been seen as a reasonable response to a marital dispute in one relationship, it may seem reasonable in subsequent marriages as well. (The best predictor of behavior is, after all, past behavior.)

While it is often useful to mislabel behavior when the labels are more positive than reality, holding unrealistic expectations about marriage can obviously have a very deleterious effect. Paul Watzlawick (1977) has called attention to this clear and present danger in his reference to the three forms of "utopia syndrome." Noting that "Utopia" was coined by Thomas Moore in 1516 as a distant island that was "Nowhere," Watzlawick has shown that the setting of change goals that are too high doom people to a lifetime of unfulfillment and frustration. Once the goals are set, some of us handle our failure to meet them as an expression of our personal inadequacy rather than the unreality of our objective. The present author has long explained depression in apparently well-functioning clients as a criterion problem: their behavior is equal to or even more effective than that of most of their peers, but the criteria they use to assess their functioning are so demanding as always to yield discouraging self-appraisals. A second expression of the utopia syndrome is crystallized in Robert Louis Stevenson's aphorism: "It is better to travel hopefully than to arrive." In Watzlawick's view, acceptance of this belief "necessitates that every fulfillment is experienced as a loss, as a profanation" (p. 303). That may explain why suicide rates rise at holiday times: there is joy in hope, but despair in the realization of that hope. Finally, the utopia syndrome can be expressed in the belief that one has learned the essential truth, but the unknowing world stands in the way of its attainment. This projection of one's shortcomings onto others is the kernel of neurosis as conceived by Adler, Sullivan, and Horney. And they stand apart from others in recognizing that the goals of treatment must rest in this life with its smelly armpits and occasional bad breath, not in some idealized beliefs about the joys of *satori* in the life that follows.

For Watzlawick, then, the goals of effective therapy must be the solution of current challenges, not the attainment of a perfect relationship. He wrote, "The limits of a responsible and humane psychotherapy are much narrower than is generally thought. Lest therapy become its own pathology, it must limit itself to the relief of suffering: the quest for happiness cannot be its task" (pp. 306–307). Thus, the couple who would strive for perfection in their marriage have taken their first steps toward divorce and despair; and the therapist who would set their sights on this unobtainable goal bears the guilt of causing iatrogenic illness.

Etzioni (1977) offered a very urgent caution in this connection. He noted that it is still true that most therapists have been trained as individual therapists, not as marriage and family counselors. This leads them to encourage their clients to seek personal fulfillment. The problem is that if one member of a dyad seeks personal fulfillment, the price of this new-found liberty is often paid by the other. In contrast, marriage therapy should help spouses to formulate expectations for and skills in mutual change, so that the process can be restrained from being beneficial to one partner at the expense of the other.

Summarizing the work of Rotter (1954, 1970), Patterson (1973) has suggested that expectations can be changed by direct verbal reinforcement or shaping during treatment, by helping the client to enter situations in which it is possible to see the outcomes that others experience, by directly suggesting alternative expectations, and by suggesting as a norm of treatment that clients seek alternative expectations and test their validity through developing new patterns of action. This approach leads naturally to a discussion of the next set of intervention procedures.

Two Levels of Behavior Change

When new labels and expectations help to generate more positive feelings and beliefs about the possibility of constructive change, the therapist is in a position to work toward instigating changes in the way in which each partner treats the other. While the possibilities for categorizing human behavior are virtually infinite, for the purpose of the present analysis it is sufficient to identify two levels of behavior. Microbehaviors are the smallest verbal and nonverbal units of any interaction. They are to the relationship what molecules are to physical objects. They generate feelings of warmth or coldness, closeness or distance. These feelings, in turn, spawn the larger units of interaction— the molar elements by which we all tend to characterize our relationships with others. They are to relationships what the properties of temperature, shape, color, and texture are to physical objects. It is assumed in this approach that microbehaviors must be changed in order to prepare relationships for molar changes, and, as is described below, different techniques are needed to accomplish each type of change.

MICROBEHAVIORAL CHANGE

Life would indeed be simple if our cognitions and our actions were essentially alike. Repeated studies, however, have shown that what we say and how we actually behave are often highly incongruent (e.g., Kenkel, 1963; Olson, 1969; Olson & Rabunsky, 1972). Recently, for example, Weiss and Isaac (1976) found that while couples' ideas about their relationship concurred with common conceptions of the "ideal marriage," their behaviors were often anything but ideal. The difference may lie not as much in their intentions as in the way they interact (Gottman et al., 1976b; Robinson & Price, 1976). These observations all point to the need to change behavior as well as to modify language and expectations. Moreover, those who have studied the relationship between beliefs and behavior (e.g., Nisbett & Valins, 1971; Weick, 1966; Zimbardo, 1966, 1969) have all suggested that a change in either beliefs or behavior can facilitate change in the other. Therefore, changing behavior is one route to take in seeking new beliefs, when this is an important change goal.

It is also true that change in marital and family experience does not come about until all parties change the way in which they act toward one another (Fogarty, 1975). Weakland et al. (1974) have stressed the importance of these changes as strongly as the case can be made in the following terms:

> Our fundamental premise is that regardless of their basic origins of etiology—if, indeed, these can ever be reliably determined—the kinds of problems people bring to psychotherapists persist only if they are maintained by ongoing current behavior of the patient and others with whom he interacts. Correspondingly, if such problem-maintaining behavior is appropriately changed or eliminated, the problem will be resolved or vanish, regardless of its nature, origin or duration. (pp. 144–145)

Whatever means are used, in the judgment of these highly regarded clinical theorists the ultimate goal of marriage therapy must be a change in the behavior of not one but both spouses.

It is possible to differentiate two levels of behavior that can contribute to marital bliss or strain. "Microbehaviors" are those high-frequency events, often occurring several times each day, that essentially communicate interest or disinterest, warmth or coldness, attraction or repulsion. Microbehaviors are thus the atomic particles that contribute to the partners' feelings of comfort or discomfort in one another's presence. Changes in these small behavioral units can go far toward changing the much more global pattern of any interaction. It has been shown, for example, that labels can be changed by a shift in the valence of these minor events of major importance (e.g., Stapleton et al., 1973). These studies manipulated ego's conception of alter and found that ego's willingness to reinforce alter was affected by the reinforcement received from alter and not by the experimentally manipulated labels. The experience shared by two parties to an interaction became their past. Pruitt

(1968) has shown that "past experience with the other person had its effect on behavior by altering the amount of [reinforcement] expected from that person in the future" (p. 147). Further stressing the value of the details of the parties' present interaction is the observation of Huesmann and Levinger (1972) that "one values future rewards less than present rewards, particularly if one is unsure about the continuation or stability of the relationship" (p. 5). Therefore, the details of interaction between two people have the power to shape their broader conceptions of one another, their expectations for the future, and their willingness to act in a reinforcing manner toward each other in the present. Fortunately, these changes appear to be under the influence of "recency" rather than "primacy" effects (Wilson & Insko, 1968), at least for nonmarried dyads; and while there are some noteworthy differences in the interaction patterns of married and nonmarried pairs (e.g., Stuart & Braver, 1973; Birchler et al., 1975), there is no reason to suppose that shifts in these microbehavioral interactions would be less effective among the married than among the single.

Whether they are easy or difficult to achieve, these changes seem to be the essential means of preparing the way for tackling the larger issues in marriage. Bateson (1972), for example, has shown that the couple's ability to deal constructively with conflict depends, among other things, on their freedom to identify conflictual issues, their capacities to discount irrelevant emotionally toned messages, their ability to adopt flexible problem-solving schemata, and the presence of a sufficient bond of commitment to allow the partners to expect future benefits from present concessions made in the service of conflict resolution. This commitment, in turn, depends upon the level of attraction that each spouse feels for the other, which, in turn, depends upon the relative balance of positive and negative experiences with one another (Brewer & Brewer, 1968; Byrne & Nelson , 1965; Byrne & Rhamey, 1965; Kelley et al., 1962; Taylor et al., 1968, 1969).

In addition to providing the basis for problem solving and conflict resolution, this reinforcement-produced attraction also builds the basis for trust, the pivot around which all social exchange revolves (Blau, 1964). We trust another when we feel that he or she will reciprocate in kind the level of investment that we make in the relationship. Indeed, without trust, we are unwilling to make any but the most casual of investments. As Brittan (1973) has described it:

> Presumably, before one enters into an exchange-relationship, we have to somehow take a jump into the unknown by committing ourselves to the other in the hope that he will reciprocate in kind. In other words, the conditions of trust precede actual exchange, yet we are told that trust itself is generated in exchange. (p. 144)

It is reasonable to suppose that each party to an interaction in which there have been disappointments will be willing to venture only small behaviors in anticipation of the development of trust, and further, that the development of trust is a necessary antecedent for more venturesome investments. Therefore, efforts to manage the microbehavioral aspects of an interaction would seem to be a most important first step toward the later goal of addressing the larger issues.

CHANGE OF MOLAR BEHAVIORS

To understand the nature of the molar dimensions of interaction it is necessary to trace briefly the logical history of relationship development. First:

> Dyadic interaction commences when two persons begin to behave in each other's presence. Each comes into the situation with certain goals in mind, certain cognitions about how these goals may be achieved, and a pattern of attitudes about the situation and the other person. Thus the person approaches the interaction with a set of motivationally relevant *plans* that serve to launch his end of the conversation. (Jones & Gerard, 1967, pp. 505–506)

These plans are the result of prior socialization, and the behavior that they produce is either accepted, redirected, or rejected by the other person. We have been told by social exchange theorists that gradually, through a process of bargaining, the two parties develop a set of norms that govern their interaction. All social relationships that develop over time develop norms for the actions of both parties (Thibaut & Kelley, 1959), and insofar as the norms provide a scheduling of privileges and responsibilities for both parties, the norms form an implicit relationship contract. Purcell (1976) has traced the way in which courting couples gradually drift toward some implicit agreements as to how decisions will be made and how privileges and responsibilities will be allocated. He believes that out-of-awareness conceptions of how spouses should interact, derived from the partners' experiences in their families of orientation, guide their early negotiations. Subsequently, they create precedents for their own bargains through their own interaction, and rather than resolving issues *de novo,* they turn time and time again to often wordless respect for the way they have done things in the past.

Major relationship contracts specify two things: (1) the ways in which each person is expected to act toward the other; and (2) and the ways in which this agreement is to be modified. Contracts thus contain both content and process dimensions. The class of behaviors that we term "macrobehavioral" are these two sets of actions—those that structure interaction and those that provide for adaptation and change of that structure. These contracts are thus the master plans of social interaction. In Carson's view (1969):

Adherence by persons to the terms of their interpersonal contracts is associated with the development of wholesome and mature interpersonal relations. It permits a maximization of joint outcomes within a context of cooperation and trust, it reduces the amount of energy expenditure required for the maintenance of surveillance and vigilance, and it encourages continuing mutual exploration and additional growth. (pp. 195–196)

Unfortunately, not all contracts are desirable in the sense that they provide reciprocal advantages at comparable costs for both parties, and therefore all contracts require renegotiation over time as a function of shifts in the life space of both parties. Some of the more restrictive elements in many contracts between spouses stem from the Old Testament view of the proper relationship between men and women, conceptions that stand in sharp contrast to current social values (Weitzman, 1975). Other problem-generating agreements result from an interplay of the maladaptive patterns of both parties. For example, Carson (1969) has suggested that contracts require renegotiation when they involve "coordinated avoidance" (p. 196)—that is, agreements to neglect important areas of interaction that might be sources of mutual gratification— or if "at least one member of the dyad is obliged to perform behaviors that are self-injurious, deviant, or otherwise maladaptive" (p. 197). In renegotiating these contracts, norms of the interaction must be made explicit, and behaviors must then be changed in conformity with the new rule structure. These behavior changes are the larger units of the marital interaction—perhaps events that occur once in a very great while, yet cast a cloud over the marriage for months on end. For example, Sue invited her parents to come along on the family vacation two years ago; Ned still feels resentful and violated, though not a word has been spoken. They need a contract concerning how plans will be made for vacations. Ned took not a second, but a third job; Sue feels undone because she never sees her "one true love." Ned thinks that he has Sue's interest at heart; she, meanwhile, regards his overtime work as a transparent excuse for putting some distance between them. They need a contract for planning how work schedules and personal priorities will be set. These are examples of the meaning of molar behavior changes accomplished through verbal agreements that take the form of new relationship contracts.

Summary

This chapter began with a review of social learning theory. It utilizes a tripartite analysis of human behavior, endorsing a position in which person, behavior, and environment are viewed as reciprocally determined. Had this chapter been written at another time in the development of psychological thought, its analysis of the need to treat cognitive and behavior-change efforts separately might not have been written. At this pivotal time, however, efforts are being made to overlook the differences between these two traditions to the disadvantage of both. Therefore, the argument put forth here has been that cognitive techniques are useful in sowing the seeds for compliance with therapeutic instigations and for reaping the harvest to the extent that the fruits of these changes must be fashioned into a new view of the relationship if they are to be maintained. It is then left to behavior-focused interventions to bear the weight of modifying the specific interaction patterns that are the potential joys and sorrows of client couples. Finally, the chapter described two techniques for changing cognitions (relabeling and the modification of expectations) and two techniques for changing behaviors (one aimed at building new daily patterns of microbehaviors and one aimed at changing larger, molar units of interaction, including the major ways in which the couple tackle the challenges in their lives over time). It next remains to describe marriages in change-oriented terms before making specific recommendations for molding these generalized treatment considerations into a cogent intervention approach. Assessment of marriages is therefore the topic of the next chapter, to be followed by recommendations for specific clinical plans in Chapter 5.

C H A P T E R 4

Assessing Troubled Marriages

DURING THEIR FIRST therapeutic session, most marriage therapy clients seek to convince the therapist that their marital stresses can be explained by one of three major conditions: idiosyncrasies in the other's behavior are generally first cited as the source of stress; this is followed by reference to some external event that has forced an otherwise well-functioning relationship off course; failing these, partners may find fault with one or more of their own personality characteristics, which are presented as the logical and unavoidable consequence of some past experience. The therapist is faced with the responsibility of redirecting the inquiry so that data on the current functioning, resources, and goals of the clients can be elucidated as a basis for the planning of effective intervention. Unless the therapist has a precise plan for the collection of assessment data, it is likely that the clients will control the fact-gathering stage of treatment, with the result being a weak or ineffective treatment approach. This chapter sets forth the guidelines for the sure-handed collection of the data basic to the planning of successful treatment.

The chapter begins by differentiating assessment of the clients' behavior as a response to identifiable external events from diagnosis, which attempts to infer durable client characteristics from observed behaviors. A preference for assessment is expressed, followed by the identification of five features that should be represented in the assessment for marital therapy. Specifically, it is argued that the assessment should be parsimonious and yield only as many data as are absolutely needed for treatment planning; it should be multidimensional to reflect relevant aspects of the broad scope of marital behaviors; it should be directly linked to specific treatment decisions; it should be situationally specific rather than assuming that clients' behavior remains constant across situations;

and because many couples terminate treatment at the conclusion of one of the first sessions, the assessment should be of value to the clients in its own right.

Based on the foregoing criteria, specific recommendations are made in the three ensuing sections of this chapter concerning the measurement of the couple's marital satisfaction and marital behaviors, identification of individual characteristics that may influence the course of therapy, and the measurement of therapeutic outcome. A great many tools are available for assessment in these critical areas. The assessment package recommended here is one that blends specific and global measures, that draws upon several different data bases, that can be conveniently and inexpensively administered, and that can be used for repeated assessment to reflect changes in couple and individual functioning in a time frame beginning before the first session and extending well into a follow-up period.

Whether or not we are aware of what we are doing, we all constantly collect data about other people, organize it into a more-or-less coherent conception of who the other person is and what we can expect of his or her behavior, and then plan our behavior accordingly in what often becomes a self-fulfilling prophesy. As clinicians we engage in precisely the same process, but it is our responsibility to do so with a much higher degree of precision than is used when we make interpersonal judgments in our private lives.

There are two broad formats for making clinical judgments. The most common process is "diagnosis," which is defined in Webster's *New Collegiate Dictionary* as "the art or act of identifying a disease from its signs and symptoms." To render an accurate diagnosis we must collect the relevant facts, understand their relationship to the available diagnostic categories, and then correctly infer the diagnosis from the presence of its pathognomic cues. Unfortunately, years of research have shown that we are not very good at collecting the needed information; that we must rely upon sweeping inferential chains to move from observation to categorization; and that we work with category systems that are far too incomplete at times and overlapping at others. For these reasons, diagnostic conclusions are often thought to be both unreliable and invalid in the sense that they are at best modestly related to the essential elements of treatment planning (Stuart, 1971c).

Clinical assessment is the alternative to diagnosis. Assessment is the process of describing the interaction between clients and the salient features of their surroundings; it relies on direct observation rather than inferences from surface cues to presumptions about underlying pathology, thereby making it more reliable; it describes productive and unproductive elements of the clients' behavior and offers immediate relevance to therapeutic planning. Clinical assessment surpasses diagnosis in reliability and validity, and it therefore serves as the foundation for the approach taken to the collection and analysis of data as a basis of the therapeutic methods described in this approach.

Five Criteria of Marital Assessment

Recent reviews by Jacob (1976) and Weiss and Margolin (1977) have summarized many of the options open to marriage therapists using a social-learning-theory approach. These options range from simple, un-structured self-report, through the use of standardized tests, to direct observation under laboratory or natural conditions. Each of these measures has a different purpose, and each approach achieves a different level of robustness. In general, Goldfried (1977) has cautioned that the field of behavioral assessment generally "appears to be at the point where the need for measures currently outstrips the available procedures . . . [and] we are faced with the danger that poorly conceived assessment procedures may begin to fill the existing vacuum" (p. 4). Nowhere is this caution better taken than in the realm of marital assessment. Therefore, the present discussion of marital assessment begins with an elaboration of the criteria that should be used in selecting materials from the broad array that is currently available.

1. *Assessment Must Be Parsimonious.* Parsimony must take its position with reliability and validity as one of the essential characteristics of a marital assessment protocol. Perhaps because of the lasting impact of the psychoanalytic approach, through which many of us learned to respect the study of the historical and intrapsychic dimensions of behavior, many clinicians share the beliefs that diagnosis is the essence of treatment itself, and that diagnosis is never sufficient unless it is complete. These beliefs have led many clinicians to delay the start of active therapy until they felt they had exhausted the supply of available data, despite the fact that much of what they collected was of dubious reliability and little of it was immediately relevant to the decisions that had to be made in planning and guiding the treatment process. Indeed, it is this sluggishness in moving treatment forward and the tendency to collect more information than is needed that may be at the root of the all-too-often-observed failure of psychotherapy to yield the hoped-for improvements.

In light of the somewhat unpredictable success of psychodynamically oriented therapy, Freud may be regarded better as one of the outstanding philosophers of human behavior than as the founder of one of the more effective means of redirecting that behavior. Freud's quest for explanations of why things happen clearly falls more in the realm of philosophers than in that of clinicians, and his relative neglect of attention to means of limiting the study of his clients to the collection of only those data that were clinically relevant differentiates his approach from those that are more effectively change-oriented.

From a social-learning-theory point of view, it is assumed that successful marital therapy does not depend upon the therapist's having a complete understanding of why the partners chose one another, why they developed the interaction patterns that have evolved during the course of their relationship, or why they decided to seek to improve or to abandon their marriages. Instead, therapists must confine themselves to a description of those aspects of the couple's functioning that they would like to maintain or enhance and those they would like to change, as well as to how they would like to arrive at a decision about whether to remain together or to separate. In short, rather than seeking *complete* information, the therapist oriented toward social learning theory seeks only that information that is *necessary and sufficient* to provide the guidance needed for the planning and evaluation of a program aimed at changing interactional behavior.

2. Assessment Must Be Multidimensional. Having entered a plea for parsimony, we must now balance that plea with a recognition of the fact that a satisfactory clinical data base must be multidimensional.

Many years ago Campbell and Fiske (1959) differentiated between convergent and divergent validity in advocating adoption of their multitrait–multimethod matrix. "Convergent validity" refers to the extent to which varied measures agree. If several assessment tools are used to evaluate a couple and their results are inconsistent, the observer cannot be sure whether the tools are unreliable or the couple's behavior is so erratic as to change significantly over time. On the other hand, if the measures agree too well, the clinician may wonder whether only a single dimension of the relationship has been measured. In contrast, "divergent validity" refers to the extent to which measures expected to assess different entities do in fact yield different results. Here the danger is that the measures will be so disparate as to address totally different phenomena. In that case, their results would not afford the clinician the multiple tests that would build confidence in a particular conclusion. Based upon these considerations, the authors concluded that an adequate assessment package must draw upon diverse measures and methods in which some tools yield overlapping results, while others are intended to assess separate aspects of the relationship.

Later, Fiske (1975) noted that in addition to using different measures, adequate assessment programs also use different observers. He contended that different observers of the same events are likely to formulate quite different descriptions of what they have seen, so that the uncorroborated judgments of just one person must be understood to have a high risk of significant bias. It is this kind of reasoning that led commentators on marital assessment (e.g., Bergin & Lambert, 1978;

Gurman, 1973; Margolin, 1977) to suggest that adequate data can be obtained only when the views of husbands, wives, and therapists are combined to formulate an impression of the couple's interaction.

The requirement that diverse methods used by varied observers be included in a marital assessment program can lead to an overzealousness in measurement that violates the essential parsimony that these judgments must also possess. Barry (1970) used the term "shotgun approach" to describe the tendency of some clinicians to use every available tool to try to arrive at a sound clinical judgment. In the recommendations for marital assessment that follow, care has been taken to reach the point of sufficient, but not excessive, levels of measurement precision.

3. *Assessment Should Be Linked to a Theory of Intervention.* Zuk (1976) and L. Fisher (1976) have observed that with few exceptions (e.g., Grunebaum *et al.*, 1969), most of the measures offered for marriage and family assessment are essentially unrelated to the services that follow. Thus, therapists are often confronted by the painful choice between attempting to translate incomplete and abstract theoretical language into the practical terms of therapeutic change (Cashdan, 1973) or of proceeding with intervention without an adequate understanding of the clinically relevant facts.

In moving from assessment to treatment, therapists are prone to make either or both of two rather natural errors. Sometimes, we tend to force our assessment in certain directions because of the availability of certain treatment tools. In keeping with the adage "To a man holding a hammer, everything looks like a nail," some therapists tend to use highly biased scanning and interpretation processes, as if to shape assessment to fit a predetermined treatment approach. For example, D. McDonald (1971) implied that physicians who believe in the value of the psychopharmacological control of mood states would be more prone than psychologists, who cannot prescribe drugs, to find clinical-level depressions in their clients. It is only through an extension of the value self-survey described in Chapter 2 that this bias can be identified and overcome. Even when they make comparatively value-fair judgments, therapists are still subject to the tendency to incorporate into their assessments some assumptions that may misdirect treatment. For example, in Chapter 7 it is suggested that open, uncensored communication may be one of the most dependable ways to do violence to marital happiness. Yet many therapists subscribe to the belief that such communication is the *sine qua non* of marital success. Accordingly, they devote disproportionate energy to identifying the minutest detail concerning who? withholds what expressions? from whom? despite the fact that effort to overcome these adaptive lapses may seriously undermine the couple's change for improved functioning.

In light of this reasoning, it can be concluded that therapists have the responsibility of purging their assessment approaches of obfuscating theoretical jargon, forced observational structures, and untested assumptions. All of the basic elements in each assessment approach must have direct and immediate bearing on the way in which specific therapeutic decisions are made in an objective manner.

4. *Assessment Must be Situation-Specific.* Mischel (1968), perhaps more than any other contemporary writer, has called attention to the situational specificity of human behavior. In the parlance of assessment and diagnostic theorists, he has argued in favor of a "state" rather than a "trait" approach. The former implies that behavior is a function of the interaction between an individual's behavior potential and the environment in which action takes place. Trait theory, on the other hand, implies that individuals behave consistently across environments because of their inherent predisposition to respond in certain ways. In calling for situationally specific assessment, Bergin and Lambert (1978) have noted that much skepticism now surrounds trait theory because it is irrelevant to the currently fashionable behavioral therapies; because it is generally believed that the testing and diagnostic routines are not helpful ways of relating to those who seek help; and because of mounting evidence that trait measures seldom generate effective treatment plans.

At least three different data sets support this conclusion. First, it has been shown in various studies (e.g., Garrigan & Bambrick, 1975; Jayaratne *et al.*, 1974; Stuart *et al.*, 1976) that changes in the behavior of children at home do not generalize to their school environment any more effectively than school-mediated changes are reflected in the child's actions at home.

Second, students of family interactions find that each family member acts differently in the company of each of the permutations of others. No one has expressed this important observation better than Laing and Esterson (1970) when, in the introduction to their classic *Sanity, Madness, and the Family*, they noted that one would find very different patterns of behavior when observing.

Jill alone
Jill with mother
Jill with father
Jill with brother
Jill with mother and father
Jill with mother and brother
Jill with father and brother
Jill with mother, father and brother. (p. 20)

If each person behaves differently—and consistently so—with each family member in the context of the home, then surely behavior is more state- than trait-governed.

Finally, Cuber's (1965) speculation that "man–woman behavior is often unique to the particular pair" (p. 54) has been borne out in a number of different studies, beginning as early as 1960 (Ex, 1960) and progressing through the 1970s (e.g., Birchler *et al.*, 1972, 1975; Ryder, 1968; Stone, 1973; Stuart & Braver, 1973; Winter *et al.*, 1973). In all of these studies it was shown that whether husbands and wives were or were not happily married, both were very likely to interact with strangers more positively than they behaved toward one another. Clearly, their pleasant and unpleasant behaviors were less a function of their traits than of their relationships to their partners in both structured and unstructured laboratory observations. As an explanation, Rubin (1972) has suggested that interactions with spouses are colored by past experiences, while interactions with strangers are history-free attempts to begin a relationship on the most positive possible footing. It can also be argued that one can treat acts of kindness offered to a stranger as a one-time experience, while those offered to spouses become implied promises of things to come—promises that many spouses wish to avoid irrespective of their level of marital satisfaction. In addition to freedom from the past and the future, spouses meeting strangers are also likely to respond more consistently with the demands of social etiquette, if only because a stranger triggers a different set of responses than those set off by a mate. Whatever the explanation, the fact that spouses treat each other very differently than they treat strangers, coupled with the situational specificity that has been observed in youngsters' behavior, contributes strongly to a state as opposed to a trait approach to marital assessment.

5. *Participation in the Assessment Process Must Be of Value to the Couple as an End in Itself.* Because couples continually evaluate their experience and adjust their behavior on the basis of these evaluations, it is important that the therapist help the clients to make these evaluations in the most constructive possible terms. Moreover, because couples often terminate therapy after the first to the fourth session (see Chapter 5), their gain from therapy may primarily be what occurs through participation in the assessment process. Because ethical considerations mandate that clients knowingly consent to participation in treatment on the basis of their shared-with-the-therapist understanding of the nature of their distress and its possible solution (Association for the Advancement of Behavior Therapy, 1977; Stuart, 1980a), they must be active and informed participants in the assessment process. Clients' active participation in an assessment process that is understandable to them is therefore both a practical and an ethical necessity. Such participation can be facilitated by an assessment process that has three important characteristics.

As a first requirement, the language used in assessment must be specific, intelligible, and acceptable to the client. Stuart (1971b) and Laner (1976) have observed that traditional clinical diagnostic language is more metaphoric than descriptive. It is better adapted to promoting a status differential between therapist and client than to informing either about the best way to help the client achieve his or her goals. Curiously, and for the wrong reasons, the less descriptive the language the greater the likelihood that the information will be accepted by the client. C. R. Snyder (1974) illustrated this fact with a rather simple study (see, too; Snyder & Larson, 1972; Ulrich *et al.*, 1963). She offered undergraduates one of four standardized handwritten diagnostic statements. The one based on a homemade inkblot was most readily accepted, followed by those based upon a locus-of-control measure, a clinical interview, and a statement of beliefs that are supposedly "generally true about people." Snyder concluded that students are more likely to accept messages based upon more mysterious data sources, distrusting their own reasoning powers and attributing inordinate power to those who can "see through" their defenses. Unfortunately, this power is better adapted to clouding their minds than to improving their self-understanding. The fact that clients accept mystery may have led clinicians to offer what was wanted, even though the statements made may have had limited relevance to the service being offered. One of the greatest contributions of social learning theory to clinical practice may be its provision of a language of behavioral description that is precise, related to treatment, and contextually derived.

Thus, *contextual relevance is the second requirement of useful assessment.* Watzlawick and Beavin (1974) have expressed as strongly as any their respect for the necessity of *in situ* assessment with the observation that "there are no objective facts outside the relationship context in which they are experienced" (p. 62). To be useful for marital therapy, all assessment data must lead the clients to a better understanding of the role that each plays in shaping his or her experience. The concept of "reciprocal determinism," as used by Bandura (1977) and discussed in the last chapter, can become an interpersonal reality only when each partner learns how to understand his or her role in prompting and maintaining the other's actions. Watzlawick *et al.* (1967) refer to this process of analysis as an understanding of the "punctuation" of an interaction as a means to promote this understanding. Building upon their logic, we can visualize the following exchange taking place the night before Bill's real estate agents' exam:

JUNE: Bill, would you please help me get dinner on the table?

BILL: Why don't you have some understanding once in a while? Can't you see I'm up to my ears in landlord and tenant rights?

JUNE: You've had six months to study for that exam. If you'd watched ten fewer football games, you would have been ready for it by now. I've worked all day and I need some help from you now, exam or not.

BILL: (*Storms out of the kitchen, grabs his coat, and heads for the door.*) I've got to get out of here or I'll go batty!

JUNE: You can get out of here all right—and you can stay out, too!

When Bill describes this interaction, he describes the way in which June's actions precede and follow his, describing a scene in which he is the helpless victim of her excesses. He might point out that (1) she blew up at him; (2) so he said he was going out for a while; and (3) she told him to stay out. June does the same. She might tell a friend that (1) he accused her of bothering him while he works; so (2) she did point out that he put off his studying until the last minute and now she needed a few minutes of his time and a little consideration; (3) to which he responded by just storming out of the house. It is only when Bill and June add one element to each of their stories that they begin to have the ring of truth. Bill should have added that he prompted June's blowup by accusing her of lacking understanding, while June could have completed her tale of woe by pointing out that she did ask for help at a time when he clearly was very tense and busy. Therefore, the clients' descriptions of their experiences are useful to them only if the therapist helps each to render more of the complete story. Instead of three-element tales— other did, I did, other did—tales of four or more elements are needed. This is the only way in which clients can be helped to learn useful things about their roles in their own interactions, and, as is shown in the next chapter, these data are available only when collected during the conjoint session.

In addition to being couched in intelligible and acceptable terms, and in addition to describing adequately punctuated interaction sequences, *assessment data that clients can use must also be positive.* When they present themselves for treatment, most couples are well versed on their complaints about one another. To provide an opportunity for them to rehash their "dirty laundry lists" can do little more than provide them with another chance to confront one another negatively, to repeat their reasons for being neither willing nor able to change, and to delay starting the process of therapeutic change. With few exceptions (e.g., Chamow, 1975; L. Fisher, 1976; Otto, 1962; Stuart & Stuart, 1973), most of those concerned with clinical assessment address client weaknesses rather than strengths (Kieren & Tallman, 1972). Zubin (1972) put it well when he suggested that "psychopathologists in the past have behaved like bookkeepers who had only red ink available" (p. 299). It is now essential that the traditional preoccupation with pathology be replaced with a new respect for the strengths and the resources for change, for only then will assessment truly serve the client's needs. This stress upon positives can be achieved through several routes. For example, helping clients to clarify their goals reinforces the belief that change is possible (R. Friedman, 1977); helping them to recognize their own resources and those of their mates can build their confidence in the feasibility of change; and helping them to attend to positives in the present can enable them to track and to learn to reinforce those things that they enjoy and wish repeated rather than dooming them to repeat the past through negative tracking and attending.

Unfortunately, as Fisher and Sprenkle (1978) have noted, "until recently a disproportionate amount of attention has been given to pathology" (p. 9). Their work and that of Kantor and Lehr (1975) and Lewis *et al.* (1976) are exceptions to this trend. Working from the "circumplex model" of the family (see below), they generated a list of 34 aspects of family functioning dealing with communication skills, cohesion, and adaptability. They obtained responses from 52% of the 600 marriage and family counselors whom they asked to rate each of these aspects. Among the items that had the greatest consensual validity for strength were basic communication skills (e.g., positive responding, attending, self-statements), supportiveness, flexibility, and negotiation skills. Among those least valued were esoteric communication skills (e.g., paraphrasing, metacommunication, and completeness of communication), the willingness to take the part of family members against others, and physical caretaking. An appreciation of resources such as these is the very essence of relationship assessment and, as will be seen in later chapters, feeds directly into the planning of specific intervention techniques.

In summary, it is ethically and pragmatically necessary to make participation in the assessment process a productive experience for the clients. This can be achieved only if the language of assessment is specific, intelligible, and acceptable to the couple; if the assessment broadens the partners' perspectives to include awareness of their own roles in shaping their interaction; and if the data collected are positive and strength-oriented. When the assessment process meets these and the other criteria outlined above (i.e., parsimony, multidimensionality, direct linkage to treatment methods, and situational specificity), the data collected as the basis for treatment can lay a firm foundation for the planning of successful intervention. In the sections that follow, specific suggestions are made of tools that are consistent with the above criteria and that meet data needs at the various stages of the treatment process. It is essential to note in this context, however, that assessment is an ongoing process that begins before the first contact with the couple and ends long after the last treatment session. The therapist who locks onto a clinical judgment early in the contact and who fails to reevaluate and modify that opinion systematically surely fails to meet a critically important responsibility to the clients (Mahoney, 1977).

Measuring Marital Satisfaction and Its Constituents

Virtually every marital treatment client and every marriage therapist seeks improvement in the client's level of marital satisfaction. Yet this universally sought goal remains as elusive as the Holy Grail because of the many problems that obstruct its measurement (Croake & Lyon, 1978). Marital satisfaction is an entirely personal experience: we each select different aspects of our marital experience for assignment of different weights at various times. Because marital satisfaction is a feeling, it is entirely subjective and may or may not ever be reflected in interpersonal behavior. So much is marital satisfaction a personal will-o'-the-wisp, that Hunt (1978) considers all attempts at its measurement projective tests, because every respondent attaches purely subjective values to every question.

Another problem inherent in the measurement of marital satisfaction is the influence of response sets like social desirability (Edwards, 1957; 1967; Glick, 1964; Nye, 1964; Straus, 1964). Marital satisfaction is both something that we all think we should have—although often not believing that we are enjoying our fair share—and something that we try to convince others we have in order to be viewed as whole and healthy persons. Cone (1967) found a significant measure of social desirability biasing Dymond's (1954) attempt to relate marital satisfaction to MMPI items. Hawkins (1968) found an original measure of marital satisfaction to be so highly correlated with a test of the respondent's social approval motivation (Crowne & Marlowe, 1964) as to add little to scores of the latter measure. Finally, using Edmonds's (1967) measure of conventionalization, Edmonds et al. (1972) concluded a correlational study based upon data from 292 married persons by noting that "the most carefully validated and widely used scale of marital adjustment, the Locke–Wallace (short) Scale, is heavily contaminated by the tendency for persons to deceive themselves and others that their marriages are 'better' than they really are" (p. 100).

Data collected in 1975 by the National Opinion Research Center and released by the U.S. Department of Commerce (1977) lend great support to the practice of taking self-reports of marital satisfaction with a grain of salt. Adults were asked to describe the level of happiness they experienced in their marriages, and it was found tht 67.4% felt that they were "very happy," 29.8% reported that they were "pretty happy," and only 2.7% reported their marriages to be "not too happy." Given our awareness of the rising divorce rate and realizing that a certain amount of distress must precede the decision to divorce, these responses from a national sample are a better indicator of the weakness of a measurement tool than of the state of marital health. While boldly claiming *marital* bliss as a nation, we may be a bit more willing to own up to less-than-picture-book *family* life. The same survey reported results of 44.1%, 32.9%, 10.5%, and 6.6%, respectively, claiming to derive from their families a "very great deal," "a great deal," "quite a bit," or "a fair amount of happiness." Whether life in families is more stressful than life in couplehood or whether we feel we can be more honest about family as opposed to marital experience cannot be determined from these data. They do, however, cast a sufficiently strong cloud of doubt over the validity of marital satisfaction measures to warrant their being taken with considerable reservation.

While some writers have advocated the inference of marital satisfaction from such individual-focused tools as the 16 PF (W. P. Jones, 1976; Meck & Leunes, 1977a, b; Singh *et al.*, 1976), the Tennessee Self-Concept Scale (Hall & Valine, 1977), and the California Personality Inventory (Gough, 1975), most clinicians and researchers prefer to use an instrument aimed specifically at relationship assessment for this purpose. By far the most widely used instrument in this area is the Locke–Wallace Marital Adjustment Inventory (Locke & Wallace, 1959). However, some believe that this instrument regards marital adjustment more as an intrapersonal state than as an interpersonal process. They also consider the instrument too narrow to apply equally well to married and to nontraditional relationships (which are becoming more common), and they view the item selection for this instrument as having been unnecessarily arbitrary. Among the doubters is Spanier (1976), who created a pool of over 300 items (in his words "all items ever used in any scale measuring marital adjustment or a related concept," p. 17), deleted items that were redundant or clearly lacked content validity, factor analyzed the remaining 200 items, administered the refined items to over 600 married and cohabiting couples, revised, readministered, and refined even further, and produced a 32-item instrument. This easily administered Dyadic Adjustment Scale yields a measure of overall adjustment, in addition to measuring consensus, satisfaction, cohesion, and affectional expression. With the permission of its author and the National Council of Family Relations, this instrument is reprinted in Figure 1.

Inspection of the items in Figure 1 reveals Spanier's concept of dyadic adjustment. He clearly believes that consensus on issues from philosophy of life to the handling of money and in-laws contributes over half of marital adjustment (17 of 32 items—items 1–15, 29, 30). Of the 32 items, 7 refer to actions that the couple may or may not take together (e.g., confiding in each other or working on a project together), 4 of the items relate to conflict (e.g., divorce threats, leaving home after fights, frequency of quarreling and of getting on one another's nerves), and 4 items refer to satisfaction with and commitment to the marriage. For some couples, and perhaps for many, these may not be the issues that account for marital satisfaction or its absence. For instance, the woman who feels that she gave up a promising career in order to remain with her husband when he was transferred to a better position may be dissatisfied not because she and her husband do not communicate well, but because she mourns lost opportunities. In the same vein, the wife who has a lasting relationship with one or more lovers may agree and communicate with her husband quite acceptably, yet she might leave him feeling suspicious, uncared for, or downright worried. In the same vein, disagreement might be rife between a husband and wife, and yet they might be blissfully happy, taking each disagreement as an opportunity for committed self-expression in quarrels that have many more positive than negative implications. Therefore, the Dyadic Adjustment Scale is not a fail-safe instrument: it may yield false positives as well as false negatives and must always be followed up with a careful clinical assessment.

Parental consensus is believed to play a role in the adjustment of children; it may play a role in marital adjustment as well. Some writers have used variants of the Role Construct Repertory Test (G. Kelly, 1955) as a means of evaluating the extent to which couples share the same interpersonal values and perceptions (e.g., Duck & Spencer, 1972; L'Abate et al. 1975; Ryle & Lipshitz, 1975; Stuart, 1975). In addition to the aforementioned opportunity to quantify the degree of similarity in the content of couples' interpersonal values, the measure also affords an opportunity to assess the similarity and difference in the structure (e.g., complexity) of their interpersonal space.

Others have measured consensus by comparing partners' scores on indices of marital satisfaction. Terman (1938), using a forerunner of the Locke–Wallace Scale, found that the satisfaction ratings of spouses correlated at the level of .81. Later studies of marital satisfaction showed correlations ranging from .45 to .80 (e.g., Coleman & Miller, 1975; Levinger & Breedlove, 1966; Margolin, 1978). Hunt (1978) even found that spouses' predictions of each other's rating of satisfaction correlated with that rating at the level of .81. Therefore, whether happy or sad, husband and wife tend to feel the same about the level of joy in their marriage.

Certainly, we all enjoy the feeling of being understood by others, and even if this feeling is illusory, it is likely to have a positive impact upon feelings of satisfaction in our relationships with others (Clarke, 1974; Lefkowitz, 1974). Booth and Welch (1978) believe that consensus tends to be issue-specific rather than an across-the-board affair, but others have found that couples tend to agree on most of the areas of strength and weakness in their marriage (Gruver & Labadie, 1975). Agreement on assets and liabilities may facilitate decision making in

Figure 1. Dyadic Adjustment Scale. Reproduced with the permission of the author and the National Council on Family Relations.

	Always agree	Almost always agree	Occasionally disagree	Frequently disagree	Almost always disagree	Always disagree
1. Handling family finances	5	4	3	2	1	0
2. Matters of recreation	5	4	3	2	1	0
4. Religious matters	5	4	3	2	1	0
4. Demonstrations of affection	5	4	3	2	1	0
5. Friends	5	4	3	2	1	0
6. Sex relations	5	4	3	2	1	0
7. Conventionality (correct or proper behavior)	5	4	3	2	1	0
8. Philosophy of life	5	4	3	2	1	0
9. Ways of dealing with parents or in-laws	5	4	3	2	1	0
10. Aims, goals, and things believed important	5	4	3	2	1	0
11. Amount of time spent together	5	4	3	2	1	0
12. Making major decisions	5	4	3	2	1	0
13. Household tasks	5	4	3	2	1	0
14. Leisure-time interests and activities	5	4	3	2	1	0
15. Career decisions	5	4	3	2	1	0

	All the time	Most of the time	More often than not	Occasionally	Rarely	Never
16. How often do you discuss or have you considered divorce, separation, or terminating your relationship?	0	1	2	3	4	5
17. How often do you or your mate leave the house after a fight?	0	1	2	3	4	5
18. In general, how often do you think that things between you and your partner are going well?	5	4	3	2	1	0
19. Do you confide in your mate?	5	4	3	2	1	0
20. Do you ever regret that you married (or lived together)?	0	1	2	3	4	5
21. How often do you and your partner quarrel?	0	1	2	3	4	5
22. How often do you and your mate "get on each other's nerves"?	0	1	2	3	4	5

	Every day	Almost every day	Occasionally	Rarely	Never
23. Do you kiss your mate?	4	3	2	1	0

	All of them	Most of them	Some of them	Very few of them	None of them
24. Do you and your mate engage in outside interests together?	4	3	2	1	0

How often would you say the following occur between you and your mate:

	Never	Less than once a month	Once or twice a month	Once or twice a week	Once a day	More often
25. Have a stimulating exchange of ideas	0	1	2	3	4	5
26. Laugh together	0	1	2	3	4	5
27. Calmly discuss something	0	1	2	3	4	5
28. Work together on a project	0	1	2	3	4	5

These are some things about which couples sometimes agree and sometimes disagree. Indicate if either item below caused differences of opinions or were problems in your relationship during the past few weeks. (Check yes or no.)

	Yes	No
29. Being too tired for sex	0	1
30. Not showing love	0	1

31. The dots on the following line represent different degrees of happiness in your relationship. The point, "happy," represents the degree of happiness of most relationships. Please circle the dot that best describes the degree of happiness, all things considered, of your relationship.

0	1	2	3	4	5	6
.	.	.	.	.	.	.
Extremely unhappy	Fairly unhappy	A little unhappy	Happy	Very happy	Extremely happy	Perfect

32. Which of the following statements best describes how you feel about the future of your relationship:

5   I want desperately for my relationship to succeed and would go to almost any lengths to see that it does.

4   I want very much for my relationship to succeed and will do all that I can to see that it does.

3   I want very much for my relationship to succeed and will do my fair share to see that it does.

2   It would be nice if my relationship succeeded, and I can't do much more than I am doing now to help it succeed.

1   It would be nice if it succeeded, but I refuse to do any more than I am doing now to keep the relationship going.

0   My relationship can never succeed, and there is no more that I can do to keep the relationship going.

nonfamilial groups (e.g., Bass, 1963; L. R. Hoffman, 1965; Maier & Hoffman, 1960). Others believe this to be true for courting (Schulman, 1974) and married couples (e.g., Bean & Kerckhoff, 1971; Kieren & Tallman, 1972). It would seem that if the couple cannot agree on the dimensions of the challenges they face, they will hardly be able to mount an effective concerted action to meet these challenges.

Perhaps the easiest way to achieve consensus is to marry someone whose perceptions, values, patterns of actions, and background are similar to one's own. This is the first of what are termed here the "boundary conditions" that affect marital satisfaction. Before briefly reviewing the literature relevant to this point, it is perhaps wise to clarify the meaning of these conditions which play such a role in facilitating the achievement of marital satisfaction or stress.

Boundary Conditions of Marital Interaction

Henry Murray (1938, 1959) may have been one of the first of the contemporary American psychologists to give boundary conditions their proper place in juxtaposition to internal states. He referred to need or stress, which is an internal motivator, in contrast to press, which is an extraindividual source of motivation. He viewed press as:

> a directional tendency in an object or situation. Like a need, each press has a qualitative aspect—the kind of effect which it has or might have upon the subject . . . as well as a quantitative aspect, since its power for harming or benefitting varies widely. Everything that can supposedly harm or benefit the well-being of an organism may be considered pressive, everything else inert. (pp. 118–119)

To be a press, the event must be currently or potentially relevant to the individual's ability to achieve personal goals. But a press need not be a reality; Murray differentiated between "alpha presses," which do exist, and "beta presses," which are possibly correct or possibly incorrect beliefs about the external world. The relationship can be viewed graphically as follows:

		Beta presses	
		Correct	Incorrect
Alpha presses	Positive	A	B
	Negative	C	D

Therefore, a wife may imagine that her husband is attracted to another woman and may react as though this other woman existed. Her belief is a beta press. If the other woman does exist, she is a negative alpha press and the beta press is realistic (cell C). Conversely, if there is no other woman, the belief is an illustration of an unrealistic beta press (cell B);

the reality is positive, but the belief is negative and incorrect. When the wife feels and in fact is loved and appreciated by her husband, she lives happily in cell A. Finally, if the wife believes that her husband has no collateral relationships, but in fact he does, her belief is incorrectly positive, but the reality is negative (cell D). Therefore, not only reality but the conception of reality has an important impact upon every individual's behavior.

The boundary conditions that affect marital interaction and satisfaction are the constellation of these alpha and beta presses. They are ever-changing. The couple can control some of these presses: for example, their selection of each other as mates, their friendships with friends and relatives in the community, where they live, and the size of their family. They cannot control others: for example, economic conditions, cultural attitudes, and some life stresses as external examples; and aging and illness as internal examples. They can, however, control the way in which they construe these events by, for instance, thinking of obstacles as opportunities. They can also control the way in which they allow these events to influence their interaction. Nevertheless, boundary conditions can predispose them to positive and joyful interactions or to negative and highly stressful experiences together. It is much easier for a well-fed couple than for a starving couple to be "happy"; yet even the starving couple can experience a range of satisfaction outcomes. By analogy, the person born with the genes for leanness has a comparatively easy time of maintaining ideal weight, but the person born with the genes for fatness can also maintain ideal weight, albeit at the expense of much more planning and effort. Boundary conditions, therefore, do not determine the success of marriage, but they do influence the content of the challenges that must be met and the energy that must be invested in the attainment of success. It is important to bear in mind, however, that freedom from all negative presses may be as harmful to the couple's chances of happiness as would be their suffering from a surfeit of such presses. Some challenge from outside may greatly facilitate their cooperation, their integration, their sense of goal and purpose, and thereby their marital satisfaction. As Lewis Coser (1969) observed some time ago, the presence of extragroup conflict can sometimes galvanize intergroup cohesion and commitment.

In order to build an appreciation and understanding of some of the boundary conditions that have a bearing upon couples' interaction and satisfaction, several such conditions are discussed here briefly.

MATE SELECTION

A number of studies have documented that "like marries like," at least with respect to sociological variables. That is, there is a higher-than-chance probability that marital partners will be similar with respect to age, race, social class origin, educational level, religious preference, and ethnic background (Kerckhoff, 1976; Stroup, 1977). There also tend to be moderately high correlations between partners on characteristics like intellectual abilities and physical characteristics like height, weight, and attractiveness (Murstein & Christy, 1976; Stroup, 1977).

Several explanations have been offered in efforts to account for the seeming predominance of the tendency for "birds of a feather to flock together." People with similar characteristics are most likely to meet. According to the propinquity theory, marriage eligibles tend to meet one another in their neighborhoods, in their churches, or at their jobs, and those who are most similar in background and characteristics are most likely to meet in these selective settings. People with similar characteristics and background also tend to be more comfortable with one another than they would be with others whose resources and interests diverge widely from their own. In addition, there is a norm favoring homogamous pairing in most communities. When suiters make heterogamous choices, they frequently meet with strong pressures to separate "before it is too late," buttressed by threats that their differences foretell the tragic end of their relationship or, failing that, forewarn their exile from their native social groups (Kerckhoff, 1976).

For the marriage therapist, the acid test of any mate-selection theory is its ability to predict marital stability. Demographers, social psychologists, and other marriage and family researchers have much to contribute on this score. For example, Norton and Glick (1976) found that religious similarity is linked with marriage stability, except that those with no religious preference are most likely to divorce. Similarity of age is also associated with marital cohesiveness, although less strongly so than religious congruence. The effect of age spread is greatest when the wife is older than her husband (Bumpass & Sweet, 1972). Some dissimilarities in education are also associated with marital instability, but these differences often vanish when other variables are controlled. For example, marriages between college-educated women and high-school-educated men are unstable, but the instability is best explained by the income level of the husband. Also, there are some data to suggest that interracial marriages are more unstable than racially homogamous marriages. While blacks have a higher rate of marital disruption than whites, Heer (1974) found that there is a higher probability of divorce in black–white marriages than in black–black unions. Those interested in need assessment (e.g., Pascal, 1974; Rogers et al., 1972) have also tended to find that similarity better predicts marital satisfaction than complementarity. The level of agreement on attitudes such as those related to family planning (Jaco & Shepard, 1975) also predicts marital stability. Finally, Patterson and Reid (1970) suggested that similarity of interests provides some marital "glue," while dissimilarity would lead spouses on separate paths for their pleasures. While some separate interests are in most instances a facilitator of satisfaction with marriage, too much of this good thing very often spells trouble for the couple.

In summary, there is a moderate amount of evidence in support of the belief that similarity in characteristics may be conducive to marital stability, with great differences often requiring adjustments just difficult enough to tip the balance toward separation and divorce. Moreover, given the fact that disparate couples must move together despite opposition from family and friends, it is also possible that their will to be different also extends to their greater than average willingness to consider and then act on divorce (Bumpass & Sweet, 1972). Therefore, similar backgrounds, values, and interests are surely factors to be reckoned with in summing over the valence of the conditions that are the boundaries of every marriage, even when full credence is given to the necessity to interpret those differences that do exist in light of their personal and interpersonal meaning to each partner rather than assuming that each difference is necessarily a barrier to marital stability. Indeed, it must be recognized that for some couples the very existence of differences and challenges that they bring may spark interest in and commitment to their marriage. In this same view, similarity may bring on a lack of interest that might quickly end a marriage for these counternormative couples.

AGE AND STAGE AS BOUNDARY CONDITIONS

Age at marriage, aging while married, and the length and stages of marriage are all time-related forces that bear upon opportunities for marital satisfaction.

Lee (1977) began one of the best recent reviews of the impact of age of marriage with the following statement:

> One of the few empirical issues in family sociology on which there is virtual unanimity is the existence of an *inverse* association between age at first marriage and probability of divorce. This relationship has been repeatedly documented by a variety of studies over a considerable period of time. (p. 493)

Lee noted too that this relationship is strongest among the young and that explanations of this association are not convincing. Bumpass and Sweet (1972) have shown through multivariate analysis that age at marriage contributes to marital stability in its own right and not as a correlate of lesser amounts of education, income, and related factors. Bartz and Nye (1970) speculated that early-marrying couples may be unprepared both socially and emotionally to assume marital responsibilities, thus explaining the fragility of their unions. In addition, Nye

(1976) has suggested that those who marry early are the most remar-riageable: cognizant of their alternative options, they may be more ready than their later-married counterparts to switch rather than to try to change their relationship. Based upon Lee's (1977) data, at least a mod-erate association between marital age and marital stability does exist. Given the observation that those who marry young and stay married appear to have a higher level of satisfaction than many who marry later, partial support is offered for Nye's (1976) hypothesis as well. Those who remain married despite the available alternative relationships may do so, as social exchange theory would predict, simply because the satis-factions mediated by the marriage exceed those expected from other possible marriages.

Hicks and Platt (1970) reviewed several decades of research relating to marital satisfaction and length of marriage, which is necessarily related to age. They noted that methodological difficulties such as dif-ferences in the number and stages of marriage studied, in the dependent variables selected, in the designs and statistical procedures used, and in sample size and representativeness make generalization across these studies hazardous. In general, however, they found a decline in marital satisfaction over time. For example, Blood and Wolfe (1960) found that wives' marital satisfaction declined from the "infant stage" until the time that the children were launched, increased slightly until retire-ment, and declined again at that point. Pineo (1961) completed a longi-tudinal study begun by Burgess and Wallin (1953) and noted a gradual "process of disengagement" between engagement and the 4th or 5th anniversary and the 20th year of marriage. While the data reported by Pineo were collected longitudinally, Rollins and Feldman (1970) re-ported some contradictory data based upon cross-sectional responses. They found a curvilinear relationship between marital satisfaction and the duration of marriage: couples reported greater happiness before and after their child-rearing stage. The problem in interpreting these and similar data, however, is that the responses were drawn from different couples at each stage of marriage. Once into child rearing, dissatisfied couples may separate, so the upward swing in satisfaction level may better reflect sampling error than a true change in the couples' satisfac-tion with their marriages (Baltes, 1968). In addition, Rollins and Cannon (1974) reported data showing that differences in the measures of satis-faction used in each of the studies account for much of their outcome differences. Working with their own new sample, they found that the Blood and Wolfe (1960) measure showed an L-shaped or steady decline in marital satisfaction, while use of the Rollins and Feldman (1970) and Locke–Wallace (1959) measures revealed U-shaped distributions. Finally, they also showed that in the two studies in which Rollins was a co-investigator (Rollins & Feldman, 1970; Rollins & Cannon, 1974), stage, sex, and stage-by-sex interaction accounted for only 4% and 8% of the variance in marital satisfaction scores, respectively. Finally, Spanier *et al.* (1975) criticized this line of research for its failure to use statistical procedures and stated that they would have tested curvilinearity. However, their effort to control for maturational, historical, and cohort effects still failed to demonstrate a clear trend in marital satisfaction over the course of marriage.

One factor that might play a role in these age-related trends is illness and exposure to life stress events such as job loss, the sense of loss when children leave home (Glenn, 1975b), and the death of friends and relatives. Using the Social Readjustment Rating Scale (Holmes & Rahe, 1967; Rahe, 1974), Frederickson (1977) showed that a small number of couples receiving therapy had undergone significantly more of these stresses during the year prior to their therapy than a comparable sample of untreated couples. To the extent that these stresses correlate with age, they may account for a goodly share of the age-related trends in marital satisfaction.

In summary, it can be said that temporal variables often play a role in predisposing couples to greater or lesser marital stability. Those who marry young may be too ill-equipped for the responsibility they assume or too preoccupied with personal and professional challenges to devote to their marriages the attention that is required. Time plays a role later on, too, as couples experience the ravages of age, illness, and a gradual loss of control of the forces that shape their lives; they may be more likely to remain together because of a shrinking range of options, but the price of their stability may be diminished satisfaction with their relationship. Therefore, a knowledge of the age of each partner can often sensitize the therapist to temporal conditions that may pose challenges that strain the effects of the best intentions that both spouses can muster.

STAGE OF RELATIONSHIP

Related to the partners' age is the stage of their relationship. It has been found that some two-fifths of all divorce actions are initiated during the first two years of marriage (see Chapter 1). The early months of a marriage are its first critical stage, a time at which husbands and wives begin to hammer out a set of rules for the many remaining days of their relationship. Given the complexity of marriage and the expectations that couples will provide for each other aid, comfort, sexual stimulation, intellectual stimulation, and much more while also doing their jobs within and outside their home, the delicate negotiation of these relationship contracts would seem to be challenge enough. But two additional factors further complicate this effort. Couples rarely if ever receive realistic, practically useful preparative education for the success-ful mastery of this developmental challenge; indeed, they are often exposed to naive and utterly unrealistic clichés that significantly limit their abilities to rise to this challenge. In addition, they must overcome all of the deceptions that were perpetrated during their courtship (Meck & Leunes, 1976) in these sensitive early months. Courtship can be portrayed as the time of maximum deception in the lives of otherwise honest and honorable people, for this is the time that each person seeks to sell—using every gimmick of good salelsmanship—his or her most valuable commodity: himself or herself. He never openly condemns her religious views during courtship but lets go both barrels on the third Sunday that she asks him to attend church with her. She has always managed to finish her work before leaving the office during courtship but suddenly has more than Hercules could manage in a day of eight far-too-short hours. She feels horrified at his cynicism about something so dear to her as her faith, equaled only by his frustration at having to spend the lion's share of his evenings alone while she catches up on office overflow. Each then wonders how he or she got into this mess, each feeling badly "taken" by the other's deception, often with little awareness of the way in which every lie has its mirror image.

Therapists seeing couples who have been recently married would do well to assess those expectations of both partners that have and have not been fulfilled on their trip down the rose-petaled aisle. The critical challenge for couples at this stage of marital development is thus one of negotiating a realistic set of privileges and responsibilities (Stuart, 1971a), a set that both will be prepared to honor until renegotiating anew.

The next critical stage in marital development occurs when the first child is born. At this time, both partners must make major readjust-ments. They are forced to give up much of the autonomy that they have enjoyed from adolescence onward. They must learn to hold personal satisfaction secondary to the responsibility of keeping their newborn alive and well. They must also renegotiate roles only recently created. Again, these are not small challenges, but the job is further complicated because most couples become parents with expectations as naive as those that preceded their marriage; they have diminished energy due to sleep loss; and they often lose sight of their own affiliative desires when preoccupied with trying to learn all that is needed for them to become effective, nurturant parents.

In most traditional marriages, the mother exercises much of the responsibility for coordinating the lives of the children. When they begin to achieve some measure of independence—as early as their first day in preschool—the mother must adjust to some measure of role loss: she is simply not as badly needed by her offspring and must find new sources of stimulation, self-definition, and responsibilities within the family. Many suburban housewives in the classical mode switch from careers as mothers to careers as chauffeurs. With the rise in women's consciousness, however, increasing numbers of women are opting out of the *Hausfrau* role and into the work world as soon as, if not before, their youngest is eligible for preschool. In either case, whether the mother remains child-centered or becomes career-focused, the children's maturation demands further role adjustments for her.

So, too, does the exodus of the youngest child from the household require the couple to reach for new patterns of interaction. When the children leave home, the couple must often learn anew how to relate to one another. If they had shared decision-making authority with their children, they must begin to make most major decisions alone; if they spent some portion of their leisure time with their children, they must learn to plan and to enjoy activities by themselves. And perhaps most important, they must learn to talk about topics of their own choosing rather than dialoguing about the children and their exploits.

For the couple that makes all of the above adjustments well, one more adjustment awaits—perhaps the most difficult of all. This is the adjustment to retirement, which requires a massive role shift by both spouses at the very time that their energies begin to ebb and they are most settled into a habitual pattern of interaction.

While much attention is currently being focused on the "passages" that men and women make as they move through the stages of their lives (Levinson, 1978), the marriage therapist must be as alert to the stages of marital development that clients are experiencing as to the stage of their personal change. Indeed, many of the pressures of relationship change may now be rationalized in the language of personal growth, greatly complicating the rehabilitative task of therapist and clients alike. Therefore, assessment of the stage of each couple's marital development often provides valuable insights useful in the planning of the service that they are to receive.

MONEY, CHILDREN, AND MARITAL BLISS

The plight of the poor has been very well documented, but perhaps not more poignantly than in the words of Parham (1968):

> Whatever else it is, being poor is being without money and the things which money can buy. Without buying power, the poor man is not fed well, housed well, clothed well, schooled well, transported well, informed well, or entertained well. . . . Probably the sense of deprivation resulting from this inability to consume in a consumer economy is the principal source of embarrassment and insecurity for the poor. If they occasionally splurge foolishly when they have extra money, part of it is because they have no

assurance there will be another time for fun within the foreseeable future. Anyway, if they saved it, their friends and relatives would need it—because the well-of-need in their present and future is in their experience, insatiable. Again, it is a mistake to see this simply as present orientation without regard for the future. The poor think about the future: they have the feeling it will be just like the past. (p. 199)

The role of the poverty line in mediating challenges or opportunities for couples is so obvious as to be undeniable (Odita & Janssens, 1977; Piven & Cloward, 1971). Indeed, Levinger (1976) cited data collected by Cutright (1971) as showing that family income is more strongly and negatively associated with divorce than any other available census variable. However, Levinger also pointed out that the relationship is not entirely simple. The husband's income is positively related to marital stability (the more he earns, the more stable the marriage), but income earned by the wife is positively related to divorce (the more she earns the greater the instability of the marriage). This relationship is further complicated by comparisons between the educational and the income levels of the spouses (see Gibbs, 1977; Levinger, 1976), and elsewhere Stuart (in press) presented considerable evidence supporting the value of employment of the wife as a facilitator of marital stability. It is also necessary to take into consideration the nature of both partners' jobs. For example, if one is a physician, the pressures, the nature of the work, and the opportunities for contact with other potential partners is great, all of which contribute to a noteworthy level of marital instability in this group (Krell & Miles, 1976; Miles et al., 1975; Perlow & Mullins, 1976). On the other hand, if one partner is a writer who spends long hours alone at the typewriter, time on the job may not be at all related to opportunities for meeting new and possibly more exciting mates.

Children also strain the family budget in many ways. For example, the birth of children requires the couple to expand to more expensive quarters at the very time that the wife often reduces her time on the job. The start-up costs for the first child often come as a shock to couples who must spend money for medical bills, furniture, clothes for the infant, and much, much more. When these economic strains of childbearing are added to the relationship costs of the "blessed event," it is not surprising that many researchers consistently find divorce-prone-ness to be positively correlated with family size (e.g., Feldman, 1974; Hurley & Palones, 1967; Laws, 1971; LeMasters, 1957; B. C. Miller, 1976; Renne, 1970). As an exception to these findings, Thornton (1977) found a U-shaped distribution: childless couples and those with large families were more likely to divorce than those with families of moderate size. Levinger (1976) and Kerckhoff (1976) both suggested that having children may be a barrier to divorce, and possibly that would explain the greater divorce-proneness of childless couples. Economic hardships experienced by the parents of large families could explain the upsurge at the high end of the continuum. For families of moderate size, the children may be an alternative source of love and stimulation for parents whose relationship is less than they desire. In fact, Luckey and Bain (1970) found that dissatisfied couples tended to view their children as their greatest or only source of "marital satisfaction," a finding that did not hold for more satisfied partners.

In conclusion, it can be said that small incomes and large families appear to be inimical to marital stability and satisfaction. However, while they may be sufficient causes for stress, they are not necessarily causes of marital dissatisfaction. For example, small incomes may not provide partners with the wherewithal to strike out on paths that might lead them apart; or the absence of enough money to buy necessities, much less luxuries, may function as a cloud that overhangs all of the couples' daily interactions, blighting their opportunity for joyful exchanges. In the same vein, being childless may provide each member of a couple with opportunities for biological and psychological fulfillment, and therefore may serve as a fragmenting rather than as a unifying force. The presence of children can likewise help to bind the couple as an expression of their generativity; or children can be the wedge that drives them apart because their relationship may not be the match of the strains of parenthood. Therefore, money and children exert an influence upon marital satisfaction and stability, but their impact is in no sense unidirectional, and every couple experiences them in very individual ways.

CULTURAL AND SOCIAL FORCES AS BOUNDARY
CONDITIONS OF MARRIAGE

While Levinger (1965) believes that couples do not always act consistently with their values, he (1976) and others (Laner, 1978; Nye & Berardo, 1973; Scanzoni, 1968) have noted the importance of cultural values in shaping the character of marital interaction. Relevant values are ethnic or social class in origin, and they affect mate selection, role allocation, and the nuances of daily exchanges between spouses. Values stem from early socialization experiences in the family of orientation of each spouse and are reinforced in almost every encounter with members of the norm-setting communities in which the spouses spend time (Grunebaum & Christ, 1976). Certain aspects of marital interaction may be dysfunctional for the couple in the view of the therapist, and yet they may be "off limits" to intervention because they are consistent with values that the couples are unwilling to challenge. For example, the wife might not seek employment because of cultural or religious proscription of the employment of women—especially of mothers—outside their homes. And yet she might experience morbid depressions attributable to the loneliness and understimulation she experiences throughout the day. Clients may be asked to state and to examine these and similar values, but direct therapeutic challenge to these beliefs may seriously injure their motivation to move forward in treatment.

Cultural values touch the structure of the couple's social experiences much as they touch every other aspect of their relationship. In a classic study (Mayer & Zander, 1966), class-related differences were found in the depth and range of spousal contacts with other members of the community. Lower-class subjects were found to have superficial contacts with more people than middle-class subjects, who had deeper contacts with fewer individuals outside their families. For both groups, marital unhappiness was significantly positively related to the willingness of spouses to disclose personal details to outsiders. One-fourth of the lower-class group as opposed to almost two-thirds of the middle-class group rated their marriages as "excellent." However, among those who did not regard their marriages as so fine, many more were disposed to seeking aid and comfort from people other than their mates. The quality of life within the marriage thus has a predictable impact upon the couple's willingness to discuss their interaction with others, and to a certain extent, extramarital intimacy may be a clear reflection of an insufficiency of opportunities for sharing exchanges within the marriage. Clearly, compensatory experiences outside the marriage can help unhappy spouses cope better with their lot, while at the same time potentially offering inviting opportunities for sharing physical as well as socioemotional intimacies. When this happens, the social network is overused as a substitute for rather than as a complement to marital interaction (McCain, 1974). When spouses share the same friends, there is less of a tendency to overuse friendships in this way (Osmond & Martin, 1978), and when they do not share friendships, the likelihood is much greater that either or both will find their next mate among those upon whose soft shoulders they have cried (Leslie, 1977). Both cultural and social factors thus provide a major set of boundary conditions that are as likely to strengthen each couple's attachment to one another as they are likely to pull them asunder.

SUMMARY

Many of the boundary conditions that strengthen or stress a marriage are beyond the control of both the couple and the therapist. Nevertheless, an appreciation of their operation can help to steer the therapist away from challenging some of the nonnegotiable givens of the marriage and toward other options of which the couple might not have been aware. While recognizing the influence of these boundary conditions, it is nevertheless essential that the therapist keep in mind the fact that these factors predispose and influence, though they do not determine, the level of the couple's marital stability and satisfaction. Within the limits of the opportunities and constraints posed by these boundary conditions, each couple can experience greater or lesser amounts of what they aspire to accomplish in their lives together. Therefore, the clinician's knowledge of the boundary conditions that set the context for each couple's interaction must be used to facilitate the enhancement of the quality of their marriage.

To aid in the assessment of boundary conditions and to fashion the knowledge gained from this assessment into a formulation likely to have an impact on treatment planning, therapists are well advised to answer the following questions. Answers should first be formulated at the end of the initial contact and should be revised in response to new information collected during the course of treatment.

Area	Assessment data	Action alternative
Mate selection	In what ways important to each spouse are the partners alike or different?	To what extent can the couple be helped to recognize and draw comfort from their similarities and to relabel differences as opportunities for growth or stimulation?
Age	To what extent are any of the couple's identified stresses attributable to the effects of aging in either or both or to differences in the rate of their experiencing the effects of age?	Can the couple be helped to change their expectations of their own or one another's behavior so that they are consistent with physical realities? Can they be helped in any way to overcome the effects of aging?
Stage	Do role shifts associated with the stage of development of the couple's marriage influence their stress level in any appreciable way?	Can discussion of the stage of the marriage "normalize" the couple's reactions? Can ways be found to compensate for changes in interaction caused by developmental stage?
Money	Is the couple's problem exacerbated by financial pressures?	Can the couple be helped to find alternative income sources, to adjust their standard of living to their resources, or to differentiate their financial woes from their relationship stresses?
Children	Do child-rearing pressures contribute to the couple's perceived stress?	Can the couple be helped to better distribute child-care responsibilities, to rely more

| | | on outside help, or to better organize family patterns to relieve the strain of child care? |
| Cultural and social forces | To what extent are the couple's adaptive efforts thwarted or aided by similarities and differences between their orientation and that of the value-shaping forces in their environment? | Can the couple be helped to adopt a shared value framework and to negotiate differences between their consensual views and those of important others in their environment? |

It is important to bear in mind that the identification of boundary conditions that contribute to problem intensity must never be allowed to lower the expectation of a positive therapeutic outcome. In fact, the existence of boundary conditions that create pressures can to some degree give the couple an opportunity to move closer together to meet an outside challenge, and couples who are beset by problems inflicted from without may be more successfully treated than those whose stress is internally generated.

Assessment of Marital Interaction

The therapist should be interested in three aspects of marital interaction: its frequency, its perceived value to the spouses, and its impact upon their commitment to one another. A naive behavioral approach would stress frequency, infer value, and generally ignore commitment impact. Therefore, in the presentation that follows, less attention is paid to the first two dimensions and more to the third.

COUNTING NEGATIVE AND POSITIVE BEHAVIORS

The essence of social learning theory is the credence it gives to the interrelationship between actions and psychological and behavioral reactions. This idea was introduced in the foregoing chapter, and it is sufficient here merely to restate the guiding principle of this approach, using the words of Thibault and Kelley (1959):

> Whatever the gratification achieved in dyads, however lofty or fine the motives satisfied may be, the relationship may be viewed as a trading or bargaining one. The basic assumption running throughout our analysis is that every individual voluntarily enters and stays in any relationship only as long as it is adequately satisfactory in terms of his rewards and costs. (p. 37)

The building blocks of relationships are therefore all of the verbal and nonverbal actions taken by both parties, as well as the manner in which each person values what is given, what is received, and such boundary factors as beliefs about alternative reinforcements available in other relationships and the costs of aborting the present relationship.

In theory, the assessment of these factors would appear to be much less challenging than the problems inherent in inferring motivations and needs in psychotherapeutic interventions. In practice, however, the challenge is formidable. Patterson *et al.* (1976), who have worked as hard and productively as any other team, call attention to several of the problems that they have encountered in generating a language for describing treatment-related interactions between spouses. They noted that the assessment must be dyadic; that the behaviors believed to be most relevant to marital satisfaction and stability are private and therefore accessible only through self-report rather than through direct observation; that couples' concerns are more often stated in the language of emotion than in terms compatible with behavioral engineering; that much of the currently available theory of marriage is equally untranslatable into objectifiable terms, while also being irrelevant to treatment; and that experimental controls to test the validity of those terms that are used for assessment are neither possible nor ethically justifiable.

In light of these limitations, the field has achieved moderate but by no means remarkable success in generating a typology for describing marital action sequences into objectifiable terms useful for treatment planning and research. Self-report, direct observation, and observation of behavior in laboratory-based analogue situations have all been used for this purpose, each with its own assets and liabilities as noted in recent reviews of marital assessment materials (Bellack & Hersen, 1977; Jacob, 1976; Weiss & Margolin, 1977):

1. Self-report has the *advantages* of being acceptable to clients, inexpensive, useful for collecting data concerning behaviors that are too personal for observation by persons other than the couple, and it tends to be sufficiently under client control so that it addresses the client's real concerns. Its *disadvantages* are that clients often fail to follow through on self-reporting for various reasons, so that the data are incomplete, the data are necessarily biased by the viewpoint of the data collector and are hence highly unreliable, and self-report data are extremely reactive.

2. Direct observation in naturalistic surroundings has the *advantages* of being collected with virtually unparalleled reliability and completeness. The *disadvantage* of direct observation is the rather great possibility that actions observed with others present may be greatly influenced by social desirability and therefore lack validity with regard to true, observer-absent behavior, in addition to being extravagantly costly.

3. Observation in a laboratory-based analogue has the same reliability and completeness *advantages* as direct observation in naturalistic
settings. It also suffers from the validity and expense *disadvantages* of the
above. However, because both task and setting are artificial, what is
observed may have even less validity than the questionable data obtained
through observing behavior in homes, offices, and elsewhere.

Self-Report Measures. Some form of self-report is used in virtually
every approach in which therapists and clients meet to discuss the
clients' state of affairs. Even though data collected by this means are
somewhat unreliable, they come closest to the pattern of conventional
social exchange and therefore tend to meet with the least client resistance. Also, they often represent the self-statements that clients are
most willing to accept and are the ones that they believe to be most
accurate. A range of tools is available for structuring self-report.

The Marital Precounseling Inventory (Stuart & Stuart, 1973) is a
multiplex form with many applications in the treatment soon to be
described. Implicit in the construction of the form are the assumptions
that (1) marital satisfaction varies as a function of the way in which each
person behaves toward the other; (2) marital interaction flows more
smoothly when the spouses have some shared but also some separate
interests and when they have formulated long-range goals that put
daily activities into perspective and help to organize long chains of
behavior; (3) change goals are more likely to be achieved when they are
specific to areas of couple's interaction; (4) each goal can best be achieved
when the spouse selecting the goal makes changes before expecting new
responses from the other; and (5) concepts like agreement and understanding are quantifiable. Completed prior to the first treatment session, the form provides ample data for planning that session, while also
helping to socialize the clients into the treatment process (see Chapter
5). Completed at the end of treatment, the form can be used as one tool
in therapy evaluation (Dixon & Sciara, 1977; Liberman *et al.*, 1976b). Use
of the data yielded by this form for treatment planning is reviewed later
in this chapter and each of the chapters that follow.

Weiss *et al.* (1973) have offered a series of self-report measures that
address critical elements in their approach. They developed a Willingness-to-Change Scale in which each partner was asked to rate on a
seven-point scale, from "much more" to "much less," the desire that the
spouse engage in activities like keeping the house cleaner or having
sexual relationships. Their Marital Activities Inventory—Alone, Together, Others—asks the spouses to indicate with whom they engage in
each of five activities like card playing, going to a museum, and discussing family problems. Finally, partners are also asked to keep a Pleasurable–Displeasurable Count, a record of the daily occurrence of pleasing
behaviors like "we cuddled in bed" and "spouse called just to say hello,"

and displeasing behaviors like "spouse drank too much" or "spouse mimics me." Patterson *et al.* (1975) indicated that they and others using their instruments reliably differentiate between distressed and nondistressed couples. Therefore, if the reports do not match the interactional facts, at least the distortions made by couples in responding to these self-report measures err in the predicted direction—the happy couples toward socially desirable expectations, the unhappy couples toward overstatement of their displeasure.

The difficulties in using standardized measures like these are that the list may not include items that are important to the couple (they do include many items that are irrelevant and therefore add to the time that couples must spend in data collections), and that the *a priori* values placed on the actions by the therapist may not agree with the clients' appraisals. These problems may offset the advantages of standardization and may prompt clients with suggestions for new items that they may not have considered. As an alternative, forms such as those used in mounting caring days (see Chapter 6) both structure the intervention and evaluate its effects. Moreover, these more "local" measures will probably be used anyway, and their use does not add to data-collection costs in the same way as the Oregon standardized forms may. Therefore, many therapists choose to use self-report measures that relate more closely to the intervention techniques that they use, rather than relying upon more standardized tools.

Role theory has provided the rationale for another set of self-report measures. After being reviewed by Parsons and Bales (1955), role theory developed rapidly in both conception and application (e.g., Biddle & Thomas, 1966), with special emphasis upon its use in marriage counseling (e.g., Kargman, 1957; Kotlar, 1967–1968; Tharp, 1963b). It has been noted that roles undergo predictable shifts in response to stage of relationship and stage of life. For example, all courting men and women have concepts about the way in which they and their intended should behave after marriage (Lovejoy, 1961; Mangus, 1936; Pfeil, 1968). Despite the fact that the interaction between the sexes that they view at home is different from that which they find in the community, most couples enter marriage expecting a somewhat traditional interaction with their mates. However, as Leik (1963) was one of the first to observe, experience tends to triumph over hope early on. Among his results was the finding that:

> The traditional male role (instrumental, non-emotional behavior) as well as the traditional female role (emotional, non-task behavior) appear [*sic*] when interaction takes place among strangers. These emphases tend to disappear when subjects interact with their own families. Particularly is this true for instrumentality, because of a dual role for mothers. (p. 144)

Thus, while he held the car door open for her and she smiled warmly before they said "I do," these and many behaviors like them may vanish as they move into the daily business of living. Levinger (1964) found that specialization takes the place of mutuality in meeting these daily challenges, and that while middle-class spouses put affection and companionship toward the top of their hierarchies of goals, the steps they take to reach these goals drift away from cultural stereotypes. Coupled with marital cooperation as a basis for this drift is a general tendency for women to move toward more masculine actions while men move toward more feminine actions as they progress through middle age (Jung, 1933; Neugarten & Gutmann, 1968). Indeed, Sedney (1977) forewarned that the person who clings to sex-role polarities when reaching middle age will hardly have the skills necessary to cope with life crises. Thus, androgyny is a life necessity as well as a dimension of the mechanics of marriage.

As suggested in Chapters 3 and 9, when marital experience matches expectation, the couple are generally satisfied. However, when hope conflicts with reality with regard to the roles that the couple play, this inconsistency can generate conflict and dissatisfaction. While it is recognized that self-reports of role expectations and behavior are fully as influenced by response set as is the measurement of marital satisfaction (Granbois & Willett, 1970), study of role relationships can shed some light on marital strengths and goals for change (Hepker & Cloyd, 1974).

Several different approaches are available for measuring role functions within families (e.g., Hurvitz, 1961, 1965; Purcell, 1976; Scanzoni, 1970). Perhaps the most widely used measure was developed by Tharp (1963a), was essentially revalidated by Barton et al. (see Barton & Cattell, 1972), and has been used as a tool for evaluating the effects of marital treatment (e.g., Tsoi-Hoshmand, 1976). The Marital Role Questionnaire solicits agreement on a five-point scale (from "very essential" to "decidedly not desirable"), with items like "The husband should be the social equal of his wife" and "Women who want to remove the word 'obey' from the marriage service don't understand what it means to be a wife." To complete its assessment of expectations, this form asks respondents to rate the importance of such dimensions of marital life as wives' helping their husbands to succeed on the job and sharing recreation with their husbands; it asks for ratings of the importance of various role activities and addresses the expected division of responsibilities for decision making. It then offers a second form measuring the enactment of these roles. The two forms together yield measures of similarity of expectation, agreement of expectation with reality, and similarity of perceived reality in areas such as role sharing, togetherness, intimacy, and parental adequacy. These ratings are made in 12 areas of marital role expectations, areas like sexual gratification, togetherness, and role sharing.

In using role-theory–derived data, it is important for therapists to control their own value biases (Abramowitz, 1977; Guttman, 1977; Magnus, 1975). The roles of women are obviously changing (Huber, 1973; Kaplan & Bean, 1977), and with them, the roles of men must change as well. What was normative a decade ago may be contrary to current norms. Against this background of change must be placed the reality that norms are subcultural phenomena that are interpreted in very personal ways. Therefore, societywide changes may or may not reach into the lives of any given couple. To be sure, however, they will interpret the values that affect their interaction differently than their neighbors interpret the same expectations. Value clarification by the therapist is therefore of critical importance if the role-behavior dimensions of the couple's interaction are included in the assessment package.

A third approach to the collection of structured self-report data is found in the work of Moos (1974). His Family Environment Scale is a means of sampling the general climate within families. The 90 true-false items in this scale take the form of the following example: "Family members really help and support one another" and "Family members often keep their feelings to themselves." These items yield 10 subscales of nine items each:

1. Cohesion
2. Expressiveness
3. Conflict
4. Independence
5. Achievement orientation
6. Intellectual–cultural orientation
7. Active–recreational
8. Moral–religious emphasis
9. Organization
10. Control

The first three of these comprise the "relationship dimensions" of family interaction; the next five make up the "personal growth dimensions"; and the final two contribute the "system-maintenance dimension." When the scale was administered to a diverse sample of 285 families, six different family types were found: expression-oriented (9%); structure-oriented (8%); independence-oriented (24%); achievement-oriented (19%); moral-religious-oriented (11%); and conflict-oriented (29%). None of these orientations is necessarily associated with either marital happiness or distress. If measured at the start of treatment along with marital satisfaction, however, identification of the type of family that each partner believes she or he has may possibly provide some leads for goals for family change that may be reflected in improved marital satisfaction.

Observational Data. Like self-reports, direct observation in office settings is always a part of therapeutic assessment. Indeed, the most valuable data that therapists collect may be those obtained through witnessing the way in which each spouse presents his or her point of view and responds to the other's presentations. Rather than being somewhat random, as is so often the case, it would be wise to focus these observations through one of the frameworks that will be presented shortly. In experimental settings, this observation may also be extended into the home either through observer presence or through the solicitation of tape recordings of home interactions. The collection and coding of these data is an expensive and time-consuming affair, which explains why they are used mostly in settings with a funding base broader than direct service. Finally, assessment through analogue means has been used for clinical purposes in research-oriented programs, but it is perhaps better adapted to efforts to learn about differences in the behavior of groups with defined properties when confronted with the standardized stimulus of the analogue situation.

When observation codes have been constructed to structure the assignment of units of interactional behavior to specific categories, Margolin (1978) has noted that the code categories are usually created on an *a priori* basis by investigators, and the resulting ratings do not correlate uniformly well with standardized measures of marital satisfaction. As a general rule, however, the codes do differentiate clinic from nonclinic samples along the dimensions of positive and negative and verbal and nonverbal behavior. Interpretation of these differences is not always easy, however. In an evaluation of one of the codes to be described below (Resick *et al.*, in press), it was found that these interpretations are often arbitrary. For example, "laugh" is classified as a positive by most investigators, but this team found it to occur frequently in conflict as a cynical expression. Conversely, disagreement is generally classed as a negative, but this group found that their *non*distressed couples used it *more*, perhaps indicating a freedom of self-expression born of trust in the relationship. In anticipation of this possible interpretive bias, Stuart (1969) asked subjects in his investigation to indicate their own on-line evaluation of their experiences together and used these evaluations only, without content codes, to evaluate behavioral patterns.

In summary, it is clear that the validity of all of the available coding systems is not yet fully established, and the cost of coding is prohibitive in many instances. Nevertheless, maintaining an awareness of the kinds of actions included in the available coding systems can help the therapist to structure his or her observations of the client. One does not have to observe negative interactions with precision when the goal is to coach the clients in positive behavior. Thus, the codes that are used to assess behavior can also serve the very useful additional purpose of defining behavioral goals; therefore, several of the currently available systems are briefly described below.

Rausch et al. (1974), for example, called for the use of the following six categories for assessment of couples' efforts to resolve conflict: (1) cognitive acts including suggestions and rational arguments; (2) resolving acts aimed at cooling the conflict or resolving the issue; (3) reconciling acts aimed at bringing the partners together emotionally; (4) appealing acts implying a request that the other accede to one's wish; (5) rejecting acts expressing coldness and nonacceptance of the other's argument; and (6) coercive acts or personal attacks that aim at forced compliance, guilt induction, or disparagement. While this is a reasonable system that certainly generates therapeutically relevant information, observer agreement with standard samples ranged from a low of only 58% to a high of 88% across categories, with an overall agreement of 77% and test–retest reliabilities ranging from .64 to .80 across categories.

In the second code system, Weiss et al. (1973) generated 19 codes for verbal interaction (e.g., agree, command, disagree, humor, and problem solving) and 11 codes for nonverbal communications (e.g., attention, laugh, not tracking, and positive physical contact) (see, too, Patterson, 1977). The verbal codes were combinable into four complex units: problem solving, problem description, and negative and positive expressions. The nonverbal interaction could also be concatenated into "negative" and "positive" categories. Two observer agreements of 90% have been reported for this scale (e.g., Engel & Weiss, 1976), suggesting that its finer categories may be more definitive than the coarser system presented by Rausch et al. (1974). However, a major problem with the Marital Interaction Coding System (MISC) is the fact that most observers collapse many of the categories to simplify the system. For example, Weiss et al. (1973) themselves collapsed the code into six categories, as did Liberman et al. (1976). Margolin (1978) collapsed them into positive, negative, and neutral categories; and when Jacobson (1977) used the system, he even omitted the neutral category from this trio. Resick et al. (in press) have done the most systematic work with this system by applying sophisticated regression analyses to evaluate which items did and did not contribute to differential patterns of observation. As a result of their pruning, several codes, such as compliance, compromise, and excuse, were omitted because of their low frequency of occurrence (Birchler et al., 1975, also eliminated these categories), and tracking was omitted because it was redundant with attention. The 17 categories preserved in the final analysis, each of which contributed to at least one of the 60 regression equations that were computed, include the following:

Accept responsibility	*Not tracking
Agree	Positive physical contact
Assent	*Positive solution
Complain	Problem description
*Criticize	Put-down
Deny responsibility	Question
*Disagree	Talk
Humor	*Turnoff
Laugh/smile	

Clinicans would do well to keep these categories in mind, particularly those marked with an asterisk, because they were the ones that best predicted marital satisfaction for men and women combined.

In a third approach, Gottman et al. (1977) asked couples to discuss items from a problem inventory in an effort to achieve consensus. They coded interaction using eight content codes: (1) problem information or feelings about the problem; (2) mind reading; (3) proposal of a solution; (4) communication talk; (5) agreement; (6) disagreement; (7) summarizing the other; and (8) summarizing self. Working from videotapes, they also coded affect from data on facial expression, voice quality, and body position. Finally, unlike the two preceding systems, theirs also coded the context of each interaction; that is, their data concern sequences of interactional events rather than simple frequency counts. Reliability data were good, with 6 of the 10 coders agreeing 88.7% of the time on content codes and 4 other coders agreeing 85% of the time on the affect codes. Using their system, Gottman et al. found, for example, that nonverbal behavior was a better discriminator between distressed and nondistressed couples than was verbal content. Specifically, the distressed couples were more likely than their counterparts to associate neutral and negative nonverbal messages with statements of both agreement and disagreement, indicating great "channel inconsistency" (p. 468) in the case of agreement. While clearly of great value and interest to the clinician, these observations are available only at the rather great anticipatable cost of a complex coding task.

Finally, Sprenkle and Olson (1978) have presented their "circumplex" model for coding interaction while couples worked on the Straus and Tallman (1971) SINFAM task. Their coarse coding system included the following categories: (1) power, or "any direction, instruction, suggestion or request intended to control, initiate, change or modify the behavior of the spouse" (p. 63); (2) creativity, or "the number of new modes of play either suggested or actually tried" (p. 64); and (3) support, or "any action intended to establish, maintain, or restore, as an end in itself, a positive, affective relationship with the other spouse; or, conversely, actions intended to punish or devalue the behavior of the other spouse" (pp. 64–65). The power code was then broken down into the categories of positive power (idea accepted), neutral power (idea ignored), and negative power (idea rejected). In the same vein, support scores could be either positive or negative. Interrater reliabilities were .92 and .97 for two power dimensions and .96 and .94 for creativity and support. Application of this system revealed that nonclinic couples used more egalitarian control strategies in crisis trials, while the clinic couples showed greater wife dominance during these interactions. Nonclinic couples also outperformed clinic couples at significant levels of control efficiency (number of successful influence attempts relative to total influence attempts), creativity (number of ideas offered), and positive supportiveness. These findings offer some initial support for the validity of the fourfold system of classification that the authors proposed, using the control and cohesion variables that they consider most important. These categories are (1) chaotically disengaged; (2) chaotically enmeshed; (3) rigidly disengaged; and (4) rigidly enmeshed. Well-functioning couples obviously fall at the intersect of these continua; they must have sufficient adaptability to cope with changing conditions and yet have sufficient organization to be able to mobilize their adaptive efforts (Hill, 1971; Wertheim, 1975).

Each of these systems has its obvious assets and liabilities. The Raush et al. (1974) code is well adapted to the study of conflict resolution but has not been evaluated beyond such situations. The Gottman et al. (1977) code is flexible and comprehensive in its attention to verbal and nonverbal behavior. However, like the Sprenkle and Olson (1978) code, whose chief merit is its high reliability and relevance to a theory of marital relations, it has not been replicated by others, so its utility in other settings remains to be tested. The code developed by Weiss et al. (1973) has been used by more researchers, albeit mostly by the trainees of its originators, with generally productive results. When reduced to the 17 categories found by Resick et al. (in press), it can be regarded as the most robust of the currently available codes for marital interaction.

In Chapter 6 and 8, evidence is presented in support of the hypothesis that well-adjusted or satisfied couples differ from their distressed counterparts on the basis of their behavior in structured situations. It is not yet clear whether the absence of positives or the presence of too many negatives is most important in differentiating the dissatisfied from the satisfied couples, but both observations have been consistently made. One explanation for the difficulty that researchers have encountered in clearly showing that either too few positives or too many negatives are the key ingredients in marital distress is that each person has a personal interpretation of each interpersonal experience. In this section, it has been shown that behaviors can be classified and counted—a frequency dimension—and that these counts can be evaluated as positive, neutral, or negative by the observers or by the couple themselves. In the next section, a model is presented for interpreting the interpersonal meaning of these high or low rates of positive and negative behaviors by either or both spouses.

UNDERSTANDING COMMITMENT TO THE MARRIAGE

Every therapist who has seen as few as 25 couples has probably seen pairs in which something like the following scenarios occur:

1. She spends years as an excessive drinker despite his protests that he will leave her unless she stops. She stops drinking only to hear him proclaim that it's too late, as he totes his suitcase out the door.
2. He begins to pack up his things to leave, professing a loss of interest in his marriage. She begins an affair, leaving just enough "accidental" clues for him to learn about what she has been doing. He then cries, protests his abiding love, and struggles madly to regain her affections. Now forewarned, she wonders whether giving up her collateral relationship might not send hubby on his way again, leaving her alone in the end.
3. She and he have a picture-book marriage: a pleasant home in the suburbs, both with interesting and rewarding jobs, two achieving children, good health, and many friends. The neighbors were stunned the day the moving van pulled up and took his half of the furniture to a bachelor apartment in the city.

In the first instance, while alcoholism may generally exert an adverse effect upon marital stability (Orford, 1976), here it appears that a seemingly negative behavior served to sustain the husband's commitment to the marriage. In the second, it appears that the feared infidelity of the wife turned ennui into fervor in a libido-flagging husband. And in the third instance, all the pie in the sky was insufficient to keep the couple together.

Outside observers would scorn the first husband and would wonder aloud why the second husband stayed in such a terrible situation. They would shake their heads in disbelief at the third couple's foolishness in bailing out of the modern American dream—a picture-book marriage. But paradoxes like these are woven into the fabric of all human existence. For example, we have all eagerly anticipated an event that paled when it was experienced, just as we have all been pleasantly surprised when undergoing other experiences that we anticipated with dread.

Therefore, it should not be surprising that exchanges that appear to be positive to casual observers, and even to the actors themselves, may have a negative effect upon the stability of the relationship, while events that appear to be patently negative have quite the reverse effect.

These relationship-specific effects of all behaviors are here defined as the "commitment value" of the actions. Part of the meaning of this term was anticipated by Levinger's (1976) discussion of cohesion. He noted that:

> It is far harder to ascertain whether a pair's cohesiveness is high than whether it is low. Outsiders to an intimate relationship do not readily discover how truly happy it is nor how bound the partners currently feel. Even insiders, the partners themselves, are not fully aware of their feelings. (p. 28)

In this sense, "commitment" refers to the extent to which each action of self can either bind the pair together or press them apart. But as it is used here, "commitment" also refers to the likelihood that the actors will behave in ways that are integrative or fragmenting for their relationship. Commitment, therefore, is expressed in both the feelings and the behaviors of all parties to every interaction at all times. In its positive expression, it draws the parties close, while in its negative expression, it forces them apart.

The commitment effect of any particular action is often very difficult to anticipate, being determined by forces of which the actors and the observers may not be aware. When therapists, as outsiders, view spousal interaction, they have a tendency to hold rather strong, somewhat naive expectations that take the form of the belief that if one will make change X, that change is almost certain to have effect X^1 on the other's commitment to the relationship. But marriage, like all of life in general, tends to be far less predictable than simple logic would predict.

Couples have ways of expressing their commitment level that are as individual as they themselves are different as people. For example, the nature of requests for marriage therapy can be studied as an index of the couple's commitment to their marriage. For some, taking a second or even a third job may be an act of intended commitment in efforts to earn more money to build a more pleasing home; but the extended absence from home that these jobs entail may be experienced by the other as a denial of commitment to the marriage, and the start of the second job may trigger defensive withdrawal and a weakening of the commitment experienced by the spouse. Therefore, the most loving of intentions do not always have the most love-nurturing effects.

Sources of Commitment. As can be visualized in Figure 2, commitment is the "fourth dimension" of marital assessment, and the aspect that may give relationship meaning to all of the events that take place in

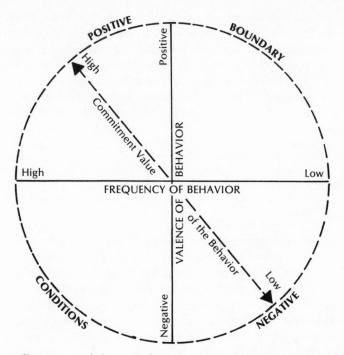

Figure 2. Illustration of the multidimensionality of the assessment of marital interaction.

marital interaction. Cuber and Harroff (1963) described five types of couples whose commitment to their marriages is maintained by very different types of behaviors: the differentiated conflict-habituated, the devitalized, the passive–congenial, the vital, and the total. He was also wise enough to recognize that couples with what many would regard as negatively classified interactions were not necessarily less likely than those engaged on positively classified marriages to be happily so. He noted that couples in each of these types of relationships report satisfaction with them, and moreover, couples in each of these types may also resist efforts to change their interactions. Interestingly, Shostrum and Kavanaugh (1971), who differentiated seven types of marriages, also found types and stability unrelated—good or bad. Apart from the attraction of satisfactions in the marriage, one may therefore wonder what forces contribute to some spouses' keeping their hands in boiling oil while others seem to flee from paradise.

One source of the variance in this decision is surely values. Zuk (1975, 1978) has referred to values favoring continuity, which would hold the couple together, in contrast to those favoring discontinuity, which would render them apart. Religion is one source of such values. Surprisingly, however, in the Catholic sample studied by McMillan

(1969), religion was cited by only 17% of the men and 15% of the women as a reason for wanting to preserve their marriage, and respect for marital vows was cited by only 15% of the men and 8% of the women as the reason for wishing to preserve their marriage. In enumerating the forces that contribute to cohesion and to commitment as used here, Levinger (1976) gave great weight to the influence of relatives and others in the immediate community; it may be that religious values have a very strong impact when they are expressed by significant others, and that in that form of expression the social pressures may replace values as the focus of concern.

The expression of these family-support values has been conceptualized as a tendency toward "familism" by Burgess and Locke (1945). They viewed as components of this tendency factors such as the feeling that people belong primarily to a family, with others being outsiders; that individual efforts should be subservient to the family's welfare; and the belief that land, money, and other resources are the property of the family. Heller (1976) has recently developed a scale designed to measure familism in the largest sense. Included among his 15 items are the following: "Married children should live close to their parents so they can help each other"; "A married person should be willing to share his home with brothers and sisters of his or her husband or wife"; and "As many activities as possible should be shared by married children and their parents." He found substantial validity for his scale as measured by other attitudes and behaviors toward the extended family, and his scale is a good index of the extent to which family and social networks reach into the interaction of the couple as predicted by Bott (1971) in her landmark research.

A second source of commitment may be the paradox of frustration as is well stated by Walster and Walster (1978). They started with the following observation by Freud (1922):

> Some obstacle is necessary to swell the tide of libido to its height; and at all periods of history whenever natural barriers in the way of satisfaction have not sufficed, mankind has erected conventional ones in order to enjoy love. (p. 213)

They then reviewed a range of writings by psychotherapists and literary figures in support of their own conclusion that:

> Although most people assume that we love the people we do *in spite* of the suffering they cause us, it may be that, in part, we love them *because* of the suffering they cause. (p. 104)

For the Walsters, then, the difficulties that spouses encounter in their relationship may be more important in helping than in hindering the level of commitment that they feel toward one another.

One set of speculations about how frustration builds commitment draws upon some assumptions about intrapsychic phenomena. Symbolized by the clichés that "The grass is always greener in the neighbor's yard" and that "Familiarity breeds contempt," novelty may stimulate interest. Disruptions in the normal flow of commitment in marriages may provide this novelty when other aspects of the interaction fail to do so. (This is one reason that couples should be encouraged to share a number of common interests that pose some stimulating challenge for them—anything from collecting the unfindable to engaging in sports in which one's performance can always be improved.) It is also possible that the threat of loss may stimulate self-doubts, and to restore balance between the cognition that one is desirable and is accepted by important others, ardent activity may be stimulated.

Social exchange theory offers a third predictor of commitment to the marriage. Thibaut and Kelley (1959) offered two concepts that bear directly upon commitment to a relationship:

> Comparison level [CL] is a standard by which the person evaluates the rewards and costs of a given relationship in terms of what he feels he "deserves." Relationships, the outcomes of which fall above CL, would be relatively "satisfying" and attractive to the member. (p. 21)

> Comparison level for alternatives is the lowest level of outcomes a member will accept in light of available alternative opportunities . . . as soon as outcomes drop below CL_{alt} the member will leave the relationship. The height of the CL_{alt} will depend mainly on the quality of the best of the member's available alternatives, that is, the reward–cost positions experienced or believed to exist in the most satisfactory of the other available relationships. (pp. 21–22)

A relationship will be stable when the experience in that relationship is consistent with expectations and when it is believed to offer more net rewards than can be gained by leaving. Commitment to the relationship can therefore be estimated through the following equation:

$$\text{Commitment} = \frac{\text{Rewards for staying} + \text{Costs of leaving that are foregone by staying}}{\text{Rewards for leaving} - \text{Rewards of staying foregone by leaving}}$$

Among the rewards for staying are the satisfactions mediated by the marriage, consistency with one's own values or those of the immediate community, comfort and convenience, and the opportunity to have continued relationships with one's children, if any. Among the costs of leaving are the reverse of these: one gives up current reinforcements and acts inconsistently with marital vows and community expectations; a measure of discomfort and inconvenience is experienced related to relocation and the strain of forming new relationships; parental relationships are disrupted; and many experience a punitive economic cost.

Among the rewards for leaving are those that one believes he or she will enjoy in either living alone or forming another relationship on a basis different from the first. But these rewards must be subtracted from those that can no longer be enjoyed in the first relationship. How strongly committed each spouse feels toward the other is therefore predictable through some psychological arithmetic; unfortunately, as with virtually every other psychological process, it is all but impossible to quantify the variables.

Curiously, it has been reported (Cole, 1976; Cole & Vincent, 1975) that those who had the happiest marriages also reported having had the fewest constraints to remain married. One can conclude from this observation that those who believe that their marriage is voluntarily stable feel more satisfied in and therefore more committed to their marriage. Abdallah (1974) reported that other potential mates look more attractive to those who are less happy in their marriage. Therefore, stability of marriage may be more sensitive to these external options than is marital satisfaction (Lenthall, 1977). It is important to bear in mind, however, that announced affairs are not necessarily a marital kiss of death, and indeed, whether or not they are known to the spouse, these "collateral relationships" (Stuart, in press) may actually enhance satisfaction with the marriage (Weil, 1975).

These suggestions do not exhaust the range of forces that affect commitment to the marriage as measured by the behavioral impact of the actions of both spouses. They do, however, reflect the cultural, personal, and relationship sources of such commitment and perhaps suggest that these factors have their effects on differential proportions at different times in the life of each married person. Through all of their idiographic elegance and their kaleidoscopic change over time, the levels of commitment that both spouses experience toward their marriage greatly affect their behavior at home and in the therapist's office.

To trace the impact of commitment, we must turn again to social exchange theory and introduce the concept of "power."[1] Emerson (1962) noted that "power resides implicitly in the other's dependency" (p. 194) and that:

> The dependence of B upon A is directly proportional to the motivational investment (value) B has in the goals mediated by A, and inversely proportional to the availability of these goals outside the A-B relationship. (p. 194)

In other words, A's power over B is proportionate to B's dependency upon A. By definition, there is some measure of interdependency in

[1]Difficulties in the assessment of spousal power are fully discussed in Chapter 9. For present purposes, the concept of power is used in its heuristic sense as an aid to understanding marital interaction. The measurement problems are discussed in the later chapter.

every relationship; therefore, every time we relate to another we give up some measure of control in our own lives. Coleman (1973) quoted Leonardo da Vinci as having said, "When you're all alone, the whole world belongs to you: when you're with another, it's only half yours." Once a relationship has begun, the threat of B's terminating the relationship is a source of power over A. As partners in an interaction never mediate resources of exactly the same value for each other, one always has slightly more power than the other because one always has more to lose from terminating the relationship than the other (Osmond, 1978). Waller (1938) was perhaps the first to recognize this phenomenon in family relationships. Subsequently, others (e.g., Eslinger et al., 1972; Heer, 1963; Powers, 1964) have developed means of measuring the differential in power that contributes to varying levels of commitment to relationships. Powers (see Eslinger et al., 1972) measured relative interest by comparing spouses' responses to 14 statements, including the following: "I believe you should live up to the expectations of your partner"; "I always try to be understanding when my partner has problems"; "It has never really occurred to me that I might lose my partner"; and "I am greatly interested in my partner." Based upon these responses, it was found that among undergraduates, males were less interested in maintaining dating relationships than were females. The responses of partners in troubled marriages are likely to point out which of the partners wants most to have the marriage go on and which would be just as happy to see it end.

Because all things are relevant in social exchange theory (Carson, 1969), so too are the forces that determine which partner has the least to lose from relationship termination. The value of reinforcements mediated by the relationship, the cost of obtaining these same reinforcements elsewhere, the extent to which these reinforcements are unique to the marriage, and the cost of surmounting the barrier forces that maintain cohesion in the relationship are all factors that affect this delicate balance. Later (Chapter 9), evidence showing that wives often get power in relationships by obtaining employment outside the home is presented. In so doing, they not only increase their value to their husbands in terms of economic contribution and greater stimulation, but they also reduce their dependence upon their husbands and open for themselves the options of independent living. Thus, when wives take jobs, very often husbands are spirited to greater ardor. In much the same way, when one spouse creates the possibility of a competing relationship, the other is often drawn more tightly toward maintaining the marriage that now exists. In contrast, when wives return to school rather than taking jobs, the marital effect of their action is more difficult to predict. As students they are absent from home and faced with much after-hours work without contributing to—and, indeed, often drawing from—the family resources. School attendance for these reasons may have a negative impact upon the husband's commitment to the marriage. However, to the extent that school attendance prefigures an opportunity for the wife to secure a better job and make a greater contribution to the family wealth, to meet other interesting men in educational settings, and to gain in personal and intellectual resources, the wife's participation in school programs can have a profound effect in increasing her husband's commitment to their marriage. The direction of the effect in both instances is determined by the impact of the wife's schooling upon the power balance between the partners.

The person with the least to lose has more power during therapy as well as in the couple's day-to-day activities. This person is usually the one who is least anxious for treatment to begin and also least willing to make an initial commitment to change. For these reasons, this is the spouse who holds the keys to the early success of therapy; he or she is the one who must therefore have the greatest expectation of realizing gains early in the treatment process.

Its effect upon commitment to marriage is the acid test of the impact of every action of both spouses. It is as important for the marriage therapist to assess commitment as it is for the physician to take the patient's temperature and measure changes in blood and urine chemistry. Unfortunately, commitment is ever-changing and always elusive. The Marital Precounseling Inventory (Stuart & Stuart, 1973) offers several opportunities to measure the partners' relative investments in their relationship. Question A asks clients to list 10 pleasing things that their spouse does. The person with the longest and most varied list is the one who receives the most from the other—and is hence the most committed. Question D asks about personal change goals and whether the spouse can help in achieving these goals; the more ways the spouse is seen as a helper, the more one is committed to the spouse. Question F asks about shared activities; the more one seeks to share activities with the other, the greater is the commitment level. Question H asks about the level of satisfaction that each enjoys in 12 areas of interaction; here, too, the greater the satisfaction level, the greater the commitment is likely to be. The same is true for scales I and J, which deal with satisfactions in communication and sex, respectively. Finally, Question L asks about commitment directly. Taken together, these items can render a rather convincing estimate of the level of commitment that each partner feels toward the relationship.

Measuring Individual Functioning

While this book is concerned with treatment aimed at enhancing marital functioning, it is essential to point out that couples are made up of pairs of individuals, and many believe that assessment for the planning and evaluation of marital therapy is incomplete unless it involves some measure of relevant individual characteristics.

Assessment of the level of depression in both partners may be the most critical "internal" measure in the armamentarium of marriage therapists. In general, depression can be seen as potentially blunting clients' willingness to engage in or to follow through on therapeutic instigations, and it can also be a sign of therapeutic failure when it follows changes that were expected to yield positive affective changes.

For example, the slowed rate of response by depressives is well documented (e.g., Beck, 1967; Becker, 1977; Liberman & Raskin, 1971). It has also been shown that depressives are more likely than nondepressives to underestimate the rate of their own positive responding (Wener & Rehm, 1975); recall more negative and fewer positive experiences (Nelson & Craighead, 1977); describe both real and imaginary relationships more negatively (Lunghi, 1977); and "catastrophize" in response to life stresses (Schless et al., 1974). These are only a few of the correlates of depression that may contribute to the association between depression and lower levels of marital satisfaction (Coleman & Miller, 1975) as well as blunt the treatment's effectiveness.

Feelings of depression are a universal phenomenon. From 16% to 20% of the American population are believed to be clinically depressed at any point in time (Weissman & Myers, 1978); therefore, between one-fifth and one-sixth of those requesting marital treatment can be expected to be experiencing a depressive state at the time of their therapy request. While depression is obviously a very complex disorder with biological (Gershon et al., 1971), situational (Lewinsohn, 1974), learning history (Benson & Kennelly, 1976; Miller & Seligman, 1975), family history (Overall et al., 1974), or other causes (Beck, 1967; Becker, 1977), a number of different measures have been found to be reliable discriminators of degrees of depression. The Hamilton Rating Scale for Depression (Hamilton, 1960) is perhaps the most widely used interview guide, and one that has reasonably adequate predictive accuracy (Knesevich et al., 1977). The 60-item MMPI D Scale may be the most widely used pencil-and-paper measure, followed by the Zung (1965) Self-Rating Depression Scale. The latter consists of 20 items of the form "I feel down-hearted and blue" and "I get tired for no reason" that are rated on a four-point scale ranging from "A little of the time" to "Most of the time." While useful for discriminating the level of depression among patients in varied settings (e.g., Raft et al., 1977), the Zung, like the MMPI, may be too heavy and pointed an instrument for the comfort of marriage therapy clients.

The U.S. Public Health Service (1977) has recently developed a General Well-Being Schedule as a generalized psychological status instrument. The scale consists of 25 items, four of which make up a cheerfulness versus depressed-mood subscale. These four items, along with a brief explanation for clients, are presented in Figure 3. Essentially a state measure because of its focus on the recent past, and dealing with only psychological as opposed to somatic and behavioral manifestations of depression, these four items nonetheless have correlated at the level of .50 with the MMPI D Scale and at the level of .62 with the Zung instrument.

These associations might be compromised somewhat when the items are presented independent of the 21 additional items in the original instrument. Nevertheless, because they can be very quickly administered, are less threatening than the more comprehensive depression scales, and have reasonably concurrent validity, these items would be very appropriate additions to a marital treatment-evaluation package. Scores indicating severe symptoms would suggest the need to address the mood disturbance of either or both spouses prior to or during marriage therapy. Conversely, neglect of a depressive problem could needlessly jeopardize the opportunity for a therapeutic success. Moreover, therapists will be interested in tracking the levels of cheerfulness and depression in both spouses as change begins to occur in their marriage. Jackson's (1957) classic assumption of a homeostatic process in families, as noted in Chapter 3, would predict that changes in the affective level of marital therapy counselees would move in reciprocal directions. While this hypothesis remains more conjecture than fact, most clinicians have observed it to occur in at least some of the couples whom they serve. Therefore, monitoring mood levels in this simple and straightforward fashion provides an inexpensive means of detecting such changes should they occur.

In addition to measuring internal change through the use of this convenient depression measure, therapists may also be interested in monitoring external behavior outside the marital interaction *per se.* Here, too, if the spouses include the quality of their interaction at the expense of deterioration in parenting, work, or leisure activities, their therapy cannot be construed as an out-and-out therapeutic triumph. In the absence of tools with established validity and reliability, the questions presented in Figure 4 are a useful means of assessing the generalization of positive changes and/or negative changes that may be associated with therapeutic modification of the couple's interaction.

In summary, it has been suggested that therapists may wish to include in their assessment for and of marital therapy, some measure of the clients' mood level. Depression is the mood to watch in marriage therapy as in sex therapy (see Chapter 11), and a number of standardized and specially developed instruments are available for this purpose. As a caution, however, therapists should be mindful of the fact that inclusion of even the most widely used standardized measures may not

Figure 3. A measure of the way you have been feeling lately.

Two of our moods—cheerfulness and depression—often have a great effect upon the way that we act. They also reflect the effects of many of our important experiences. It is important for your therapist to know from time to time just how you have been feeling. Your cheerfulness would be a sign that you are reacting very positively to the changes that have been taking place both in your therapy and in other areas of your life as well. Your depression obviously has the opposite meaning and is something that your therapist may wish to help you with at the same time that you receive help with your marital problem. The following four questions have been taken from the General Well-Being Schedule developed by the United States Public Health Service. Your thoughtful answers to them will help both you and the therapist to understand your current feelings. Thank you for taking the time to provide this valuable information.

Name: _____   Date: _____

1. How have you been feeling in general? (During the past month)

    1 _____ In excellent spirits

    2 _____ In very good spirits

    3 _____ In good spirits mostly

    4 _____ I have been up and down in spirits a lot

    5 _____ In low spirits mostly

    6 _____ In very low spirits

2. Have you felt so sad, discouraged, hopeless, or had so many problems that you wondered if anything was worthwhile? (During the past month)

    1 _____ Extremely so—to the point that I have just about given up

    2 _____ Very much so

    3 _____ Quite a bit

    4 _____ Some—enough to bother me

    5 _____ A little bit

    6 _____ Not at all

3. Have you felt downhearted and blue? (During the past month)

    1 _____ All of the time

    2 _____ Most of the time

    3 _____ A good bit of the time

    4 _____ Some of of the time

    5 _____ A little of the time

    6 _____ None of the time

4. How *depressed* or *cheerful* have you been? (During the past month)

0	1	2	3	4	5	6	7	8	9	10
Very depressed										Very cheerful

Figure 4. Parenting-Work-Play Scale.

While you are concentrating on change in your marital relationship, it is also important to keep track of your experiences in three other essential areas of your life: your relationship with your children, your work experience, and your enjoyment of leisure time. Please take a few moments to answer the following questions so that you and your therapist can understand your current experiences in these broader areas of your life. Thank you very much!

COMPARED WITH THE WAY THINGS WERE IN THE PAST, HOW WOULD YOU RATE YOUR EXPERIENCES IN THE FOLLOWING AREAS OF YOUR LIFE *DURING THE PAST MONTH?*

	Much more than usual	More	Same as usual	Less	Much less than usual
I. Parenting					
A. The time that I spend with my children now is . . .	5	4	3	2	1
B. The satisfaction that I derive from spending time with my children is . . .	5	4	3	2	1
C. My spouse and I agree about the way to manage our children . . .	5	4	3	2	1
D. My children respond positively to me . . .	5	4	3	2	1
II. Work					
A. I enjoy my work now . . .	5	4	3	2	1
B. I do quality work now . . .	5	4	3	2	1
C. My confidence about my future on this job is now . . .	5	4	3	2	1
D. I receive positive reports about my work from peers and superiors . . .	5	4	3	2	1
III. Leisure					
A. I enjoy my leisure time now . . .	5	4	3	2	1
B. My active leisure time (sports, hobbies, reading) compared with my inactive leisure time (watching television) is now . . .	5	4	3	2	1
C. The time that my spouse and I spend together in leisure time activities is now . . .	5	4	3	2	1
D. I enjoy the leisure time that my spouse and I spend together . . .	5	4	3	2	1

improve the meaningfulness of the assessment outcome (e.g. Kostlan, 1954; Meehl, 1959; Stuart, 1971c), and therefore, the use of these tools should not take the place of sensitive and careful direct observation by the therapist.

Assessment of Treatment Outcome

As mentioned earlier, the therapist has an ethical responsibility to plan and continuously monitor the effects of the services that are offered and to share the results of this analysis with the clients at appropriate times during the contact (Association for the Advancement of Behavior Therapy, 1977; Stuart, 1980a). This means that some form of outcome evaluation must be built into any comprehensive treatment package.

All too often this assessment of treatment effects is limited to the casual question, "Do you feel that things are improving for you?" Several studies (e.g., Garfied et al., 1971; Lieberman et al., 1973) have shown, however, that therapists and clients alike make judgments about therapeutic effects through rose-colored glasses. For example, clients participating in a marriage enrichment program studied by Venema (1976) made very few of the predicted changes and yet rated their treatment experience positively. If the predictions were not utterly wide of the mark, the clients surely were. In another study (Jenkins, 1976) efforts to change specific interaction behaviors between spouses failed, but they rated their marriages as better nonetheless.

Rather than asking clients how they felt about treatment in global terms, Sigal et al. (1976) asked about new problems after treatment terminated. They found that treated clients experienced more new problems than their nontreated counterparts. Findings such as this lead to the conclusion that when treatment results are assessed, the measures used must be sensitive to deterioration as well as to improvement. Lambert et al. (1976) have offered a broad conception of deterioration that includes not only a worsening between two sessions that exceeds expectation, but also the lack of expected improvement that other untreated individuals are known to experience. Unfortunately, a goodly percentage of clients undergoing individual psychotherapy (Bergin & Lambert, 1978) and marriage and family treatment (Gurman & Kniskern, 1978) are found to suffer a worsening of their condition following treatment, rather than merely missing out on opportunities for improved functioning.

Treatment effects can be assessed through global or specific measures. Global measures are appealing because they are easy to construct and convenient to administer; they are also most likely to yield positive results and most likely to yield judgments that are shared by clients, therapists, and others (Cappon, 1964; Garfield *et al.*, 1971; Koegler & Brill, 1967; Landfield *et al.*, 1962; Strupp *et al.*, 1969). However, it is difficult to interpret their meaning because different raters attend to different data from different points of view, so the evaluator is never certain about how much and of what kind of change was observed by what people and under which conditions.

When treatment effects are measured through the use of symptom-related indices, agreement among raters is often disappointingly low (e.g., Garfield *et al.*, 1971; Gibson *et al.*, 1955; Lewinsohn & Nichols, 1967; Nichols & Beck, 1960). When the indices are standardized, norms are available for external comparison of results. This advantage is at least partially offset, however, by the fact that the standardized scales may not be relevant to the client's goals in treatment nor to the therapeutic methods being used. In light of these considerations, it may be best to include some global measures as well as some behaviorally specific measures of the changes sought by clients and their therapists. The global measures address the question: Does the client appear to be feeling and functioning better? The specific measures address the question: Are these global changes attributable, at least in principal, to changes that were the goals set for the treatment that was offered?

One means of evaluating treatment outcome is to answer each of the following questions in order, as suggested earlier by Stuart (1976a):

1. Did one partner agree to treatment?
2. Did both partners agree to treatment?
3. Did one partner make a reasonable number of the requested behavior changes?
4. Did both partners agree to make a reasonable number of the requested behavior changes?
5. As a result of these changes did one partner feel more committed to the relationship?
6. As a result of these changes did both partners feel more committed to the relationship?
7. Did one partner maintain the behavior changes made during treatment?
8. Did both partners maintain the behavior changes made during treatment?
9. Did one partner sustain increased feelings of commitment to the marriage?
10. Did both partners sustain increased feelings of commitment to the marriage?

Treatment that fails to engage the couples in treatment or to promote compliance with instigations for behavior change is clearly ineffective intervention. So, too, is treatment that produces behavior changes that consistently fail to promote greater commitment to the relationship, sustained behavior change, and positive commitment.

In addition to answering these specific questions, therapists may also wish to evaluate treatment outcome using a goal-assessment technique. Goal attainment scaling and the so-called problem-oriented record were both introduced in 1968. Goal attainment measures the extent to which the positive change goals established in a treatment undertaking have been realized (Kiresuk & Sherman, 1968), while the problem-oriented record measures the reduction in problems noted at the outset of treatment (Weed, 1968). Both systems have in common the identification of either standardized or individualized lists of weighted problems or goals, delineation of successive approximations of these goals, and periodic rating of client behavior in each of the goal areas. Because it is believed that problem scanning may exacerbate behavioral problems, and because the positive orientation of goal attainment scaling is more consistent with the thrust of treatment based on social-learning-theory principles, the latter approach is described here.

Kiresuk and Lund (1977) presented goal attainment scaling as the construction of a rating grid. Along the abscissa are listed up to five goals; along the ordinate are five approximations of these goals, ranging from the best treatment outcome anticipated, through an average expected outcome level, down to a worst likely outcome level. The authors suggested that the contents of the form be negotiated between therapist and client(s). Lombrillo et al. (1973) listed as possible benefits of this approach that it offers the therapist a conceptual basis for treatment planning; mobilizes the client's adaptive resources; and permits the establishment of realistic goals that are formulated in light of the client's intentions, abilities, and life space, while at the same time permitting a summing over clients' treatment outcomes for treatment purposes. A sample goal attainment scale for marital treatment is presented in Figure 5.

Inspection of this generalized form reveals some assumptions about the treatment that is being evaluated. Because it is *marital* therapy, its inherent assumption is that a willing commitment to remain married is its goal. Of course, it is recognized that for some couples, remaining married may be the last desirable outcome. But marriage therapy must be evaluated in terms of a marriage-enhancement/marriage-maintenance goal, and if a high proportion of its clients divorce instead of staying married, a name change for the therapy may be in order. The form also reflects a belief that to realistically achieve a renewed, hopeful commitment to the marriage, both spouses will be required to ask for the changes that they desire; to follow through on the changes that they are asked to make; and to prompt and acknowledge the change efforts of their spouse. Each of these is an element in a set of rela-

Figure 5. Generalized Goal Attainment Scale for marriage therapy.

X = level at intake (date:)
A = test after four weeks (date:)
B = test after eighth session (date:)
C = test at treatment termination (date:)
D = test at follow-up (date:)

Make marks in red for husband rating
Make marks in blue for wife rating

Score summary
Test   Husband   Wife
Intake
A
B
C
D

	1. Commitment to marriage	2. Expressed desire for change	3. Follow-through	4. Prompt mate's change effort	5. Acknowledge mate's effort
Scale attainment levels					
Very poor level of treatment success (−2)	Decision by one spouse to divorce, no discussion	Refusal to state change is possible	Failure to interact with mate in any way	Continued acts that prevent change by mate	Continued complaints in old terms
Level of poor treatment (−1)	Decision by one mate to divorce after discussion	Negative requests for change	First effort frustrated, no repeat	Maintain unfriendly distance from mate	No comment on effort by mate
Neutral level of treatment success (0)	Shared discussion leading to stay/divorce decision	Some vague but positive change requests	Partial follow-through on commitments	Maintain reasonable closeness	Comment on absence of negatives
Moderate success with treatment (+1)	Shared decision to stay with some expressed hope	Some specific and positive requests	Commitments met	Attempt to "change first" to help mate make changes	Comment on new positives
Marked success with treatment (+2)	Shared decision to stay with great hope	Many positive and specific requests	Commitment level met and exceeded	Mate's most difficult requests met before expected change by mate	Strong and regular comments on new positives

tionship-management skills that all couples must have. Those achieving higher levels of these skills are believed to have the best opportunity for long-range success, and therefore making a change at these levels is believed to be the best outcome that therapy can offer.

In addition to this generalized goal-attainment scale, therapists can construct specific scales measuring change on each dimension of a unique treatment program offered to each couple. The scales might be communication, behavior exchanges, problem-solving behavior, shared activities, sexual interaction, or any other goals of the treatment that is offered. Used alone or in conjunction with the more generalized approach illustrated here, these specific goal-attainment scales can play a valuable role in treatment planning and evaluation.

Kiesler (1977) has, in fact, noted no less than 14 advantages accruing to the use of goal attainment scaling, compared with its relatively minor disadvantages. Among its positives are its relevance to the client's individual goals; its economy; its sensitivity to both improvement and deterioration; its specificity and quantifiability; and its suitability for data collection from therapist, clients, and significant others. Its disadvantages stem from its inconsistency with more global psychotherapeutic approaches inimical to objectification and its evolutionary status from a methodological standpoint. For example, item weighting is still somewhat arbitrary, and the level of abstraction of alternative outcomes must be formulated without available standards. Nevertheless, Kiesler (1977) and this writer strongly recommend the use of goal-attainment-scaling approach both as a means of putting the treatment process more under the control of the clients and as a means of evaluating the treatment outcome for comparative purposes.

Moving down the scale of standardization, but at the same time up the scale of convenience, readers may be interested in considering the generalized treatment evaluation form presented in Figure 6. The form begins by asking clients to restate their therapeutic goals and to evaluate the relevance and effectiveness of their treatment to this goal. It then asks clients to evaluate several moods in themselves and in their mates. Inclusion of these measures of internal as well as external change has been recommended by Bergin and Lambert (1978). Next, the form asks clients to itemize changes in their own behavior and that of their mate, allowing for identification of both positive and negative evaluations of these changes. Gurman and Kniskern (1978) recommended the use of procedures like these as a means of sensitizing evaluation to both improvement and deterioration. Finally, the form asks clients to rate some dimensions of their treatment experience. To partially minimize a halo effect, these are phrased negatively and require rejection of the statement to offer a positive evaluation. The form is brief, taking about 10 minutes for completion, and provides invaluable information that can be discussed during the session in which it is completed. It alerts therapists to clients' reactions to treatment in terms that permit immediate accommodation. For example, finding that clients do experience change, but that they regard these changes as steps in the wrong direction, should lead either to reframing the changes (relabeling) with the client or to altering the course of treatment. In the same vein, asking clients to evaluate the quality of their interaction with the therapist can lead to adjustments in the techniques of service delivery. As with goal attainment and scaling, when obtained "on line"—that is, at two- or three-week intervals during treatment—these data can have a powerful impact upon the effectiveness of the service that is being offered.

As an epilogue to this discussion, it should be noted that pre–post change scores are not necessarily regarded as the best indices of treatment effectiveness. There are a number of serious problems with this approach, as noted by several teams of researchers (e.g., Cronbach & Furby, 1970; Fiske, 1971; Manning & DuBois, 1962; Mintz, 1972). Specifically, these investigators have found (1) that repeated measures share measurement error, making differences hard to interpret; (2) that a statistical artifact, "regression toward the mean," increases the likelihood that clients who are worse off at the start will show greater improvement at the end of treatment; and (3) that posttreatment measures tend to be more related to the client's level of functioning at that time than to actual differences in the level of functioning before and after therapy. For these reasons, the use of "residual change scores" is recommended (Green et al., 1975). In this procedure, estimates are made of the predictable level of change based upon pretreatment functioning: Treatment is effective to the extent that these expectations are realized. Inclusion of standardized measures for which norms of "healthy" functioning exist is another way of measuring change objectively. This approach has been strongly recommended by Bergin and Lambert (1978).

Estimating the Probability of a Positive Treatment Outcome

While none of the other published materials describe or evaluate a treatment approach that is identical to the one presented here, several published reports do make use of approaches related to social learning theory. It is important for therapists to be apprised of the probability of success through these methods so that they are able to meet their ethical responsibility to share this information with clients (Stuart, 1975, 1980a) and to make their own assessments of the likelihood that therapy will be beneficial to their clients.

Stuart and Roper (1979) have offered an extensive review of the results of these treatments, and their findings are only briefly reviewed

Figure 6. Treatment Evaluation Form (client[s]).

You are participating in a process intended to help you to achieve some important personal-change goals. While the therapist can make some important and valuable judgments about the effectiveness of the service that is being offered, you are the expert in the final analysis. It is you who are the best judge of whether you are making good progress toward your goals and should continue on the present course or whether you would feel more confident about achieving and maintaining your goals through a somewhat different approach. Therefore, I would like to ask you to take a moment to answer the following questions. Please try to base your answers on the way that you have been feeling and functioning during the *past two weeks*. You may have had some very good days or some very bad ones; please answer these questions in terms of the way in which you have felt in general during this time. Thank you for your help in helping me to help you.

1. Name(s): _____   2. Date: _____

3. Please list your three most important goals when you started treatment. Then please indicate the extent to which you feel your treatment has addressed each goal and the extent of change that you have experienced in each area.

	With respect to this goal my treatment is:			My progress toward this goal has been:			
Your goal	Very relevant		Not relevant	Great		Moderate	None
a. _____	3	2	1	5	4	3	2	1
b. _____	3	2	1	5	4	3	2	1
c. _____	3	2	1	5	4	3	2	1

4. Along the top of the space below are words describing some common feelings. For each one, please indicate how truly each word would have described you during the past year. Then indicate how truly each word would have described you during the past two weeks.

	Feel calm	Feel content	Feel self-confident	Feel optimistic
During the past year				
Very true	1	1	1	1
Sometimes true	2	2	2	2
Rarely true	3	3	3	3
Almost never	4	4	4	4
During the past two weeks				
Very true	1	1	1	
Sometimes true	2	2	2	
Rarely true	3	3	3	
Almost never	4	4	4	

	Feel calm	Feel content	Feel self-confident	Feel optimistic
During the past year				
Very true	1	1	1	1
Sometimes true	2	2	2	2
Rarely true	3	3	3	3
Almost never	4	4	4	4
During the past two weeks				
Very true	1	1	1	1
Sometimes true	2	2	2	2
Rarely true	3	3	3	3
Almost never	4	4	4	4

6. Please list below the most obvious changes that you have observed in your own behavior and that of your spouse since you began treatment. Then please estimate the extent to which you consider this to be a change in the right direction.

	A very positive change		Neutral	A very negative change	
a. My own behavior changes					
1. _____	5	4	3	2	1
2. _____	5	4	3	2	1
3. _____					
b. Changes in my spouse's behavior					
1. _____	5	4	3	2	1
2. _____	5	4	3	2	1
3. _____					

7. Finally, I would very much appreciate your evaluating several aspects of the service that you have received. You will find listed on the left five statements. Please indicate how true you feel each one is for your treatment experience.

	Very true	Somewhat true	Neutral		Untrue
a. I have not been able to state my case.	5	4	3	2	1
b. Therapist ignores my feelings.	5	4	3	2	1
c. I don't understand what I am expected to do.	5	4	3	2	1
d. I don't agree with some of the things that I am expected to do.	5	4	3	2	1
e. I don't follow through very well on the things I am asked to do.	5	4	3	2	1

THANK YOU VERY MUCH. I will use this information to try to improve the service I am offering you. It may encourage me to continue with the same treatment or to think about ways to change the focus of our efforts. In either case, I shall discuss with you the things that you have told me on this form, and I do appreciate this help.

here. Three types of research designs have been used in this research: analogue, single-subject, and group. Analogue studies generally bring into laboratory settings couples who may or may not identify themselves as facing marital distress. They are then exposed to assessment and/or intervention procedures in an effort to identify components of marital stress and potentially effective treatment techniques. For example, Eisler *et al.* (1973) attempted to demonstrate the reliability and practical utility of videotape assessment of marital interaction. In the same vein, Carter and Thomas (1973) demonstrated the adequacy of instruction for specific communication changes by couples, with electronic feedback signals contributing little to the partners' more human, social feedback system. In general, studies such as these have heuristic value, but their telling problem is the issue of whether couples' experiences in the laboratory have any bearing upon their interaction at home.

Studies of clinical intervention are much more closely related to the critical questions posed by therapists. Table 1 summarizes the data from a representative sample of studies published through the past decade. There it will be seen that the earliest studies in the social-learning-theory tradition (e.g., Stuart, 1969; Patterson & Hops, 1972; Stern & Marks, 1973) offered several advantages over case studies in the psychotherapy literature. Their techniques were more precisely defined; they relied upon objective outcome measures; and they collected their data continuously throughout the treatment process and included some follow-up evaluation as well. Because they lack experimental controls, like the analogue studies, these case reports are only heuristically valued. They have, however, spawned more complete treatment packages (e.g., Azrin *et al.*, 1973; Patterson *et al.*, 1975; Stuart, 1975; Weiss *et al.*, 1973). Thus, while the "product level" (Paul, 1969, pp. 44–48) of these case studies has tended not to be very high, their results supported the development of more ambitious programs.

Single-subject designs were the next evolutionary stage for research in this area. For example, Azrin *et al.* (1973) offered their clients three weeks of "catharsis counseling" followed by "reciprocity counseling." They reported a favorable result for their focal treatment, but the strength of their conclusion is flawed by a number of methodological problems. For example, because the focal treatment was always preceded by the placebo, it is not clear whether the focal treatment would be effective if offered alone. In the same vein, the fact that daily data were collected from couples who knew that change was expected of them clearly established a strong potential for reactive bias in the core outcome data. Hickok and Komechak (1974) used a partial reversal (B–A–B) design to evaluate use of a token economy in services to a distressed couple. However, because the positive effect did not reverse,

Table 1. Review of selected outcome studies of effectiveness of behavioral marital treatment[a]

Stuart (1969)

Subjects: 4 couples "on the brink of filing for divorce"
Length: 7 sessions in 10 weeks
Format: Conjoint
Design: Case study
Techniques:

1. Couples taught to initiate behavioral change in effort to socialize them into treatment approach.
2. Each spouse asked to request 3 positive, specific behavior changes of other.
3. Couples taught how to make requests effectively.
4. Couples taught to monitor compliance and that of spouse with therapeutic instigations.
5. Communication skills built through behavioral rehearsal and coaching.
6. Behavioral contracting taught as means of structuring behavior exchange.

Outcomes:

1. Self-reported increase in average daily hours of conversation, frequency of sexual interaction.
2. Improvement in marital satisfaction on inventory adapted from Farber (1957).

Follow-up:

1. At 24 and 48 weeks, self-reported conversation and sexual behavior changes maintained.
2. Also changes in global rating of marital satisfaction maintained.

Patterson and Hops (1972)

Subjects: 1 couple with prior training in parenting
Length: 9 sessions in 9 weeks
Format: Conjoint
Design: Case study
Techniques:

1. Weekly reading assignments (Lederer & Jackson, 1968).
2. Evaluation of videotapes of own interaction.
3. Modeling and supervised practice of nonaversive interaction.
4. Training in pinpointing requested behavior changes.
5. Training in *quid pro quo* contracting techniques.

Outcomes:

1. Improvement in 3 classes of problem-solving behaviors in coded laboratory observation.
2. Based on home observation, no change in aversive behavior, but increase in husband–wife interaction time.
3. No changes in self-reported pleases, displeases, or positive thoughts.

Follow-up:

1. Home observation revealed no change in aversive behavior but maintenance of increase in husband–wife interaction time.

---

[a] Reprinted with the permission of Academic Press from R. B. Stuart & B. L. Roper, Marital behavior therapy: A research reconnaissance. In P. Sjoden, S. Bates, & W. S. Dockens (Eds.), *Trends in behavior therapy.* New York: Academic Press, 1979.

Table 1 continued

Azrin, Naster, and Jones (1973)

Subjects: 12 couples recruited from college counseling service or through mail solicitation

Length: 14 sessions in 7 weeks

Format: Conjoint

Design: Case study with catharsis counseling followed by reciprocity counseling (replicated A-B design)

Techniques:
1. Catharsis counseling procedure consisted of talk about feelings about marriage and completion of daily marital satisfaction ratings.
2. Reciprocity counseling: (*a*) spouses listed 10 satisfactions given and received at home, with reciprocity discussed in sessions; (*b*) spouses listed other desired interactions; (*c*) spouses trained to give verbal response to positives received; (*d*) training in compromise in 3 problem areas, with training in contracting; (*e*) training in making requests and in adding positive statements to negative messages; (*f*) training in generalization of contracting skills to new problem areas; (*g*) couples were asked to read marriage manual (Ellis, 1966) and to discuss their ratings of sexual activities; and (*h*) daily ratings of marital satisfaction (in 9 problem areas) exchanged and discussed throughout reciprocity counseling.

Outcomes:
1. Self-report marital happiness scale response higher for reciprocity than for catharsis counseling, with 96% of clients reporting greater happiness at end as opposed to beginning of reciprocity counseling.
2. Average happiness ratings were greater on each of 9 areas of scale during last week of reciprocity counseling than during 3 weeks of catharsis counseling.
3. In test of specificity of effect of the procedure, happiness scores were greater in 6 problem areas after direct counseling.
4. In test of generalization, scores were higher in 6 noncounseled problem areas during reciprocity as opposed to during catharsis counseling.
5. None of the 12 couples separated or divorced.

Follow-up:
1. At 1 month, marital happiness scale scores of 88% of couples were higher than at start of reciprocity counseling.
2. At 4 months, all but 1 of the couples remained married and together.

Stern and Marks (1973)

Subjects: 1 couple considering separation; wife having "severe obsessional rituals"

Length: Apparently 10 sessions over 5 weeks

Format: Conjoint

Design: Case study

Techniques:
1. Training in how to request and list desired behavior changes.
2. Training in verbal contracts on *quid pro quo* model.

Outcomes:
1. Decrease in wife's rituals, with increase in productivity.

Table 1 continued

2. Increase in husband's involvement in home improvement and in interaction with wife.
3. Increased frequency of sexual activity.

Follow-up:
1. At 6 and 12 weeks, wife's rituals remained lower and her productivity higher; husband's home improvement efforts lower, but conversational involvement was sustained.
2. Sexual activity declined, but was higher than at start of treatment.
3. At 1 year, couple separated, but wife's rituals remained under control.

Hickok and Komechak (1974)

Subjects: 1 couple considering divorce
Length: 10 weeks
Format: Conjoint and individual, cotherapy
Design: B-A-B design with B = token economy, A = no-token economy
Techniques:
1. Orientation through observation of family interaction and discussion of behavior control.
2. Instigation to cue and emit positive behavior and omit negative responding.
3. Token system exchanged time out of house for physical intimacy or sex.
4. Assertion training for husband, who also received instructions about appropriate sexual behavior.

Outcomes: Self-reported steady increase over all phases in tokens received by wife for sexual interaction and by husband for baby sitting while wife was out of the house.

Follow-up: At 2 months, wife not leaving house as much and enjoying time with husband more; increased rate of sexual contact maintained, and husband assuming more responsibility for child care.

Wieman, Shoulders, and Farr (1974)

Subjects: 1 couple referred by university counseling center
Length: 20 sessions over 24-week period
Format: Conjoint, cotherapy
Design: Multiple baseline design over 3 target behaviors
Techniques:
1. Orientation to principles of reciprocal reinforcement.
2. Selection of 3 target behaviors by each spouse—1 easy, 1 moderate, and 1 difficult—with instructions to exchange behaviors in that sequence.
3. Communication training consisting of "feeling talk" and "empathetic listening" instruction.
4. Instruction in sexual skills, including mutual pleasuring, sensate focus, and mutual masturbation.

Outcomes:
1. All 3 target behavioral exchanges were successful, based on self-report.
2. Improvement noted on Locke–Williamson Marital Adjustment Scale (Locke & Williamson, 1958) and on Conjugal Life Questionnaire (Guerney, 1964).

Table 1 continued

3. Spouses reported general improvement in quality of their lives together, with husband reporting abatement of distress due to ulcer problem.
4. Multiple baseline results suggest that intervention accounted for most behavioral changes.

Follow-up: Informal data at 4 months indicated maintenance of adequate sexual activity, communication change, and rate of exchange of "little" positive behaviors.

Patterson, Hops, and Weiss (1975)[b]

Subjects: 10 "moderately distressed" couples
Length: Average of 6 sessions
Format: Conjoint, cotherapy
Design: Case study, with couples treated separately as pairs
Techniques:
1. In baseline sessions couples listed pleasurable and displeasurable behaviors and attempted problem-solving negotiation.
2. Couples asked to read Patterson (1971).
3. Spouses trained to recognize pleasing and displeasing behaviors, and to increase rate of pleasing behaviors offered in "love days" procedure.
4. Training in pinpointing and discrimination as means to operationalize expectation.
5. Training in listening, paraphrasing, information gathering, and problem-solving communication.
6. Training in specifying and contracting for behavior changes.

Outcomes:
1. In laboratory problem-solving exercise, facilitative behavior increased and disruptive behaviors decreased.
2. In self-report, husbands and wives both reported increase in pleasing behaviors, while husbands, but not wives, reported decrease in displeasing behaviors.

Follow-up:
1. At 3 to 6 months, for 5 of 10 couples reported by Weiss, Hops, and Patterson (1973), marital satisfaction, as measured by Locke–Wallace Scale (1959), increased.
2. For same couples, desire for change in spouses' behavior decreased, but there was no significant change in amount of time spent together.
3. At 1 to 2 years, 2 of the 7 located couples were divorced and 4 of the 5 remaining couples "seemed to be happier" and reported fewer conflicts.

Harrell and Guerney (1976)

Subjects: 60 couples recruited from a university community
Length: 8 weekly 2-hour sessions for treatment group; assessment only for no-treatment group
Format: Conjointly in group (3 couples per group)
Design: Experimental, with random assignment to treatment or control group

---

[b]Includes data from Weiss, Hops, & Patterson (1973).

Table 1 continued

Techniques:
1. Weekly homework assignments consisting of reading and skill-practice exercises.
2. Training in expressing opinions and feelings and in listening and summarizing partner's message.
3. Partners identify a relationship issue and pinpoint their specific behavioral input or contribution.
4. Partners generate several specific alternative behavioral solutions and *then* evaluate the alternatives.
5. Partners agree to implement, and later renegotiate, a contract (approximately 2 per couple) around the exchange of 1 alternative behavior each.

Outcomes:
1. Treatment group outperformed control group on the following measures:
   a. Adequacy of skills at 2 of the 5 steps in a laboratory conflict negotiation task.
   b. Self-report of adequacy of solutions reached in laboratory conflict negotiation task.
   c. Decrease in negative verbal behaviors (interrupt and "put-down" statements) in laboratory task.
2. Treatment and control group did not differ on the following measures:
   a. Adequacy of skills at 3 of the 5 steps in laboratory conflict negotiation task.
   b. Change on Handling Problems Change Score (Schlein, 1971).
   c. Changes of perceptions of marital satisfaction on Marital Adjustment Scale (Locke & Williamson, 1958), the Family Life Questionnaire—Conjugal (Collins, 1971), the Satisfaction Change Score (Schlein, 1971), and "perceived rate of relationship change" on Relationship Change Scale (Schlein, 1971).
3. Control group outperformed treatment group in that positive behaviors ("agree" and "approve") decreased for treatment group in laboratory task.

Follow-up: None

Liberman, Levine, Wheeler, Sanders, and Wallace (1976)

Subjects: 4 couples in behavioral treatment group, 6 in "interactional" comparison group (all were clients at a community mental health center)

Length: 8 weekly 2-hour sessions; 1 follow-up session after 1 month

Format: Conjointly in groups

Design: Quasi-experimental due to consecutive rather than random assignment of couples to behavioral versus comparison group

Techniques:
1. Fee deposit returned contingent on attendance.
2. Presentation of therapeutic rationale.
3. Training in discriminating and graphing pleasing behaviors and recording pleases on daily basis throughout treatment.
4. Presentation of "Tenderness" film (Serber & Laws, 1974) depicting physical affection and verbal feedback.
5. For comparison group mainly:
   a. Catharsis, ventilation, sharing of feelings.

Table 1 continued

b. Discussion of insight into marital relationship.

6. For behavior therapy group only:

   a. Behavioral rehearsal, modeling, prompting, and feedback to build communication skills.

   b. Behavioral contracting using holistic model.

   c. Massage exercise.

   d. Weekly homework assignments, including assigned reading (Human Development Institute, 1967).

Outcomes:

1. Behavior therapy group complied with more assignments.

2. Behavior therapy and comparison group did not differ on the following measures:

   a. Number of pleasing behaviors given and received.

   b. Number of daily shared activities.

   c. Marital Activities Inventory (Weiss *et al.*, 1973).

   d. Marital Precounseling Inventory (Stuart & Stuart, 1973).

   e. Partners' estimates of own and each others' desires for change (Willingness-to-Change Questionnaire; Weiss *et al.*, 1973).

   f. Marital Adjustment Test (Locke & Wallace, 1959).

   g. Consumer satisfaction with treatment.

   h. Observations of spouses' touching each other during sessions.

   i. Problem-solving responses, problem description, and positive verbal behavior in laboratory problem-solving sessions as measured by Marital Interaction Coding System (Weiss *et al.*, 1973).

3. Behavior therapy group outperformed comparison group on following measures:

   a. Increase in congruence or mutual understanding (Willingness-to-Change Questionnaire; Weiss *et al.*, 1973).

   b. Exchanges of more "looks" and smiles during sessions.

   c. Decrease in negative verbal behaviors (Marital Interaction Coding System; Weiss *et al.*, 1973).

   d. Fewer negative nonverbal responses and more positive nonverbal responses during problem solving (Marital Interaction Coding System; Weiss *et al.*, 1973).

Follow-up:

1. One couple in each group temporarily separated after treatment termination.

2. At 2 and 6 months, groups did not differ on spouses' estimates of partners' desire for change, with both improved over pretherapy (Willingness-to-Change Questionnaire; Weiss *et al.*, 1973).

3. At 2 and 6 months, groups did not differ in congruence or mutual understanding (Willingness-to-Change Questionnaire; Weiss *et al.*, 1973).

4. At 2 and 6 months, groups did not differ on Marital Adjustment Test (Locke & Wallace, 1959), with both improved over pretherapy.

Jacobson (1977)

Subjects: 10 couples solicited through newspaper ads

Table 1 continued

Length: Treatment group received pre- and posttherapy assessment interviews and 8 treatment sessions while waiting-list control received only pre- and postassessment sessions

Format: Conjoint

Design: Experimental, with random assignment to treatment or to control group, plus multiple baseline design for 4 or 5 treated couples

Techniques:

1. Signed treatment contract.
2. Each spouse recorded data at home on 2 behaviors of partner for 2-week baseline and during treatment.
3. Reading assignment: Patterson (1971).
4. Instruction, feedback, modeling, and reinforcement with regard to minor and then major problem solving.
5. Nightly problem-solving sessions and behavioral recording as homework.
6. In-session discussion of home data and problem-solving practice.
7. Instruction in holistic behavioral contracts.

Outcomes:

1. In laboratory problem-solving task, experimentals emitted more positive and fewer negative responses.
2. Experimental couples showed greater improvement on Locke–Wallace (1959) than controls.
3. Multiple baseline data suggested contracting effective in promoting specific behavioral changes.

Follow-up: One year after treatment, Locke–Wallace (1959) scores for experimental couples were marginally higher than at posttest.

Dixon and Sciara (1977)

Subjects: 7 couples participating in university extension course on marital improvement

Length: 8 weekly 2-hour sessions

Format: Conjointly in group

Design: Case study, with multiple baseline designs for each couple

Techniques:

1. Spouses listed 10 satisfactions given and received at home and discussed reciprocity.
2. Development of skills in nonjudgmental, behaviorally descriptive communication about daily satisfaction ratings on modified Marriage Happiness Scale (Azrin, Naster, & Jones, 1973).
3. Training in negotiation of behavioral exchanges in areas covered by Marriage Happiness Scale with group sharing and feedback.
4. As maintenance procedure, couples helped to pinpoint which workshop procedures were most effective.

Outcomes:

1. Increase in commitment to and optimism about marriage on Marital Precounseling Inventory (Stuart & Stuart, 1973).
2. Improvement in weekly satisfaction ratings on modified Marriage Happiness Scale (Azrin et al., 1973) in areas of affectionate interaction, communication with spouse and children, and/or family interaction.

ASSESSING TROUBLED MARRIAGES   125

Table 1 continued

---

3. Some support for specificity of effect of treatment procedures as reflected in multiple baseline data from 3 couples.

Follow-up: None

Jacobson (1978)

Subjects: 32 "moderately disturbed" couples solicited mainly through advertisements

Length: Initial interview plus 8 weekly 1–1½-hour sessions for treated couples

Format: Conjoint

Design: Experimental, with random assignment to 1 of 3 therapists and 1 of 4 conditions: (*a*) a behavioral program using good faith contracts (GF group); (*b*) a behavioral program using *quid pro quo* contracts (QPQ group); (*c*) a nonspecific treatment condition (NS group); and (*d*) a waiting-list control condition (WL group)

Techniques:

1. Good faith (holistic) group: Treatment techniques duplicated those used in the experimental group in Jacobson (1977).
2. *Quid pro quo* (partitive) group: Treatment techniques identical to those of good faith group except that couples were taught *quid pro quo*, instead of good faith, behavioral contracting.
3. Nonspecific group: Techniques were intended to be roughly equivalent to behavioral treatments on such factors as attention, expectancies, credibility, therapist activity level and directiveness, and rationale for treatment, and to differ from the behavioral treatments in that specific instructions in problem-solving and communication skills and contingency-contracting procedures were excluded.

Outcomes:

1. No differences due to therapist or therapist–treatment interaction on the 4 outcome measures.
2. In laboratory problem-solving task, both behavioral groups combined emitted less negative, and more positive, verbal behavior than either the WL or the NS group; considered separately, each behavioral group was superior to each control group on negative and positive verbal behavior with the exception that the GF, but not the QPQ, group outperformed the NS group on a decrease in negative verbal behavior.
3. Both behavioral groups (combined and separately) improved more than either the WL or the NS group on self-reported marital satisfaction (Locke & Wallace, 1959).
4. No differences between the GF and QPQ groups or between the NS and WL groups on positive negative verbal behavior in laboratory problem-solving tasks or on the MAS (Locke & Wallace, 1959).
5. The 3 treatment groups did not differ from each other and improved more than the WL group on ratings of marital happiness in 12 areas (subscale of Marital Precounseling Inventory; Stuart & Stuart, 1973).

Follow-up: Some average of 1-, 3-, and/or 6-month follow-up data on the MAS (Locke & Wallace, 1959) indicated that the combined behavioral groups maintained posttest superiority over NS group.

---

it is not possible to tell if the clients simply responded to nonspecific factors in the treatment situation or if the changes mediated by the use of tokens was so strong as to be resistant to extinction when the token system was removed. Wieman *et al.* (1974) and Dixon and Sciara (1977) used multiple-baseline designs to test the value of behavioral exchanges and a version of the reciprocity treatment developed by Azrin and his associates. In what are perhaps the best-chosen single-subject designs for research in this area, these researchers found a slight tendency for the results to generalize across measures. Here, again, it is not possible to tell whether this tendency is the result of the power of forces inherent in the treatment situation not specifically related to the focal methods or of the power of the techniques to induce generalization.

Liberman *et al.* (1976a) made use of a group design in which a small number of couples was assigned consecutively (but not randomly) to either behavioral or interactional conditions. Unfortunately, it is clear that these conditions have much in common, that the therapists and clients in the behavioral condition were markedly overburdened, and that the data collection protocols were so demanding as to possibly have an adverse effect upon the meaningfulness of the results. This study showed no difference in outcome between the two treatment programs, a finding perhaps best explained by their overlap. While this study used groups of six couples each, Harrell and Guerney (1976) assigned 60 couples to treatment featuring either behavior therapy or communication training. Statistically significant differences on 4 of 13 dependent variable measures favored the behavior therapy group. A number of reporting problems make these data difficult to interpret. Perhaps the most serious problem, however, lies in the design of this research. As is apparent from the foregoing chapters of the present volume, communication training is at least an implicit and most often an explicit dimension of behavioral interventions. Therefore, the dichotomy posed in this and other similar projects is artificial and may best be approached as an analysis of the efficacy of one component of a comprehensive package as opposed to the results achieved through following the total program. Finally, generalization from this research is also hampered by the fact that as in some of the studies cited earlier (e.g., Dixon & Sciara, 1977; Azrin *et al.*, 1973), it used nonclinic couples as subjects, drawing a cloud over the immediate relevance of these findings for typical couples seeking counseling.

In the only study to date combining group and single-subject designs, Jacobson (1977) randomly assigned 10 couples either to focal behavior therapy or to a minimum treatment waiting-list control group. Using a covariance design, he found that couples receiving the focal treatment emitted more positive and fewer negative responses in a laboratory problem-solving task and reported greater marital satisfaction than their minimally treated counterparts. Unfortunately, the multiple-baseline data presented by the author lead to equivocal conclusions about the effectiveness of the intervention. In a subsequent study, Jacobson (1978) attempted to improve upon the first. The two behavior therapy groups in this research contrasted *quid pro quo* or partitive contracting procedures with good faith or holistic contracts. The two contrast conditions were an attention placebo and a waiting-list control. Unusual care went into the design of this research, which included three therapists, measures of clients' evaluations of the therapists, and independent ratings of the credibility of the service offerings. The results were generally positive in that the behavioral groups performed better than the waiting-list group on the four measures, which included use of the MISC (Weiss *et al.*, 1973) for coding negative and positive verbal problem-solving behavior; marital satisfaction ratings (Locke & Wallace, 1959); and marital happiness ratings in 12 areas (Stuart & Stuart, 1973). Only on the self-report measure of happiness in various areas did both behavioral groups fail to outperform the nonspecific group. The failure to find differences in outcome attributable to therapist or therapist × treatment interaction in client and student credibility ratings of treatment and therapist is taken to suggest that the positive results of the behavioral groups may be attributable to the relevant treatment ingredients.

Jacobson (1978) is to be commended for the following features of his study: (1) the use of multivariate analysis of covariance, which minimizes capitalization on chance and statistically controls for any pretest differences; (2) treating couples' rather than individuals' scores as the unit of analysis; (3) the effort that went into creating a credible nonspecific control group as well as the rather thorough specification of its content; and (4) the attempts to assess the credibility and equivalence of the three therapists and the three treatments on all but the experimentally manipulated differences. While not without its minor flaws (e.g., the small sample size and the absence of suitable explanations for the findings of no difference on some measures), this stands as probably the most carefully conceived study of its kind in this important area.

Elsewhere (Stuart & Roper, 1979), the measurement and statistical design features of research aiming to validate the productivity of the social-learning-theory approach have been discussed. Because research in this area is incredibly demanding when contrasted with laboratory research or with studies conducted in controlled environments, such as schools and hospitals, or studies of interactions much less complex than marriage, the total volume of reported results has been slow to develop. It does, however, exceed the rigor of research devoted to assessment of the outcome of nonbehavioral interventions, despite the fact that it has yet to achieve optimal standards of excellence. Given the paucity of research and the uncertain results produced by those studies that have been undertaken, the strongest conclusion that can be drawn from this literature at this time is that there appears to be fairly strong support for the application of these methods in the relief of marital distress. In no sense, however, can the results of this decade of research be interpreted as offering clinicians a strong and unequivocal mandate for the application of these methods. The implication of this conclusion is not that other methods are to be preferred; few if any have achieved even the limited research status found here. Instead, it is suggested that

1. The social learning theory approach to marital treatment must be regarded as being in a developing experimental status.
2. Therefore, clients should be told that the treatment they are to receive must be regarded as being in a stage of development.
3. Care must be taken to evaluate carefully each phase of the services offered, as well as the general therapeutic outcome.

To do less would not be in keeping with either the spirit or the letter of the current guidelines for ethical practice (Association for the Advancement of Behavior Therapy, 1977; Stuart, 1980a). In the same breath, it should be stressed that *every other currently employed marriage therapy program faces exactly the same strictures,* and no other program can as readily fulfill the third requirement.

Therapists seeking to meet these requirements can review the assessment recommendations found above and elsewhere (e.g., Stuart & Roper, 1979). Several recent volumes also present excellent summaries of the alternative single-subject designs that are available (e.g., Hersen & Barlow, 1976; Jayaratne & Levy, 1979). Responsible clinicians will study and selectively employ both these assessment and design materials in order to provide themselves with the feedback necessary for the proper evaluation of the services they render—feedback that is most useful when received during rather than after treatment.

SUMMARY

In this section recognition was given to the need for every therapist to evaluate the outcome of treatment offered in every instance. A range of alternatives was noted at the start of the section, after which suggestions were made for using several different techniques. A straightforward monitoring of client compliance and feeling change is the most direct approach available. The use of goal attainment scaling is suggested as a second technique because it permits on-line monitoring of the progress made toward selected relationship enhancement goals. A consumer evaluation scale was also presented as a direct means of soliciting the clients' organized appraisal of the progress of their treatment.

All of these techniques can, of course, also be supplemented by read-ministration of the individual- and couple-functioning measures described in earlier sections of this chapter.

This section concluded with an evaluation of the outcomes reported during the decade beginning in 1969, when the first report of a systematic application of social learning theory to marital treatment appeared. A review of this literature confirms the view that this approach is still in its infancy, and that clients have a reasonably good chance of achieving a positive therapeutic outcome, but that because therapeutic success is by no means assured, particular attention must be paid to the evaluation of therapeutic outcome using a broad array of materials to structure this assessment.

Conclusion

Implicit in the recommendations made in this chapter is the assumption that there is no "one true cause" of any human problem (Bakan, 1968). Therefore, the goal of assessment in marriage therapy is to explain not how the problem began but how it can be successfully managed. Recognizing that the assessment process must be efficient yet detect resources for change and areas needing change in many aspects of the clients' behavior, suggestions have been made for the collection of specific, treatment-related data through a process that can be beneficial to the clients even if they do not go beyond the first assessment stage of treatment. Also implicit in this approach is a recognition that much of the clients' interaction can be influenced by the boundary forces of their relationship, and that behaviors that might be considered highly aversive to outside observers may be relationship-maintaining for the clients themselves. Therefore, the therapist must be sensitive to the context and to the relationship meaning of all of the facts that are amassed during the assessment process.

It must be recognized that although marriage therapy has a tradition of at least 50 years as a formal activity, the adequacy of assessment devices has not kept pace with the proliferation of methods and the growth of the clientele. Therefore, several less than perfect instruments must be included in any contemporary assessment package. The recommendations made for this program are summarized in Table 2, indicating the assessment tools along with indications of their purpose and desirable timing. Therapists who prefer the use of other instruments, such as the MMPI, the 16 PF, or the California Personality Inventory, may wish to replace the recommended mood measure with one of these. Those who include in their counseling a specific effort to restructure role relationships may wish to include either the Inter-

Table 2. Recommendations for instruments to be included in a package of materials for the planning and evaluation of marriage therapy

Purpose	Instrument	Recommended schedule of use
To assess internal state with an interpersonal focus	Dyadic Adjustment Scale (Spanier, 1976; see Figure 1)	Prior to first session, four weeks after start of treatment, prior to treatment termination, and with all follow-up inquiries
To aid treatment planning	Marital Precounseling Inventory (Stuart & Stuart, 1973)	Mailed to clients for completion before scheduling of first treatment session; again at final session
To assess interactional behavior changes within the marriage	Standardized forms such as the Oregon forms (Patterson *et al.*, 1973) or localized measures such as those included in Chapters 6 through 12	Weekly as they apply to the instigated changes associated with each stage of treatment, and as probes during follow-up inquiries
To assess internal state with an intrapersonal focus	Cheerfulness–Depressive Mood Scale of the General Well-Being Schedule (U.S. Public Health Service, 1977; see Figure 3) or MMPI D Scale	Prior to first session and at monthly intervals thereafter during treatment, and with all follow-up inquiries
To assess behavior changes outside the marital relationship	Parenting–Work–Play Scale (see Figure 4)	Prior to second session and at monthly intervals thereafter during treatment, and with all follow-up inquiries
To evaluate treatment progress	Goal Attainment Scale (see Figure 5)	Completed *during* first session and reviewed every third session thereafter
	Treatment Evaluation Form (see Figure 6)	Completed during final treatment session
	Dyadic Adjustment Scale (see above)	Pre–post comparisons give some measure of improvement in reported marital satisfaction
	Marital Precounseling Inventory	Provides data on additional changes to be made during follow-up or maintenance stage of therapy

personal Checklist (ICL) (Leary, 1956) or the Tharp (1963a) Marital Role Questionnaire as measures of interactional behavior. In addition, those working in psychiatric and community mental health settings may wish to add instruments that have particular relevance to these settings (e.g., Hargreaves *et al.*, 1977; Waskow & Parloff, 1975). Inclusion of measures like these will clearly add to the cost of assessment, measured in both client and therapist time. However, in this era of aroused consciousness of the rights of clients (Stuart, 1980a), the cost of *not* attending to the requirements of systematic treatment planning and evaluation greatly outweighs the cost of collecting the necessary data.

Therapists can do a great deal to increase their clients' willingness to provide the necessary information. First, it is essential to explain to clients the relevance of all of the data that are requested. Second, it is essential to *promptly* feed back to clients the therapist's impression of the data that are provided. This does not mean confrontation with the full load of negative implications that can be drawn from these data; it does mean finding constructive ways to review strengths and to translate negative data into goals for change. Third, it is essential for the therapist to prompt clients to collect relevant data between sessions. The completion of forms like the goal attainment scale can easily be accomplished in the 10 minutes prior to selected sessions and/or during sessions. When clients are asked to monitor their behavior between sessions, however, planned telephone calls from the therapist can do wonders in improving the completeness of the records that are presented. Rather than using compliance with monitoring instigations as a test of clients' motivation, therapists should use the thoroughness with which clients comply as a test of their own therapeutic skills; low levels of compliance signal weak clinical skills, not weak clients. Finally, it is essential for the therapist to follow up all data collection procedures, not only with acknowledgment, but with pointed efforts to feed the data back into the service offered to the couple in ways that are explained to them.

When these requirements are met, therapists can gain a reasonably accurate and complete picture of their clients' functioning over time. The next chapter presents guidelines for therapeutic structuring, and the remaining chapters of this book present means of carefully using the data that are collected in the process of assessing troubled marriages.

C H A P T E R 5

Structuring the Therapeutic Process

Many clinicians agree that effective treatment requires the willing collaboration of a therapist who is skilled in interpersonal behavior and clinical technique and one or more well-motivated clients seeking reasonably precise changes in their life situation(s). Unfortunately, researchers have great difficulty in agreeing on which therapist and client characteristics, which treatment maneuvers, and which therapeutic structures contribute to the best therapeutic outcome—itself a subject of considerable controversy. Clinicians cannot await the consensus of the researchers before mounting treatment programs because clients are seeking help even though the care givers may not have reached closure on the best methods to use.

This chapter offers a rationale for a treatment structure that is time-limited, structured, historical, and goal-directed. It develops a role model for therapists that calls for active mediation and reeducation, and it develops a model of compatible roles for clients. Clients in marital treatment are viewed as experts on the nature of their goals, but as learners in the steps needed to assist them in reaching those goals.

In the next section of this chapter, suggestions are made for adapting these techniques to the needs of several special client groups: couples about to be married, separated couples, and those who are divorced. In each instance the basic theory remains the same, but the context and some of the techniques are altered. The chapter concludes with recommendations to aid the therapist in adhering to the recommended stages of treatment, stages that closely conform to the natural history of the development of intimate, long-term relationships.

Many of the recommendations made in this chapter are substantially documented. Little research has been done in other areas in which decisions must be made. In every instance some data can be cited that are contrary to the recommendations made here. In every instance, too, some of the reader's clinical experience will be contrary to the recommendations. Readers are urged to seriously consider the adoption of these recommendations when using the therapeutic approach recommended here, only because the recommendations are optimal for the present approach, not because they have any claim to being the ultimate clinical truths. Subsequent research and clinical experience may call for a revision of the recommendations made here. Meanwhile, because the therapeutic enterprise must go on, ethically responsible choices must be made in the context of less-than-perfect data, and these recommendations are certainly worthy of serious consideration by those interested in developing or perfecting skill in the clinical application of social learning theory.

Clients who enter any form of treatment have no guarantee of success in achieving even the most legitimate of therapeutic goals despite their having the most optimal of all personal resources for behavior change. Bergin (1966), followed by Stuart (1971c), noted that the psychotherapy literature describes a two-way street: some clients improve more than chance, others remain the same, and still others deteriorate. Recently, Gurman and Kniskern (1978) found that marital therapy clients show some chances of improvement, no change, or a worsening of their lot when their treatment experiences have ended.

Several factors contribute to the likelihood of therapeutic gain or loss. Successful treatment appears to depend upon the salubrious interaction of therapist and client characteristics, treatment techniques, the timing of service delivery relative to the stage of the distress, and the supportiveness of both the treatment and the extratherapeutic (home, work, community, etc.) environments. Effective treatments tend to share a set of common characteristics (e.g., Allen, 1977; Frank, 1961; Harper, 1959; Marmor, 1976; Shoben, 1949; Stieper & Wiener, 1965; Torrey, 1972). For example, the service must be offered for the primary benefit of the client, although it is recognized that both therapist and client gain from the encounter. The therapeutic environment must offer sufficient support to encourage the client to express his or her concerns, and suggestions for changes to meet these challenges must be presented tactfully and in such a manner as to be understood by and acceptable to the client and others whose behavior must also change in the service of goal attainment.

The attempts of theorists to single out one of the elements in this complex interaction as *the* necessary and sufficient ingredient of effective treatment have generally been unsupported by the findings of researchers. For example, Frank (1961) and Goldstein (1962) very persuasively called attention to the role of expectancy in therapeutic results. However, a decade of research has failed to show that realistic expectations are any more powerful than any other element of the treatment process in predicting therapeutic success (e.g., Gomes-Schwartz, 1978; Martin & Sterne, 1975; Wilkins, 1973). Others have viewed the therapeutic relationship as being the *sine qua non* of successful treatment (e.g., Bordin, 1959; Schaffer & Shoben, 1967; Strupp *et al.,* 1969), attributing to it the power of a *necessary and sufficient* condition for positive treatment outcomes (e.g., C. R. Rogers, 1957). While there has been some support for this assumption in research undertaken by leaders of the client-centered therapy movement (e.g., Traux, 1963; Traux & Mitchell, 1971), the empathic, warm relationship described by Traux and Carkhuff (1967) and scaled by Lennard and Bernstein (1960) has been found to be not only an *insufficient* but at times an *unnecessary* element in successful treatment (e.g., Beutler *et al.,* 1972; Garfield & Bergin, 1971; Morris & Suckerman, 1974; Mullen & Abeles, 1971; Sloane *et al.,* 1975). This finding may be attributable—at least, in part—to clients' recognition that the relationship they enjoy with their therapist is tantamount to the "purchase of friendship" (Schofield, 1964), and that the rules governing the therapeutic relationship differ little from those obtaining in any other "naturally occurring relationship" (Rotter, 1970; see, too, Kell & Mueller, 1966; Mueller, 1969). Thus, neither expectancy nor a benevolent interpersonal encounter can be regarded as a panacea for those undergoing emotional stress.

With the first few chapters of the book on effective treatment still undergoing painstaking revision by therapists and researchers around the world, it must be admitted that much of the effort expended by clinicians in their service-delivery efforts must be guided by some rather arbitrary decisions about the treatment process. The approach taken here accepts with caution many of the conclusions that are the consensus of clinicians and researchers, recognizing that no one—even no combination—of these guarantees successful outcomes. For example, it is presumed that clients who expect to gain from treatment are more likely to do so than those who enter therapy believing that it will not be helpful. In the same vein, it is presumed that therapists' abilities to motivate clients to follow through on instigations are proportionate to their interpersonal skills. These and many of the other general assumptions about the ingredients of effective therapy apply to the present program. In addition, however, it is believed that the delivery of effective services in this model requires four rather special prerequisites. While these assumptions can be challenged on clinical and/or research grounds—in common with every belief in the lore of human services—those wishing to make use of the stages of treatment to be described later are urged to plan conjoint, short-term, structured, and goal-directed treatment offerings. Because it is recognized that subsequent research may call for the revision of these assumptions, the rationale for each will be explained before we move into a discussion of the roles of therapist and client.

Assessment Should Be Conjoint

It is probably safe to say that virtually every marriage therapist has seen at least some spouses separately, either with or without conjoint sessions. Unfortunately, no research addresses the question: Are separate interviews with individual spouses a help or a hindrance to marital therapy outcome? Regarding treatment that is all either individual or offered in conjoint or group formats, Gurnam and Kniskern (1978) found:

> When conjoint, group and concurrent–collaborative marital therapies, all of which involve both spouses in treatment in some manner, are considered together, the rate of deterioration is only half of that accruing to individual therapy, i.e., 5.6%, 11.6%. (p. 9)

As it is practiced in diverse approaches, conjoint marital treatment thus appears to offer some safeguard against client deterioration. A number of studies have in fact shown that couples treated conjointly outperform those who undergo separate treatment (e.g., Beck, 1975; Freeman *et al.*, 1969; G. S. Greenberg, 1974; Miaoulis, 1976; Wattie, 1973).

Some therapists may argue it is important to see married clients separately at least some of the time, if not attempting to offer treatment that is entirely "separate but equal." These therapists tend to identify with orientations such as the psychoanalytic approach, which is keyed to individual change and essentially lacks assessment and intervention techniques for dyads. They would argue that therapists must be privy to all the facts if they are to be effective, believing further that the presence of the spouse inhibits each person from telling the whole truth. They believe, too, that the distress of the partners is a product of their separate intrapsychic functioning; therefore, remedies for the distress can be truly achieved only through individual intrapsychic change. Finally, they feel that the engineering of conjoint treatment is difficult because of the small likelihood that both partners will be either willing (e.g., Leslie, 1965) or able (e.g., Freedman & Rice, 1977) to continue in treatment.

In response to the first point—the belief that truths will be missed if all contacts are conjoint—two thoughts should be considered. First, it can be argued that we are all intrinsically biased in our reports of our own experiences, constantly editing our disclosures either intentionally or inadvertently to create the desired reaction in ourselves and others. Therefore, the truths told in individual sessions may involve much distortion. If this is true, it is through direct observation of the couple's interaction that the therapist can come closest to a true understanding of their relationship. In other words, treatment based upon the clients' self-reports is very likely to be misguided, while treatment based upon observational data is likely to be better adapted to the clients' situation as it actually exists (Haley, 1963a; Minuchin *et al.*, 1963). Second, it can be suggested that any data provided by one spouse without the knowledge of the other is essentially useless for clinical purposes. For example, if Sue tells the therapist that she is having an affair with her husband's closest chum, the therapist has two unenviable choices: to enter into collusion with Sue at the expense of the opportunity to be honest with her husband or to become the harbinger of the sad news, breaking faith with Sue while at the same time risking great injury to the therapeutic relationship with her husband. This point has been rather well made, albeit humorously, in the following advice to those who would thwart their therapists:

> Use this one only if the marriage counseling is helping in spite of all your efforts to the contrary. Call your therapist from a phone booth and tell him you want an individual session with him, but that you don't want your spouse to know. Tell him there are some things you just can't say in front of your spouse, but don't want him to feel hurt or left out. If your therapist refuses to see you individually, end the conversation by saying, "OK but you won't tell Larry I called will you?" (Adelson & Talmadge, 1976, p. 94)

In short, it is contended here that the only therapeutically relevant data are those that are available from observation of the couple's interaction during sessions, information that is produced in a totally open and aboveboard exchange between all concerned. Therefore, it is a good idea to *include both spouses in every treatment session.* This is especially true of the early meetings when the therapist has two missions: to structure the clients' roles in treatment and to gain the information needed to plan the intervention.

In addition to these negative reasons for treating couples conjointly, some very important positive reasons can be offered. First, it is the mission of the social-learning-theory approach to train couples to emit the desired behaviors in the natural context of their lives (C. H. Patterson, 1973; Rotter, 1954, 1970). As they will of course interact conjointly outside of treatment, it is reasonable to expect that they will learn to improve their skills more effectively if their skill-building training is offered conjointly. When spouses are seen together, the therapist is able to combine the "interaction" and "instigation" therapies described by Kanfer and Phillips (1969), greatly increasing the likelihood that the instigations will be followed between sessions. In addition, by intervening with both spouses directly the therapist increases the likelihood that the instigation will be conveyed and understood. That is, if the therapist sees only one spouse, he or she must influence that person to interact with the other spouse in a particular way. If the technique is unsuccessful, the therapist cannot know whether the maneuver or the execution was at fault. On the other hand, if the instigation is delivered to both spouses by the therapist, at least some of the uncertainty about treatment failure can be reduced and corrective action can be taken. Furthermore, were the therapist to help one spouse change his or her behavior in order to induce changes in the actions or reactions of the other, the rights of the other would be compromised to the extent that the other spouse might not concur in the value or direction of the changes.

In response to the suggestion that conjoint treatment is often impractical, two responses can be made. First, if it is true that therapeutic risks are greater in single-partner intervention, it may be in the clients' interest to offer treatment only under the conditions that are most likely to prove helpful rather than to offer a less defensible service. Second, therapists who are fully committed to rendering only conjoint marital treatment can be expected to have a high rate of compliance with the request that both spouses participate. Very often one spouse—typically the wife—calls to request treatment. She may say that her husband is unwilling to participate. However, if the therapist follows several steps, the involvement of the husband is almost always possible. First, the wife should be offered a brief rationale for the necessity of her husband's cooperation, for example, that all marital problems are the work of both partners and that problems can be effectively understood and resolved only when the views of both partners are available. Should the husband still refuse, the therapist can suggest that the wife relay the request from the therapist that the husband participate in at least the first session so as to offer his guidance as to how the treatment should progress. In such a session, the husband can participate in goal selection, protecting his right of self-determination should he elect not to participate in treatment. Finally, if the husband still refuses to join in the process, the therapist should, with the wife's prior consent, contact him directly. During this conversation, the therapist should repeat for the husband the rationale for his involvement, after which a brief summary of the intervention program should be offered and the husband should be reassured that he need not return to treatment after the first session if he so chooses. It is the rare husband indeed who resists this onslaught!

As a final note to this section, it is worthwhile to point out that while conjoint interviews should be the norm of marital treatment as represented here, there is at least one special situation in which individual contacts with spouses can prove to be beneficial. There are times when personal pride, consistent failure to accurately interpret the meaning of important communications, or preoccupation with a personal problem may obstruct the clients' efforts to express sufficient commitment to one another to permit their strong participation in the treatment process. When this happens it is helpful to see both spouses separately for 10–15 minutes in order to identify and neutralize commitment to the change process. The content of these brief encounters should be limited to discussion of the interviewee, and the spouse should not be discussed. After both partners have been seen individually, it is then helpful to bring them together for a conjoint session, which is begun by the therapist's stating (if true) that each person separately reconfirmed his or her commitment to work toward an improved relationship, followed by the request that each restate this commitment to the other. The value of contacts such as these is that the therapist can gently confront each person with his or her perception of the client's resistance without exposing the client to the risk of loss of face before the spouse. Used in this planful way, exceptions to the conjoint therapy rule can significantly improve prospects for a favorable treatment outcome.

Treatment Should Be Short-Term, Ideally Time-Limited

In addition to the finding that conjoint treatment may be more effective than service to spouses separately, it has also been found that short-term treatment often offers greater benefits than treatment of longer duration.

In 1939 Alfred Adler (1964) advocated that practice of offering clients from 8 to 10 sessions, but this recommendation was not generally accepted, no doubt because of the dominant role played by psychoanalytic theory in American therapeutic practices at that time. However, the exigencies of treatment during World War II forced experimentation with short-term treatment techniques (e.g., Grinker, 1947; Gutheil, 1944; Prugh & Brody, 1946). Although it was considered merely "first aid" (Baker, 1947) and an ineffective means of promoting lasting change (Fenichel, 1954), interest in short-term treatment continued to smolder during the rest of the decade, with applications generally limited to clients with situationally induced problems or clients believed to be too limited in ego strength to gain from the greater demands of long-term treatment (W. U. Snyder, 1950).

During the 1950s some *ex post facto* and some experimentally designed studies began to appear. In the former category, D. S. Cartwright (1955) and J. W. Taylor (1956) both attempted to analyze the outcome of psychotherapy from closed records. Both found that the clients who had been in treatment the longest showed the greatest improvement. Obviously, however, this type of research suffers from many design errors, not the least of which is the fact that clients who undergo dynamically oriented therapy and remain in treatment for longer periods receive more positive evaluations from their therapists than those who leave treatment before the therapist is ready for their departure. In support of this view, Nichols and Beck (1960) realized that the "gains" reported by undergraduates who had participated in an average of 14.7 interviews were those most clearly subject to therapeutic bias. Conversely, when tighter experimental designs were used, differences between the benefits of short- and long-term treatment became more difficult to discriminate. For example, Pascal and Zax (1956), using the best of the comparatively soft criteria available at the time, compared the results of treatment averaging 10, 60, and 183 sessions and found minimal differences.

The quality of research improved during the 1960s, and with it came a growing respect for the benefits of short-term approaches. Shlien et al. (1960, 1962) compared the results of client-centered therapy offered for an average of either 20 or 37 sessions. While not including behavior-change measures, their results indicated a greater improvement in the level of congruity between self-concept and ideal self-concept for those undergoing shorter as opposed to longer therapeutic contacts. However, because they found that the clients undergoing a time-limited Adlerian therapeutic program did not differ significantly from the level of change experienced by clients receiving long-term client-centered treatment, they concluded that the effect of time limits is mediated by the rationale of the treatment offered. That same year Lorr et al. (1962) reported that they could find no significant differences in outcome experienced at seven different Veterans Administration mental hygiene clinics by 133 patients who were randomly assigned to semi-weekly, weekly, or biweekly sessions when they were assessed by a complex battery of measures 4, 8, or 12 months after the termination of their treatment.

Stimulated by Malan's (1959, 1963) findings based upon a very well-designed study showing that short-term treatment could be highly effective, the 1960s were to witness a rapid increase in the number of studies reaching either neutral (i.e., length of treatment time does not predict outcome) or positive (i.e., short-term treatment results are superior) conclusions in wide-ranging settings (e.g., S. Adams, 1967; Muench, 1964; Reid & Shyne, 1969; Sarason et al., 1966; Strupp et al., 1969). As a result of these findings, the decade of the 1970s began with theorists like Garner (1970) and Wolberg (1971) advocating the use of any of the 73 different short-term approaches described by Small (1971), and with reviewers like Meltzoff and Kornreich (1970) suggesting that there is "very little good evidence that time in therapy past some undefined point brings commensurate additional benefits" (p. 346).

During the present decade, interest in short-term treatment has remained high (e.g., Katz et al., 1975; Malan et al., 1975; Miaoulis, 1976;

Negele, 1976; Oldz, 1977; Straker, 1977; Stuart & Tripodi, 1973). It appears that the pendulum has now swung from the dominance of long-term treatment before World War II to the present recognition of the favorable benefit–cost ratio results of short-term treatment. This spirit is well captured by the results of Cummings's (1977) recent review of the results of treatment offered at the Kaiser–Permanente Clinics: he found that for 85% of the patients seen, active, innovative short-term treatment was *more effective* than long-term treatment, while longer-term treatment was actually deleterious for from 5% to 6% of the clinic patients.

How can we explain these counterintuitive findings suggesting that we may actually offer too much of a good thing? First, it has also been shown that many of those entering treatment expect short-term therapy (Bent *et al.*, 1975) by active therapists (Slaney, 1978). Also, a number of studies (e.g., Fiester & Rudestam, 1975; Garfield, 1971; Noonan, 1973; Sarason *et al.*, 1966; Stieper & Wiener, 1965) have shown that therapy clients generally remain in treatment for an average of fewer than 10 sessions, often with quite significant benefit. Therefore, it may be that treatment that is consistent with the client's expectations may be more effective precisely because it is congruent with those expectations. Moreover, it is possible that longer-term treatment offerings may imply for the client that the therapist believes that the level of the existing problem is greater than the client believed, thereby undermining the client's adaptive resources.

It is also possible that most of the benefit that treatment can offer is derived during the first 5–10 sessions. In support of this idea, Stuart and Tripodi (1973) found that delinquents and their families who were offered treatment with a 90-day limit began to manufacture problems that justified treatment continuance, a device not tried by those whose treatment was limited to either 15 or 45 days overall. Sigal *et al.* (1976) found this effect to extend even beyond the end of treatment; their longer-term, dynamically treated subjects reported more problems after therapy than their early terminations reported. Finally, in planning treatment duration, therapists seem to be more guided by their own theoretical commitments than by their clients' needs (Frank, 1961). That is, therapists subscribing to theories that call for long-term treatment tend to see their clients as needing many sessions; early terminations are most often client-initiated, suggested by the therapist only upon very strong "resistance" from the client. Conversely, therapists subscribing to short-term or crisis-oriented treatment tend to conceptualize client needs in terms of fewer sessions. In either event, it is the therapist's beliefs rather than the client's distress that may exercise the greatest influence upon early notions of the ideal treatment duration for any given client. Given the fact that clients generally enter treatment because of some acute stress, casual treatment that does not offer immediate help may permit the situation to worsen, to the client's detriment, and may also be only marginally defensible on ethical grounds because of its great expense and intrusiveness (Association for the Advancement of Behavior Therapy, 1977).

On the positive side, there is reason to believe that the setting of short-term limits on treatment may help clients to mobilize their resources quickly and efficiently, with sufficient time to deal with the treatment-eliciting life crisis. In this vein, M. Cox (1978) observed that "timing is always significant. Patient and therapist must know when the end is, because only then will they know when 'just before the end' is" (p. 157). The time limit may help clients to organize their adaptive efforts along the one ubiquitous dimension of all human experience: time. Aware of the passage of time, they may be cued to use a rapid, more effective schedule for problem-solving efforts, rather than a more passive and therefore less productive problem-solving strategy. In support of this possibility, social psychologists (e.g., Benton et al., 1972; Stevens, 1963) have found that time limits in bargaining situations have two effects: they emphasize the fact that the session may end with no product, and they emphasize the fact that new efforts are expected.

Just as a time limit would seem to motivate the client to make more appropriate use of the treatment situation, so, too, does it appear to tend to increase the activity and awareness of the need for planfulness of the therapist. Phillips and Wiener (1966) stressed this dimension of time limits in the following words:

> Time is emphasized here because it is immediately cogent, assessable, and clear. It lends an immediacy and sharpness and it brings an urgency to planning that makes structuring inevitable, so that there is less drifting and improvisation in therapy. (p. 5)

The structure of treatment is therefore its next important dimension.

Treatment Should Be Highly Structured

Frank (1962) noted some time ago that when clients enter treatment, their thoughts about their problems and possible avenues of solution are generally in a muddle. Naturally, if they clearly visualized a possible fruitful course of action, they would follow it; their client status is an expression of the difficulty they are experiencing in defining their problems in solvable terms, in planning appropriate action, and/or in following through on a plan of attack once it has been formulated. To help them cope with this distress, Frank believed that almost any organized approach by the therapist could be helpful, so long as the therapist's organization is employed as a means of helping calm the furies of the client's chaotic thoughts, feelings, and actions. This sense of organization is powerfully conveyed through the manner in which the therapist structures the treatment that is offered.

The Adlerians (Ansbacher, 1972) have long recognized the need for structure in treatment, particularly in therapy of limited duration. Haley (1969a) humorously offered a prescription for therapeutic failure with the admonition "be passive, be inactive, be reflective, be silent and beware" (p. 78). Recent studies have shown that structured therapies are more easily learned by clinicians (Rappaport et al., 1973), while also being more consistent with client expectations than less structured approaches (Bent et al., 1975). Structured approaches also tend to relate theory, assessment, and technique more closely, so that they tend to be far less random and more to the point. Zuk (1976) has bemoaned the fact that therapists are more apt to portray the logic of their procedures as artistry than to take responsibility for the scientific validation of the premises and evaluation of their results. When the intervention is structured, as illustrated by the work of Strong (1975), specific assumptions can be tested, as can the relative contributions of various elements in the approach. Moreover, structured therapies have generally been shown to be more effective than the less predictable approaches (e.g., Paquin, 1977; Phillips & Wiener, 1966; Stieper & Wiener, 1965; Valle & Marinelli, 1975), as well as less likely to result in deterioration. This last conclusion was phrased by Gurman and Kniskern (1978a) who found that the therapist who was most likely to promote client deterioration was one who:

> does relatively little to structure the guiding of early treatment sessions; uses frontal confrontations of highly affective material early in therapy rather than reflections of feeling; labels unconscious motivation early in therapy rather than stimulating interaction, gathering data or does not actively intervene to moderate interpersonal feedback in families in which one member has very low ego strength. (p. 11)

Therefore, the provision of an appropriate therapeutic structure may at least rival the importance of positive therapist and client expectations and the provision of a facilitative therapeutic relationship in promoting the attainment of therapeutic goals.

Four conditions should be met if marital therapy is to be adequately structured. First, the treatment must be goal-directed: virtually everything that transpires between the therapist and clients should be done in the service of one or more of the agreed-upon goals. Second, the therapist's role should be precisely defined in a manner that is consistent with the overall rationale for the service that is being offered. Third, the clients, too, should have defined roles. Effective short-term treatment demands that the clients' participation be as goal-directed as that of the therapist. Finally, the intervention procedure should be conceptualized as a series of independent yet interrelated stages that build clients' skills cumulatively. The stage formulation provides both therapist and clients with a master plan of the therapy, a plan to which either can refer to evaluate the level of progress made and the steps that remain to be completed. Because of their importance, each of these elements is discussed in detail.

TREATMENT GOALS

For at least two reasons, the treatment literature offers sparse specific discussion of the formulation of treatment goals: considerations in goal determination are inherent in the theories of behavior that underlie the various approaches; and respect for the individual (idiographic) dimensions of human distress may outweigh the importance that clinicians give the more general (nonmothetic) dimensions of the problems brought to their attention. Nevertheless, the essential structure of treatment depends heavily upon the formulation of agreed-upon change goals. For Bandura (1977), goals are behavioral standards against which individuals assess the consequences of their own actions. For Kazdin (1975), the statement of therapeutic goals requires an answer to the question: "What behavior is to be changed in the stimulus conditions specified?" (p. 66). Building upon the thrust of both writers, the goals for treatment can be understood to consist of:

1. Specification of some target behaviors.
2. Specification of the conditions under which these behaviors are to be emitted.
3. Specification of some measure of personal and/or social change that is expected to result from the emission of the target behaviors under the specified conditions.

Goals thus concern what is to be done? under what conditions? with what results?

To be adequate, *goal statements must be precise*. But Haley (1977) has declared:

> Problems, whether one calls them symptoms or complaints, should be something one can count, observe, measure, or in some way know one is influencing. (pp. 40–41)

However, very often clinicians accept as goals events that are in fact the consequences of behavior changes. For example, "improving the quality of the marriage" is an indirect consequence of some specific action changes by both spouses. Often, too, therapists accept as goals very global statements that are not amenable to measurement. For example, "inducing the partners to act more responsibly" does not describe measurable events: "inducing the partners to attend to each other's conversation more consistently" does describe behaviors that could be measured objectively.

Adequate goal statements *must also call for positive changes*. Rotter (1954; C. H. Patterson, 1973) recognized that most therapeutic approaches call for the elimination of problem behaviors by, for example, suppressing "neurotic" functioning. He, along with Kazdin (1975), recognized, however, that no clearly effective strategy now exists for response suppression. Behavioral suppression involves eliminating behaviors that, presumably, are being prompted by their antecedents and maintained by their consequences. The individual is therefore asked to resist stimulation to act and to forego the attainment of reinforcements without having been taught either how to modify the conditions that potentiate action or how to obtain reinforcements through acceptable means. Therefore, the *primary* goals of treatment must always be positive, even though the *secondary* goals might be negative. For example, the secondary goals of the treatment of an alcoholic wife married to an abusive husband might be a reduction in her drinking and in his violence; the primary goals, however, must be an increase in interactions that they both experience as pleasurable.

In this same vein, the goals for treatment must address behavioral changes that help the clients to *modify the circumstances that appear to be conducive to their problem behaviors*. In another context, Stuart (1980b) has suggested that an "indirect" approach has more to offer than a "direct" approach in the treatment of problem eating. In an indirect approach, an individual who eats in response to boredom would be helped to learn assertive actions that would lead to more stimulating experiences, which, in turn, would be expected to reduce the urge to eat. A direct approach, on the other hand, would begin by trying to suppress problem eating despite the fact that the client's life is impoverished from a reinforcement standpoint. Sound practice would therefore call for indirect methods first, followed. if necessary, by a direct approach. With the drinking and abusive couple mentioned above, indirection would call for changing the quality of their interaction first, and then dealing directly with the alcohol consumption and the violence.

Researchers at the Mental Research Institute at Palo Alto have conceptualized this difference by contrasting "first-order" and "second-order" goals for change. In coining this vital distinction, Watzlawick, *et al.* (1974) used the following illustration:

> A person having a nightmare can do many things in his dream—run, hide, fight, scream, jump off a cliff, etc.—but no change from any one of these behaviors to another would ever terminate the nightmare. *We shall hence-*

forth refer to this kind of change as first-order change. Waking, obviously, is no longer a part of the dream, but a change to an altogether different state. *This kind of change will from now on be referred to as second-order change.* . . . Second-order change is thus *change of change.* (pp. 10–11)

For example, if Harry and Mary quarrel over how often to have sex, directing them to have sex once or 15 times weekly would not solve their problem, which is not one of the content (frequency of sex) but rather one of process (learning how to decide on the frequency of their sex). Clients are more apt to accept and to understand first-order change directives, but these are the instigations that are least likely to achieve the desired results.

Harry and Mary have had a sexual problem for many years. Harry has characteristically withdrawn, while Mary has played the role of the unhappy pursuer. To ask them to have sex often before overcoming some of Harry's hesitations and before helping Mary to learn how to initiate sex in a more sympathetic, less threatening manner would be a serious error of timing. Timing errors, along with goal selection at an inappropriate level, can seriously undermine the therapeutic potency of any clinical directive.

Goals that seek first-order change when change of the second order is needed, as well as goals calling for behavioral suppression rather than broader situation change, are often "trivial" in that they lead to short-lived if any behavior change. M. Cox (1978) used this term in another way, which points to the fourth criteria of therapeutic goals. He regards the therapist's attempt to discount the client's stated goals as "trivializing," a maneuver that can seriously undermine the client's motivation for change in the therapeutic environment. The topic of resistance or countercontrol is dealt with later in this chapter; for the present, it is important to note that much of what is termed "resistance" on the part of the client is often little more than "rejection of the client's goals" by the therapist. Combs *et al.* (1971) have noted:

People are *always* motivated if they are forever engaged in seeking self-fulfillment. Indeed, they are never unmotivated unless they are dead. To be sure, they may not be motivated to do what some outsider believes they ought or should . . . [but motivation] is always there, "given" by the very nature of the life force itself. (p. 76)

Following this reasoning, it can be assumed that all people are always motivated to do something; the challenge of therapy is to help the client develop productive patterns of action in the service of the socially constructive goals that they select. Goal formulations must therefore be *based upon the concern that the clients bring to treatment.*

For example, a couple requesting help with problems related to his involvement with other women and her chronic depression must receive intervention aimed at relieving these stresses. The therapist should express an understanding of these goals, then describe a treatment approach that seeks positive changes through defined methods. In this way, the couples' goals are accepted, reshaped, and used to help provide the motivation needed to influence their acceptance of the treatment program. As another example, when a couple come for help with a child-management problem, but it is apparent to the therapist that each is trying to use the child as an ally in a marital struggle, the couple's criterion should still be met. The therapist does this by recognizing their concern about improving their child's behavior but suggesting that first they must develop reliable means of defining their goals for the child's behavior and of reinforcing each other's efforts to cue and to reinforce those behaviors. In this consensus-building effort, the therapist often finds ample opportunity to deal constructively with marital issues as an intermediary goal en route to helping the couple realize the longer-term goal of changes in their child's actions.

Many researchers have found that clients are more likely to accept changes when they feel that they have had some say in goal selection. For example, it has been shown that subjects tolerate exposure to aversive events more readily when they believe that their compliance is voluntary, whether in a social psychology lab (e.g., Averill, 1973; Kanfer & Seidner, 1973) or in a cancer ward (Langer *et al.*, 1975); residents in homes for the aged exercised greater responsibility for self-care when they believed that they could choose to do so (Langer & Rodin, 1976); volunteer subjects tended to outperform those who were required to participate in experiments (Gordon, 1976); and students did better in the classes that they chose (Liem, 1975) and in reading programs that they chose to join (Kanfer & Grimm, 1978) rather than in classes and programs that they were constrained to join. Therefore, at least the illusion of choice seems to minimize resistance while strengthening the motivation to change; and in treatment situations, the choice must be real rather than an illusion if the demands of professional ethics are to be fulfilled (Davison & Stuart, 1975; Stuart, 1979b).

Finally, treatment goals must also be *modest*. It has been observed that it is:

> the "real," "big" or "basic" problems that many therapists and patients expected to be changed by therapy. Such goals are often vague and unrealistic, however, so that therapy which is very optimistic in concept easily becomes lengthy and disappointing in actual practice. (Weakland *et al.*, 1974, p. 113)

Treatment is only a small aspect of the complex lives of the couples who turn to it for help in redirecting and redesigning their interaction. It can help to make modest changes, but it cannot remake the people nor their lives. Therefore, the therapist must resist acceptance of the couple's request for changes that go beyond the power of the method. For example, the husband of the wife who has announced her plan to leave may ask that the therapist help him regain his wife's love. That the therapist cannot do. It is possible, however, to learn from the wife what changes she and her husband might make to ease some of the pressure that she feels, and then to help them both make the prescribed behavior changes. The therapist can do no more to "light the unhappy wife's fire," and to undertake to do so would be a grossly overstated promise of what treatment could possibly offer.

Acceptable therapeutic goals are thus specific and positive, call for new behaviors that can change the situations that are conducive to problem behaviors, are consistent with the clients' initial requests for help, and are modest. Fundamental to all of these criteria is the general objective of behavior change as the immediate goal of treatment, with change in feelings being the later effects of these behavior changes. Both the social learning approach and the interpersonal approach seek therapeutic changes in this sequence. For example, the following is the fundamental premise of the Mental Research Institute group (Weakland *et al.*, 1974):

> Regardless of their basic origins and etiology—if, indeed, these can ever be reliably determined—the kinds of problems people bring to psychotherapists persist only if they are maintained by ongoing current behavior of the client and others with whom he interacts. Correspondingly, if such problem-maintaining behavior is appropriately changed or eliminated, the problem will be resolved or vanish, regardless of its nature, origin or duration. (p. 145)

In line with the theory of reciprocal interaction (Bandura, 1977) described in Chapter 3, it is assumed here that when people learn to change their behavior, they earn different feedback from themselves and others; this feedback and the reinforcement that it engenders, in turn, serves to trigger changes in feeling states. The statement of treatment goals must therefore initially specify behavior changes, with changes in affect expected to follow as the longer-range consequences of the attainment of the initial goals.

Finally, it is important to note that the preliminary goals of treatment must be negotiated during the *first* therapeutic session (Haley, 1977). For the reasons indicated above, agreement on goals offers clients the advantage of having tangible proof that the therapist believes their goals can be met. Just as importantly, this early goal statement helps to focus the content of treatment sessions and the clients' intersession behavior. In addition, recognition of both initial and long-term goals helps the clients to realize that their major concerns are not being overlooked as they are asked to work on successive approximations of their major behavior-change objectives. As the initial and intermediary goals are achieved and/or as the couple's interests in the original long-term goals change, the statement of therapeutic objectives can and should be renegotiated. In one study in which goals were integrated into formal contracts for change in the behavior of all members of the families of predelinquent youths (Stuart et al., 1976), it was found that therapists renegotiated contracts with families as often as four or five times during treatment, each contract averaging some six months (Stuart & Lott, 1972). As life evolves, so, too, should the goals of treatment aimed at improving its quality.

DIMENSIONS OF THE ROLES OF THE THERAPIST

In this active approach to treatment, as in the interpersonal approach (Haley, 1963a, b, 1977), the therapist has the responsibility of controlling the therapeutic interaction. It is the job of the therapist to create a therapeutic environment that facilitates the clients' acceptance of change-inducing instigations as much as it is the job of the therapist to render instigations wisely, to evaluate the effects of the intervention, and to use this evaluation-produced feedback to redesign the methods that are used. The power that the therapist must use to do these jobs well must be developed through interaction with the clients, and the needed authority is often *gained or lost during the first half of the first treatment session.* The couple enter treatment with their own ideas about how the therapist can be of help: they often wish to specify not only the goals of treatment but also its method. The therapist must weigh each element of these prescriptions, accepting those believed to be conducive to change and redirecting others that are likely to be barriers to change. A clear understanding of the important dimensions of the therapeutic role can immeasurably assist the clinician in structuring a role that is likely to lead to the desired changes in the clients' actions and reactions.

The first dimension of the therapist's role is that of *mediator.* While Zuk (1966, 1967, 1976) has stressed the importance of this "go-between" function, Hurvitz (1974) has noted that even when therapists do conform to this strong expectation of their clients, they:

> generally do not explicitly acknowledge or report their intermediary function because it cannot be justified on the basis of the traditional theory and practice of psychotherapy based upon a dynamic unconscious and the resolution of unconscious conflicts through interpretation and insight. (p. 145)

Perhaps another reason for our retreat from formal acceptance of the mediational role is a hesitance to accept the Solomonic responsibility of judging right and wrong in the lives of the distressed couple. If this is the case, the caution is misdirected because the mediational role in marriage therapy carries no such responsibility.

In business and labor negotiations, arbitrators have more power than mediators (I. Bernstein, 1954; Elkouri, 1952; Johnson & Pruitt, 1972; Trotta, 1961). Arbitrators can subpoena witnesses and documents, thereby gaining access to considerable information before rendering binding decisions; the data base of the mediator, on the other hand, is limited to the information that the parties wish to share, and the mediator's decisions are no more than nonbinding recommendations. The arbitrator's rulings have the force of law; the mediator's recommendations gain their force from the quality of the negotiating environment that is created, from the accountability of having to bargain in relative good faith after having made a public commitment to do so, and from the fact that the mediator's recommendation makes it possible for the parties to make concessions without loss of face.

The marriage therapist functions as a mediator. The couple, upon entering treatment, generally have some fairly clear idea about what concessions each will have to make in order to restore balance in their relationship. It is the job of the therapist to enable each person to state his or her desires, to bargain with the other for the exchange of requests, to help each person develop any lacking skills that may be necessary for delivery on the agreements, and to monitor follow-through. To do these things, the therapist must maintain neutrality despite the spouses' efforts to use the intrinsic instability of the three-person conjoint therapy group to form coalitions (Haley, 1963a; G. W. McDonald, 1975). The therapist must also be sure to attend to the process through which the couple attempt to negotiate a solution to their difficulties, allowing the clients to determine the content of their new agreements. In this vein, the therapist must function in a distinctly educational capacity, combining the mediational role with an effort to enhance the clients' skills in formulating attainable goals.

Accordingly, the second dimension of the therapist's role is that of *reeducation*. Many contemporary descriptions of the treatment process stress its educational component. For example, Strupp *et al.* (1969) defined the therapeutic relationship as educational by saying: "The therapist teaches and the patient learns. As a teacher, the therapist is an expert: the patient is a student" (p. 3). In the same vein, Combs *et al.* (1971) described the therapeutic process in educational terms as follows:

> The process of helping is a process of problem solving that is governed by what we know of the dynamics of learning. Helping people discover more

effective and satisfying relationships between themselves and the world is an exercise in learning. In that sense all helpers of whatever school are fundamentally teachers. (p. 176)

Unfortunately, while many clients view the therapist as a "prime behavior changer or teacher," this is a role from which the therapist "has been deposed, or which he has never assumed in many psychotherapeutic theories" (Stieper & Wiener, 1965, p. 7). It is a role that is central to the effectiveness of the approach that is being recommended here.

Essentially, all of treatment is a teaching and learning experience for all parties. The therapist learns through the clients' experiences much as the clients learn by following therapeutic directives. At least five different dimensions of the treatment experience are directly educational for the client. The first two areas of teaching content were described in Chapter 3: they are the help that the clients receive in learning how to shift perspectives or to decenter in order to gain a more accurate description of their marital interaction and the help that is given in the use of new vocabulary to relabel experience.

The clients are also taught the rationale that underlies the intervention that they are about to receive (Allen, 1977; Torrey, 1972). The therapist should accomplish this early in the first session in order to communicate the aura of competence that may contribute to the development of positive expectations. The therapist can accomplish this by using several minutes at the start of the meeting to explain the general approach to be used. It is important to include in this description a mention of the experimental model that will be used in attempts to evaluate efforts to reach each goal. According to this model:

1. One client states the goal.
2. The other client asks for any needed clarification, then either agrees to work on reaching the goal or offers another suggestion.
3. When both have agreed that the goal is important, they and the therapist generate a list of possible goal-attaining steps.
4. From this list of alternative options, the clients work with the therapist to fashion an action plan that includes a means of measuring compliance.
5. Based upon the level of compliance and how the couple report that they feel about their efforts, they will continue, modify, or abandon this effort.

It is important for the clients to understand that they will have specific action plans and prompt means for evaluating the effects of their efforts, so that they will always be in control of the thrust of these efforts, with the therapist serving as facilitator and resource.

The next two things that clients learn in treatment are how to modify intrasession behavior and then how to generalize from the session to their extratherapeutic environments. Therapists first offer a rationale for instigations that are recommendations for specific behavior changes. Included in the rationale is some prediction of the benefits of compliance with the instigation. The instigation is then typically followed with modeling, then coaching or guided practice, to the extent that the target behaviors are producible in the treatment setting. For example, the therapist may feel that Marge and Alex exchange too many "dirty positives." Marge might say, "I do appreciate the way you offer to wash the dishes—whenever I complain that I have a serious headache," while Alex is likely to respond, "It's always a pleasure to be able to help when you don't feel that you can hold up your end of the bargain." Marge expresses a positive (appreciation of help from Alex) but includes a barb (the implication that she must be at death's door before he offers his assistance). Alex responds in kind with a positive (his interest in helping) and a put-down (the implication that Marge does not honor her commitments). During the early part of the session, the therapist can offer deserved recognition for their participation in the treatment process, thereby modeling "clean positives," stressing these words as potential mnemonic devices that will help them to make later use of the concept. The couple can then be asked to practice giving clean positives in the treatment session, with feedback first from the therapist and then from each other. The therapist then rounds out the in-session training by instigating their use of positives between sessions, asking both to make a commitment to use, acknowledge, and record the use and acknowledgment of this new communication tool.

Unfortunately, much of the emphasis in marital treatment focuses upon the couples' behavior during therapy sessions. This is important because, as Carkhuff and Bierman (1970) have noted, whatever clients practice most in therapy they are most likely to carry with them into their real world. However, while the clients are easily observed and influenced during sessions, their interaction in the presence of the therapist may have little relevance to their relationship when they are alone and unobserved. Rotter (1970) made this point very succinctly in the following terms:

> While it is true that analysis of the patients' interaction with the therapist can be an important source of learning, it is unsafe to overemphasize this as the main vehicle of treatment. Many times improvements seen by the therapist are improvements or changes that take place in relation to the therapist or the therapy situation, but the patient discriminates this situation from others and generalizes little to other life situations. (p. 237)

It is therefore a major task of the therapist to teach the couple some techniques that they can use to increase the likelihood that they will use at home, over time, and across situations, the relationship-management skills that have been learned in their therapy.

As an epilogue to this discussion of the educational component in marital therapy, it is important to indicate one content that is not included in this approach. In his discussion of the social learning approach, Rotter (1970) stressed the irrelevance of introspective insight to the solution of most clinical problems:

> It is usually believed that what the patient lacks most is insight into himself, but it is likely that in general what characterizes patients even more consistently is lack of insight into the reactions and motives of others. (p. 223)

It may be clearer to reserve the term "insight" for "self-reflection" and to use the term "understanding" to denote an appreciation of the dimensions of one's reciprocally determined interactions with others. The cultivation of insight often requires a confrontational assault on the client's self-descriptions and self-explanations, followed by his or her reluctant acceptance of an unflattering label for prior actions. The cultivation of understanding, on the other hand, is a more benign process in which the client is helped to determine goals, to describe present behavior in light of the stated goals, and to plan alternative actions as needed. Because understanding is oriented to positive goal attainment and because it does not involve any negative labels, it is less likely to generate the resistance that so often accompanies insight-inducing interactions. Indeed, confrontation is usually a desperation measure by the therapist, one that is better adapted to expression of the therapist's frustration than to facilitation of change in the client. Moreover, confrontation also tends to model the use of terminal language and an aggressive approach to goal attainment, both of which are often already overrepresented in the client's repertoire.

A third dimension of the therapist's role is acceptance of the responsibility to *direct the couples' goal attainment efforts with consistency and firmness*. This dimension of the role is somewhat in contrast with certain interpretations of the general treatment literature. While many clinicians believe that their relationship with the client should be sufficient to produce needed change, as noted earlier, this approach assumes that the relationship between therapist and clients facilitates the latter's acceptance of clinical instigations, with outcome of treatment being in large measure dependent upon the quality of the prescriptions given. Also, while many clinicians believe that the couple should essentially have complete control of the therapy, as noted above, this approach recognizes that the couple have primary responsibility (with editing feedback from the therapist) for choosing the goals of treatment, while the therapist (with editing feedback from the spouses) has primary responsibility for selecting intervention methods.

These assumptions underscore what might be termed the "executive" functions of the therapist. Interestingly, this position is consistent with the early writings of Carl Rogers, founder of the client-centered school of psychotherapy. In 1959 he wrote:

> It has been our experience to date that although the therapeutic relationship is used differently by different clients, it is not necessary nor helpful to manipulate the relationship in special ways for special kinds of clients. (pp. 213–214)

Cashdan (1973), too, believed that "the therapist's tactics are governed not so much by the client's utterances as by a plan that transcends the specific case" (pp. 4–5). In other words, there is an interplay between the client's wishes and the therapist's careful judgment about which actions would be in the client's best interest. The therapist who would sacrifice a professionally responsible sense of therapeutic process at the whim of the client is one who clearly does not take seriously enough the tenets of the approach that he or she is committed to using.

There are several times when the influence of the therapist is challenged, two of which bear special mention. The first pertains to the desire of many clients and therapists alike to discuss problem histories. In the most recent edition of their highly regarded book *A New Guide to Rational Living,* Ellis and Harper (1975) have expressed their belief that this obsession with history has risen to the level of being one of the most serious underpinnings of neurotic patterns of behavior:

> Perversely enough, one of the most important psychological discoveries of the past century, emphasized by both the psycho-analytic and the conditioned response (or behaviorist) schools of thinking, has proved most harmful to many individuals: the idea that humans remain most importantly influenced, in their present patterns of living, by their past experiences. People have used this partially sage and potentially helpful observation to create and bolster what we call Irrational Idea No. 8: The idea that your past remains all-important and that because something once strongly influenced your life, it has to keep determining your feelings and behavior today. (p. 168)

Indeed, the therapeutic corollary to this mistaken idea is the belief that in order to develop an effective means of helping clients achieve their current goals, therapists must have a complete understanding of the client's problem history.

There are many problems with history taking. First, much of what is told as history and believed to be true is at best a semirealistic, imaginative reconstruction of the past. Indeed, several empirical evaluations of the truth of historical statements attest to their inaccuracy (e.g., King, 1958; Orlansky, 1949; Stevenson, 1957; Szasz, 1964). Second, clients' accounts of the past are generally slanted in two directions: they are more apt to stress past failures than past successes; and the speaker is likely to describe himself or herself more as the victim of others than as a coconspirator in the unhappy events of the past. Taken together, these biases have the effect of reinforcing the client's pessimism about the prospect of future change while also building rationalizations to support resistance to change. In fact, it can be argued that the client's primary motivation for telling about past events is to do something in the present that will affect the therapist's behavior in the future. In other words, not only is the veracity of historical detail suspect, but the material is often edited for effect as a form of social engineering. Third, when confronted with history, the therapist can make few facilitative responses. It is possible to challenge the facts, but the client is the expert because only he or she was there. It is possible to suggest reinterpretations of the past, but the therapeutic value of these reconstructed ideas has in no sense been established. Discussion of the past has, for example, been associated with therapeutic outcome, but not with therapeutic success (e.g., Gomes-Schwartz, 1978; Sloane et al., 1975). Finally, discussion of the past diverts attention from the current issues, delays therapeutic progress, and is inconsistent with the action orientation that many clients expect from their treatment.

For these reasons, the taking of histories is discouraged, except under certain limited and highly specific circumstances. Such an approach is consistent with such present-oriented psychotherapeutic approaches as the Adlerian method. Speaking for that school of thought, Pew and Pew (1972) have written:

> We want to know only enough past history to identify present convictions and guidelines. Themes that are discovered in marital history are related to here and now problems and events. Recounting the past injustices is discouraged because both past and future are fictions; they are not concrete reality. Attempts by marital partners to discourage themselves or each other by reliving the past or anticipating the unknown future are pointed out until they catch themselves, an "aha" experience. (p. 199)

In line with this reasoning, several criteria can be identified for the therapeutic use of incursions into the past:

1. It is more desirable to limit therapeutic planning to a present-oriented data base.
2. When the past is introduced into the treatment session, emphasis should be placed upon past successes in a strength-oriented scanning for resources that can be used as a foundation for constructive efforts in the here and now.
3. Every question concerning the past should stress the role of the client, downplaying the roles of others.
4. An immediate, goal-oriented interpretation should be placed upon all remembrances of things past.
5. Discussion of the past should always be used as reinforcement of client's efforts to deal constructively with the planning of goal-directed behaviors rather than being a last resort in a search for explanations of current nonaction.

In short, discussions of the past can have a paralyzing effect upon therapeutic progress, and every mention of the past must be directly related to constructive planning efforts (see, for example, Stieper & Wiener, 1965, p. 129).

The lure of the past is a powerful influence on clients' interview behavior. They, like the therapists, are part of the current culture, so they too share the romance of psychohistory. For the therapist, the past can hold considerable interest; for the client, the past holds some of the keys to current failure. Unfortunately, the therapist occasionally aids and abets a common form of resistance by the client when it takes the form of defensive switches from present to past frames of reference. The two times when this resistance is most likely to occur are when therapy begins and when therapeutic breakthroughs are about to occur, for these are the times when the client's fear of change tends to be greatest.

It is also incumbent upon the therapist to exercise firm direction when client resistance is observed. Some amount of resistance is inevitable whenever one person attempts to influence another (Brehm, 1966), and this resistance often takes the form of spontaneous countercontrol measures (Davison, 1973). In addition, the idea of change is intrinsically fear-arousing, and "the patient's avowed willingness to cooperate notwithstanding, he also has a large investment in maintaining the status quo" (Strupp et al., 1969, p. 4). Compounding these ubiquitous sources of resistance is the fact that change in marital therapy means incurring all the risks of moving closer to another person. Huesmann and Levinger (1972) noted that while many people deeply desire the rewards of greater closeness with others, they also experience a fear of this closeness. They observed that "It might cost little to be stood up by a blind date, but it would be quite hurtful to be rejected by someone dear" (p. 4). Aronson (1969), too, has pointed out that familiarity breeds reward, but with it the capacity to hurt. Distressed couples are experts on the experience of hurt at each other's hands, so both can be expected to resist the very changes that they have come to therapy to accomplish. Moreoover, there is also the system-maintaining effect that Haley (1963a) has described so well:

> People in relation to each other tend to govern each other's behavior so that their relationship remains stable, and it is in the nature of governors that they act so as to diminish change. Implicit in this way of looking at relationships is a premise which might be called the first law of human relations: When one individual initiates a change in relation to another, the other will respond in such a way as to diminish that change. (p. 222)

It is therefore clear that many couples would rather fight than switch, and they often work toward neutralizing rather than facilitating the efforts of the therapist to promote change. The therapist is thus faced with the challenge of resisting the clients' efforts to move to the side or backward rather than moving ahead.

With the model of the client that emerges from this understanding of the forces that promote resistance, it is clear that the therapist who would be helpful must possess great skill in resisting a couple's unproductive efforts. This resistance requires the provision of reassurance, redirection, and repetition of the needed directives—the three "R's" of this dimension of the therapist's role. Cashdan (1973) has offered what he terms the "immediacy rule," according to which he leads "the client to the present whenever he is mired in the past and into the therapy room when he gravitates to events outside of it" (p. 71). Haley (1973), too, has noted that the "marital couple in difficulty tends to perpetuate their distress by attempting to resolve conflict in such a way that it continues" (p. 221). For that reason, he admonished the therapist to redirect the couple's problem-solving efforts, because if left to their own devices, they would worsen rather than improve matters.

It is generally safe to assume that when the couple in active distress wish to talk about the content of a disagreement, the proper focus should be on the process of their exchange. Conversely, when they choose a process, the odds are strong that only a content-oriented discussion would advance their cause. For example, when Alice complains about Hal's broken promises and she wishes to flail him about her specific disappointments, it is a good bet that progress can be made only through discussion of the process through which he makes and breaks commitments. If he is pressured to make a reluctant or unrealistic promise, clearly the responsibility for its nonfulfillment is only partly his. On the other hand, if the couple ignore the specifics and wish to talk about the process, there is a strong possibility that what is needed is agreement about who did what to whom. When the level of distress is lessened and the couple are truly working on relationship enhancement, they will deal with both process and content issues at one time; however, until that time the therapist is well advised to be ever ready to help them shift perspectives, whichever start they make. This is not done in the spirit of manipulation or playfulness; it is, in fact, the expression of the deepest responsible concern of the therapist for attainment of the couple's treatment goals.

Three additional dimensions of the role of the therapist also warrant special mention. First, it is important to remember that the *therapist always serves as a model for the clients*. Every gesture and every word have the potential for being guides that the clients may imitate. Questions direct the spouses' attention to areas that the therapist considers relevant and important. The style of questioning and making statements is often viewed by the clients as a prototype of the way in which they are expected to behave. Even nonverbal gestures have prompt value. Therefore, the therapist must maintain a constant self-vigil over the example that is being set by his or her behavior.

Related in significance to this modeling function are two additional therapeutic roles described by Zuk (1976; see, too, Garrigan & Bambrick, 1975). The therapist sometimes functions as a "side-taker" in order to lend weight to the position taken by one partner or the other. He or she does this in order to upset a pathogenic balance. For example, if the partners disagree about whether they should or should not move to another city and are paralyzed by this inability to overcome an inertia maintained by power-equal positions, the therapist might side with the partner wishing to move just to promote problem-solving discussion that might or might not result in a decision to relocate. The goal of this side taking is not to influence the content of the decision; it is intended to have an impact upon the process of decision making.

The therapist also occasionally serves as a "celebrant." In this role, the therapist, in effect, officiates at some rite of transition in the family and lends the mantle of community recognition to its occurrence. For example, the decision of the partners to stay together or to separate is an example of the kind of action that the therapist, in effect, consecrates, thereby making it "official" and therefore more binding.

In concluding this discussion of the role of the therapist, it is necessary to introduce two notes of caution. The role called for in this approach is that of mediator, reeducator, and director of perception, planning, and action—clearly a very active role. Should the therapist become too active, however, several dangers are imminent. It is important to remember that the treatment must be based upon the clients' selection of goals and the clients' acceptance of plans and the clients' evaluation of outcomes. It is the responsibility of the therapist to elicit, to attend to, and to respect these client-produced data. The therapist is one member of the triad and is obliged to provide some of the motive force, while the couple's hands are on the helm. In addition, the educational role of the therapist requires that the clients be taught the techniques needed for planning and carrying out the means for determining and attaining their own goals. Therefore, the therapist must assume a progressively *less active* role after teaching the skills needed for mastering each stage of treatment. Therefore, at each stage, one might *direct the first efforts, coach the second series, and merely give feedback about the couple's efforts thereafter.* Such an approach has the added advantage of helping the clients to attribute to themselves the ability to manage their relationship constructively. It has been shown that when clients attribute to the therapist, drug, or other dimension of the clinical situation the power to solve their problems, they are far less likely to maintain the change than would be true if they self-attributed this power (Davison & Valins, 1969; Kopel & Arkowitz, 1975). Therefore, great attention should be paid to this building of a sense of self-efficacy (Bandura, 1978) in the couple.

DIMENSIONS OF THE CLIENTS' ROLE

As cited by Watzlawick (1964), Genet, in his play *The Balcony,* portrayed a judge as saying to a young girl who stood accused of being a thief, "You have to be a model thief if I am to be a model judge. If you are a fake thief, I become a fake judge." And to the executioner, "Without you I would be nothing." And again to the young girl, "And without you, too, my child. You are my two perfect complements. Ah, what a fine trio we make!" The judge expressed the essential truth of all human interaction: NO actor can perform independently of the supporting cast. Therefore, the therapist can do no better in the job of helper than the clients are proficient at receiving help. Therefore, to increase the strength of the client's performance, the therapist has the responsibility of doing some very important role casting.

For the treatment methods recommended here, ideal client behavior meets the following criteria:

1. The couple regularly attend scheduled appointments.
2. During sessions the couple should
   a. attend to therapist-modeled behaviors;
   b. accede to therapist directives concerning *positive* interaction during the session;
   c. participate in the definition of long-range and immediate treatment goals and plans for behavior change;
   d. agree to only those instigations with which they truly intend to comply;
   e. participate in the evaluation of the effects of the treatment-mediated interaction changes.

3. Between sessions the couple should
   a. complete all tasks to which they consented during the treatment sessions;
   b. complete any written or other records of changes in their own and/or one another's behavior.

Because of their virtual universality in all behavioral approaches, all but one of these elements of these clients' roles need no discussion. However, item 2b, which calls for sustaining a positive interaction during treatment sessions, does merit some discussion.

The therapeutic approach represented here is built upon efforts to teach the clients new ways to describe their marital experience, to plan self-responsible methods of changing their interaction, and to evaluate their marriage on the basis of their actual experiences with one another. As has been indicated, the goals for change must be positive and must be accomplished within a relatively brief time frame. Taken together, these various requirements support the need for a highly structured treatment approach. As one of the requirements of this structure, *everything that transpires during sessions* must work in the *service of goal attainment,* and extraneous prompts and reinforcements for counterproductive actions must be all but eliminated. Therefore, the therapist is called upon to take pains to see that ideally everything that happens in the session facilitates goal attainment. To accomplish this, the therapist must (1) use the process language of goals rather than the terminal words inherent in a "problem-oriented" approach; (2) prompt positive exchanges between the partners; (3) reinforce positive exchanges whenever they occur; (4) model a strength-oriented approach to describing and planning changes in the couple's interaction; and (5) redirect clients' negative interaction into positive channels whenever hostile exchanges occur. These tasks stand in sharp contrast to some of the cathartic therapy techniques that call for "letting it all hang out" during treatment sessions. As a general rule, clients tend to be far too well practiced in their interpersonally destructive, ineffective, hostile maneuvers, whether the snide put-down or the highly animated frontal attack. To permit, much less encourage, these to occur during sessions can have little more than the adverse effect of legitimating and thereby strengthening them for the clients. Therefore, the treatment session must provide a novel learning environment for the couple, an environment that is qualitatively different than that in which they have recently played out the drama of their lives. This must be an environment built of controlled exchanges that consistently reinforce rather than weaken the couple's bonds of commitment, indeed a truly positive and facilitative environment.

To participate in such an experience, distressed couples must often quickly learn to use skills with one another that tend to be lacking in their relationship, yet present in their interactions with others (see Chapter 4). The fact that these responses already exist in their repertoire eases the task of the therapist, which is more one of retraining the partners to generalize these often well-practiced public skills back into their private marital interaction. In this, as in all other learning situations, consistency of experience facilitates skill acquisition; therefore, every exchange in treatment should be consistent with the positive skill-building focus of the therapeutic approach.

The couple are unlikely to act spontaneously in these positive ways, which are frequently inconsistent with the stressful interaction that brought them for help; therefore, the therapist must do several things to increase the likelihood of these constructive responses both before and during the therapeutic experience.

Several authors (e.g., Heitler, 1976; Goldstein, et al., 1966; Orne & Wender, 1968) have recommended induction of the client's role in a process that might be termed "anticipatory socialization for treatment." These techniques can be used to help clients anticipate warmth in the therapist (R. P. Greenberg, 1969; Greenberg et al., 1970) and to help build the positive expectations that Frank (1961) and Goldstein (1962) consider so important for therapeutic success.

Several different kinds of approaches have been used for this purpose. The Marital Precounseling Inventory (Stuart & Stuart, 1973) described in Chapter 4 has a role-prestructuring effect. The form asks clients to identify the strengths and those aspects of their partner's behavior that they find appealing. It also asks clients to think in terms of positive and specific change goals, emphasizing attention to the ways in which a change in the actions of one can facilitate changes in the reactions of the other.

Audiovisual materials have been used for this role-training procedure. Truax and Wargo (1969) used a videotape to structure the roles of hospitalized outpatients in psychotherapy. Long (1968) used a filmed model for role structuring. Finally, Stuart (1980b) has prepared an audiotape specifically for the purpose of preparing couples to participate in the type of treatment that is advocated here. This tape includes a brief statement of the treatment rationale, "advice" to the clients as to how they can gain maximal advantage from their treatment experience, and several vignette models of clients' successful handling of several therapeutic challenges. This tape can be sent to clients prior to their first interview, can be played in the waiting room before they meet with the therapist, or can be incorporated into the first session.

Several teams of researchers (e.g., Hoehn-Saric et al., 1964; Sloane et al., 1970) have used a two-part, pretreatment, role-induction interview to achieve many of the same purposes that are the target of the audiovisual materials. In part, this interview is faith building, but its role in helping the client to learn desired role behaviors is more important than its inspirational aspect. While evaluations of the long-term results of treatment using and not using this procedure have not shown significant differences (e.g., Liberman *et al.*, 1972), this may—in part at least— be because the service offered was far less structured than that recommended here. In an even more ambitious program, Warren and Rice (1972) used four half-hour interviews (following the first, second, sixth, and ninth sessions) to teach clients productive role behaviors and to encourage them to introduce their major concerns during therapy sessions. While only inferential, one could suggest three different possible sources of gain stemming from this interview method. First, the extratherapy interview may be more neutral than treatment *per se*, and therefore it may not elicit the same defensiveness as might appear during actual treatment; this lowered resistance may facilitate role learning. Second, more repetition of the instigations may lend weight to them. Finally, this interview, like the Marital Precounseling Inventory and the audiovisual materials mentioned earlier, may offer more highly structured and clearly stated role-induction messages than are likely to be offered by the therapist, who is, at the same time, concerned with management of the specific content and process issues in treatment.

Whatever techniques are used, it is the responsibility of the therapist to facilitate the clients' constructive use of the treatment time being offered. As Schofield (1964) has recognized, an effective therapeutic relationship involves effective actions by all parties, and this relationship "is not a spontaneous one but rather a controlled, circumscribed [and] and limited one" (p. 108). This helpful collaborative relationship will be much more likely to materialize only if the therapist tells the client what to do (Fiester & Rudestam, 1975) rather than hanging back and waiting for opportunities to reinforce constructive behaviors that might never occur before the client loses interest in treatment altogether.

A PRECISE CONCEPTION OF TREATMENT STAGES

A conception of treatment stages is for the therapist and clients what a road map is for a driver and the passengers in the car: it is a precise guide for the directions to be followed, and one that all can use to keep their efforts headed in the chosen direction. As with a road map, however, in which detours are sometimes necessary because of road disrepair or because the driver learns of interesting side trips along the way, the stage sequence should be considered an ideal but not an absolutely necessary framework. Indeed, the stage model offered implies a certain overlap of steps. For example, communication and behavior-change instigations are intrinsic in the first (caring days) stage of treatment.

There will be times when the clients come with a specific request for help in later stages of treatment, and in the therapist's judgment it may be necessary to accede to this request if the clients' participation in treatment is to be assured. But as they are presented here, the stages of treatment correspond closely to the stages of relationship development, and to deviate from the prescribed sequence too far or too often can seriously undermine the prospects for long-term success. Therefore, the therapist may be well advised to explain to couples asking for services appropriate to a later stage the advantage of taking a slightly indirect approach that will buffer their chances for attaining their well-chosen goals.

A theory of stages gives the therapist guidance in knowing what to respond to immediately, what to defer until later, and what to ignore entirely (Ford & Urban, 1963). Cashdan (1973) believes that a theory of stages is essential to effective intervention because it "provides the consistency and continuity that form the basis of therapeutic growth" (p. 101). Indeed, virtually every systematic approach to therapeutic intervention structures the therapist's behavior with a theory of stages, whether the therapy is psychoanalytic, (e.g., Fenichel, 1954; Greenson, 1967), psychotherapeutic (e.g., Rogers, 1958; White, 1956; Wolberg, 1965), interpersonal (e.g. Cashdan, 1973), or group (e.g. Rose, 1977; Yalom, 1970) in orientation; and whether it addresses change in marriages (e.g., Liberman *et al.*, 1976) or families (e.g., Cleghorn & Leven, 1973; Foley, 1976; Mueller & Orfanidis, 1976; M. A. Solomon, 1977).

Some of the stage theories are comparatively simple. For example, Carkhuff and Berenson (1967) offered only two stages: the first involving "downward and inward" movement as the therapeutic relationship is developed; the second being "upward and outward" as the client develops the ability to function independently and more effectively. Others offer more elaborate thories. For example, Cashdan (1973) suggested that treatment progresses through five stages as follows: (1) "hooking," in which "the therapist is transformed from a relatively distant and removed professional figure into someone who is perceived as warm, caring and involved" (p. 42); (2) clients' attempts to use this relationship manipulatively and maladaptively; (3) therapeutic "stripping" of these maladaptive strategies; (4) the emergence of adaptive interactional behaviors; and (5) "unhooking" or termination. Clearly, Cashdan's approach places the therapist–client relationship at the center of the treatment process. Other theories are more descriptive of stages through which the clients' relationship with one another evolves during treatment. For example, in describing the reactions of the families of schizophrenics to treatment, Mueller and Orfanidis (1976) observed the following stages: (1) an initial resistance to treatment that must be overcome by convincing the family that not the identified patient alone but all members of the family are the targets of intervention; (2) dissolution of the fusion between one of the parents and the identified patient; (3) repair of the sense of alienation experienced by parents at the loss of the pathological tie to the identified patient; and (4) solidification of the marital unit as a dyad and reinforcement of the independence of the identified patient.

The stage theory that provides the structure for the approach used in this book focuses upon the teaching objectives of the therapist or the learning goals of the clients rather than upon the therapist–client or client–client relationship. A truncated description of the stages is presented in Figure 1. All of the remaining chapters offer a rationale for the instigations recommended at each stage of the intervention.

As an overview, the first two items in Figure 1 are designed to prestructure roles for the client and to fashion a therapeutic contract (see below). The caring-days procedure is the first step in treatment because it is recognized that distressed couples tend to offer each other few and weak positive reinforcements; that they need an opportunity to experience the power of positive change early in treatment; and that the changes that they are likely to be willing to make are quite small. Therefore, the caring-days procedure starts treatment by asking clients to identify and deliver to one another a number of small, daily positive behaviors. Extensive social psychological research (e.g., Benton *et al.*, 1972; Chertkoff & Conley, 1967) has shown that bargaining proceeds best when begun with small requests. In addition, the warmth and commitment that a week of these successful exchanges can generate can go far toward building the trust needed for more open expression (Taylor *et al.*, 1969) and for commitment to a more energetic process of change (Bateson, 1972). Huesmann and Levinger (1972) have made two very important observations that support the importance of building trust through immediate exchanges and that place these exchanges at the forefront of therapy. On the first point, they noted:

> Irrespective of the depth of involvement, an individual often anticipates rewards in a dyadic interaction long before they occur. Yet even when the future rewards are higher than the present rewards, a person does not always emphasize the future over the present. This occurs because of a discount on the future. One values future rewards less than present rewards, particularly if one is unsure about the continuance or stability of the relationship. (p. 5)

This view provides an incisive justification for a "change-first" approach as a means of building some trust in the relationship as well as in the treatment process. On the second point, Huesmann and Levinger (1972) noted that "Each person learns about the other's probable future actions from the nature of his past actions" (p. 6). Because the real-life recent

Figure 1. Outline of the sequence of intervention techniques in the social-learning-theory-based approach to marital treatment.

Technique	Criteria for moving to next step
1. Completion of Marital Precounseling Inventory (Stuart & Stuart, 1972).	1. First appointment not scheduled until completed forms have been received.
2. Explanation of rationale of treatment, including its short-term, conjoint and structured format, with relationship-enhancement skills taught before attempts are made to deal with conflict and other problems.	2. Agreement to either a written or a taped verbal therapeutic contract (Stuart, 1980a).
3. Introduction of caring-days technique, in which small, high-frequency, conflict-free behaviors are exchanged daily by both spouses.	3. Six or more caring behaviors should be exchanged daily for at least one week, leading to a slight increase in commitment to the relationship experienced by both spouses and a belief by both that changes in behavior can produce changes in feelings.
4. Introduction of communication-change techniques, including: (a) listening skills; (b) self-statements; (c) "how" questions; (d) clarification; and (e) positive feedback.	4. Each spouse should demonstrate the ability to accurately paraphrase the other's self-statements, in addition to being able to request and acknowledge change constructively.
5. Introduction of contracting procedure including: (a) training in adoption of "two-winner" bargaining set; (b) selection of strategically important positive and specific change goals; and (c) formulation of "holistic" contracts for the exchange of groups of important behaviors rather than "tit-for-tat" agreements.	5. The couple should successfully negotiate and put into practice agreements for the exchange of more important behaviors, some of which may have been the object of conflict in the past.
6. Introduction of the "powergram" (Stuart, in press) procedure for the allocation of decision-making authority, followed by training in problem-solving skills.	6. Both spouses should agree to areas of sole, shared, and mutual authority, and then use this allocation as the basis for identifying problems, generating alternatives, and selecting, implementing, and evaluating solutions.
7. Introduction of training in conflict containment through the identification and suppression of some conflict triggers, the exercise of skill in maintaining conflicts at the issue-specific level, and management of the expression of anger in ways respectful of the norms of the marriage.	7. The frequency and intensity of conflict should decrease, as should the time necessary for the couple to accomplish reconsolidation after a disagreement. Both should experience an increase in trust and a willingness to risk change in a more flexible, less defensive interaction.
8. Introduction of strategies for maintaining the changed interaction, including anticipation of the possible sources and dimensions of future conflict, the development of resources for aiding conflict containment, and the use of a periodic reassessment of the strengths and goals of the interaction.	8. Both spouses should be able to successfully complete discrimination and action training exercises as methods of anticipatory socialization for their lives together after treatment termination. Appointments should be scheduled for post-therapy follow-up sessions at 3- and 12-month intervals.

actions that brought the clients into treatment are likely to have been negative, the positive expectancy needed to provide the motive force for building positive expectations and goal-attainment skills depends upon a revitalized history of some current positive exchanges. Finally, it has also been found that relatively frequent expressions of affection are associated with marital adjustment (Morse, 1973), so that changes prompted by participation in the caring-days technique have value in their own right.

Consistent with the recommendations of Nunnally *et al.* (1975), the next stage of treatment is concerned with building the partners' skills in *selected* types of communication. Specifically, the couple are taught how to listen, to make requests, to acknowledge the granting of their requests, to ask facilitative questions, and to request and offer both clarification and positive feedback. Without the ability to do these things, the couple will be hard-pressed to bargain for more meaningful behavior exchanges. Indeed, Nemeth (1970) has stressed the importance of clear communication to the success of any bargaining venture, as well as the virtual impossibility of effective bargaining when the parties are limited to ambiguous message exchanges.

The next stage of treatment (item 5 on Figure 1) involves training the partners in the skills needed for negotiating realistic agreements for the exchange of important behaviors that each desires from the other, followed by the delivery and acknowledgment of these sought-after exchanges. The importance of these exchanges is well stated by Wills *et al.* (1972) in the following words:

> For relationships in an advanced stage of distress, the spouses may well label their difficulties as feelings of hostility and disrespect for each other, but the genesis of this hostility may lie in a cumulated series of dissatisfactions over relatively simple instrumental actions (as well as in personal insults and rejections), and the ultimate stability of the marriage may depend upon the problem-solving techniques used to deal with this source of displeasure. (p. 23)

With the ability to negotiate specific agreements and a relationship that features a marked increase in positive exchanges, the couple are now ready to progress to that level of treatment termed by the Minnesota Couples Communication group (Nunnally *et al.*, 1975) the "identification of rules." In this instance, however, the rules pertain to the allocation of responsibility for decision making, and the couple are offered help in generating their own decision-making system. Aided by this new set of proactive, prospective agreements, the couple take a major step toward increasing the positive predictability of their relationship.

Item 7 in Figure 1 specifies the need to train the couple next in techniques useful for containing conflict when it arises between them.

While many couples begin therapy by asking for help in harnessing one another's rage, this approach makes the assumption that they are fighting with good cause and will fight less only when some of the conflict triggers are quelled and when they have opportunities to gain more positive attention from one another. Therefore, efforts to deal with conflict are postponed until after the component skills have been acquired.

It is at this stage that the couple might be offered counseling for any problems in sexual adjustment (see Chapter 11). It is here assumed that the desire to engage in close, loving sexual interaction is a consequence of the attachment generated by a constructive relationship. Therefore, even when the treatment-initiating request is for sex therapy, this service is postponed if the necessary marital strengths are not apparent.

Finally, maintenance skills are taught as a way of helping to increase the likelihood that the couple will generalize the skills learned in treatment to new challenges in their interaction during the months and years following the end of treatment. These techniques are discussed in Chapter 12.

Some Suggestions for Making This Treatment Program A Reality

The foregoing sections have described an active reeducation treatment model offered to couples conjointly for a brief period of highly structured service. Included with the rationale for each of the features of this approach were suggestions for making it a reality. This final section of the chapter, dealing with the structure of treatment, offers several suggestions for service delivery techniques that generalize across stages and objectives and are aimed at augmenting the ethical stature and general effectiveness of the marital treatment enterprise.

1. *To help reduce treatment time, it is essential that the first session be highly productive.* In traditional approaches, not only the first but actually the first few sessions are often allocated to data collection primarily and to socializing the client into the desired treatment role secondarily. In these approaches, active intervention usually awaits the completion of these two important steps. The present approach, on the other hand, is designed to begin active intervention shortly after the start of the first session. This approach is akin to the first-session goals described by G. F. Jacobson (1971) for use in outpatient therapy settings:

> Whenever he can, the therapist accomplishes . . . during the first hour . . . a working diagnosis, tentatively formulates his treatment plan, and begins the treatment intervention. (p. 145)

Two measures mentioned earlier help to make these goals a reality in the present approach. First, the clients are asked to listen to an audio-tape that defines their roles in the treatment process (Stuart, 1979a). Second, the clients are asked to complete the Marital Precounseling Form (Stuart & Stuart, 1973), which provides the therapist with an overview of their self-assessed strengths and treatment objectives prior to the first meeting.

Traditional therapists tend to begin the first session with a proba-tive question that the client is expected to answer despite a lack of familiarity with the therapist's expectations of how he or she should behave. In this approach, the therapist is encouraged to speak first, recapitulating in two or three minutes the essence of the treatment rationale as presented on the presocialization tape. The therapist is thus allowed to establish his or her identity before the clients are asked to leap into the unknown and thereby reduces their anxiety to a certain degree. This approach also increases the probability that the couple's early responses will be consistent with the general thrust of the treat-ment, allowing the clinician to establish an early, positive control of the intervention process.

The therapist next asks the spouses to tell each other some of the positive things that each noted about the other's behavior on the pre-counseling form. It is wise always to ask that the first statements be made by the spouse whose list of positives is longest and most varied. That partner will provide a more positive model for the other than would the spouse who appeared to have fewer positive things to say. As each positive is offered, the therapist can subtly begin communication training by asking the speaker to clarify exactly what is liked and by asking the listener to acknowledge the positives that are being offered. This small interchange offers a microcosm of the general treatment approach: the therapist potentiates positive behaviors selected by the clients; the clients emit, refine, acknowledge, and reciprocate these posi-tive actions.

Next, the therapist can offer a (a minute or two) précis of the larger behavior-change goals noted on the couple's completed forms, indicat-ing that these challenges will be approached after some headway has been made on some steps that logically must be taken first. It is then timely to ask the clients to identify the items that they would like to use as a start on their caring-days list as described in the next chapter. This discussion generally rounds out the first session, by the conclusion of which several very important things have happened: (1) the therapeutic roles for the clinician and the couple have been established: (2) all have agreed on a general format for intervention; (3) the first behavior-changing instigation has been begun; and, hopefully, (4) the couple have begun to develop a greater sense of commitment to each other and a greater appreciation of the possibility of immediate change. To reinforce each of these achievements, it is often very helpful for the therapist to telephone the couple three or four days after the first session to prompt them to follow the caring-days instigation, to reassert his or her interest in their progress, and to offer any well-deserved positive reinforcement for those changes that have already taken place.

2. *To make the goals and methods of treatment absolutely clear, the therapist should offer the clients a treatment contract, at least in words, and ideally in writing.* Stuart (1980a) has reviewed the ethical desirability of a written treatment contract as a means of protecting the clients' right to informed consent and as a means of defense of the therapist should the clients allege that this vital right has been abridged by the treatment they have undergone. At least two kinds of contracts are useful. Figure 2 presents a rather general contract that specifies the privileges and responsibilities of the therapist and clients, without specifying specific intervention goals. This form is useful as a further means of reinforcing conceptions of the rationale and roles of treatment. Elsewhere, Stuart (1975) has published a form for a much more challenging contract, one that provides specific information not only about the treatment method and its general effectiveness, but also about specific goals, techniques, and criteria for evaluating therapeutic outcome. Completion of this form, which generally takes as long as a complete session, is a second highly effective way to launch the intervention in that it offers a very systematic framework through which therapist and client can achieve consensus on the specific thrust of their work together. Finally, it can be pointed out that the use of both of these forms requires the clients' signatures. Working on a project described above (Stuart *et al.*, 1976), Levy (1977) found that clients' initials on written lists of the instigations they are asked to follow greatly increases the probability that they will follow through as directed when this technique is contrasted with the simple verbal communication of therapeutic directives. Therefore, the use of formalized contracts is as much a therapeutic expedient as it is a response to the guidelines for ethical service delivery (Association for the Advancement of Behavior Therapy, 1977).

3. *To evaluate his or her role performance, it is helpful for the therapist to make an audiotape of every session* and to evaluate the tapes when treatment results do not appear to be matching expectation. When the therapist explains that the tape is being made only as partial insurance of good-quality service, with the added potential benefit of its being available for feedback use during the treatment process (e.g., Andes, 1975; Bergner, 1974; Shoffner, 1977), couples are all but certain to agree to having the session taped, and the therapist need keep no more than one prior session for each couple, thereby permitting the use of a single tape for each pair.

Figure 2. A generalized contract for marital therapy.

It is understood that Mr. and Ms. _____
have expressed interest in one or more of the following goals (please check):

____ To decide whether or not to continue their marriage.

____ To improve the quality of their interactions.

____ To plan ways of renegotiating their commitment to each other to permit opportunities for more independence.

____ To plan ways in which their marriage can be amicably dissolved.

It is understood that they are not both equally committed to the above goal(s) and that neither is entirely certain about what action to take at this time. Therefore, they agree to the following:

1. They will participate in all treatment sessions jointly.

2. They will in person, on the phone, in writing, or by any other means tell the therapist only those things that are already known to the other.

3. They will express their goals for change in their relationship.

4. They will agree to make changes very thoughtfully and will thus follow through on any commitments so made.

5. They will participate in the process of collecting and analyzing any data needed to monitor and evaluate the effects of all clinically relevant interaction changes.

It will be the responsibility of the therapist to help the clients to identify their goals, to plan ways in which their goals can be achieved, and to evaluate the general effectiveness of these changes. The therapist agrees to see the couple for _____ sessions at a fee of $_____ per session. At the end of the first session, the therapist agrees to offer the couple a prognosis. Each three sessions thereafter, the therapist will help the couple to evaluate their progress. At the end of the stipulated number of sessions, the therapist agrees to conclude treatment if the treatment has not met reasonable expectations. Treatment will also be terminated if the goals have not been achieved prior to the targeted number of sessions. Conversely, treatment contacts will be extended for a designated period of time if the results appear to warrant their continuance.

Date:

Husband:

Wife:

Therapist:

With the tapes in hand, the therapist can review the past session should the current session indicate client noncompliance with instigations, discouragement with the rate of progress being made, uncertainty about what is expected of them, or any other results or process-oriented concerns. In reviewing the tapes, the therapist may wish to make use of the Allred Interaction Analysis for Counselors (Allred & Kersey, 1977). This is a rather simple coding system in which seven therapist behaviors and two client behaviors are described. The therapist behaviors are (1) educates; (2) gathers information; (3) interprets/confronts ; (4) seeks alternatives/recommends; (5) supports; (6) equivocates; and (7) detaches/aggresses. The two client behaviors are works and resists. Allred and Kersey described three uses for this system, which has acceptable reliability and some indication of face and concurrent validity. First, therapists can track the relative frequency with which they use each of the defined behaviors. Consistent with this approach, heavy use should be made of categories (1), (4), and (5). It is also possible to compute a therapist–client talk score by dividing the number of times the clients speak into the number of observations of therapist's talk in all seven categories. Third, it is possible to calculate a functional–obstructive ratio by dividing the number of observations in categories (6) and (7) into the sum of observations in categories (1) through (5).

Whether the Allred instrument is used in a formal self-feedback approach or the therapist's monitoring of the tapes is done more casually, the making, retention, and occasional review of these tapes is an excellent means of maintaining the quality of the therapist's behavior in a highly ethically responsible fashion.

As a final suggestion aimed at increasing the therapist's correct understanding of the impact of his or her efforts upon the clients, it is possible for the therapist to offer the clients, at the conclusion of each treatment session, a brief session-evaluation form. A form was developed for this purpose in a project in which graduate students offered family-oriented behavior therapy to delinquents and their families (Stuart *et al.*, 1976). At the conclusion of each session, the clients were handed one card asking questions including the following:

1. Did the therapist begin the session by asking me about my success with recommendations made the previous week?
2. Did the therapist respond to my experience by praising my success and/or by suggesting ways in which I could have a better experience in these areas next week?
3. Was the therapist generally positive in responding to my comments in the session?
4. Did the therapist make suggestions for positive changes in my behavior in a way that helped me to understand exactly what I am being asked to do and how it is likely to prove helpful?
5. Were these suggested behavior changes relevant to my goals for my sake and for my treatment in general?
6. What are the major things that I have learned from this session?
   a. _____
   b. _____
   c. _____

7. What have I been asked to do differently this week?
   a. _____
   b. _____
   c. _____

Working together in answering these questions helps the clients to reach consensus and to consolidate the gains from each session. Sharing their conclusions with the therapist provides an opportunity to overcome any misunderstandings. In addition, candidly and objectively reviewing the therapeutic process models for them a useful relationship-management technique while also strengthening the rapport between therapist and clients. Therefore, many gains can be made from use of the last five minutes of each treatment session for this purpose.

4. Resonating with the therapist's efforts to manage his or her role in treatment, it is *also important to make certain that everything the clients are asked to do is consistent with the general objectives of treatment and that their compliance is consistently monitored.* The Treatment Planning Worksheet and the Master Case Record form presented in Figures 3 and 4, respectively, are aids in this direction. On the first of these forms, it will be seen that the therapist begins by noting the goals suggested by the husband, the wife, or both. Then, in Section II, the therapist can restate these goals as needed (perhaps to make them more positive and specific), relating these reformulations to the clients' original requests. The techniques used to achieve these goals can then be listed, with brief note being made of when the instigation was begun and the results achieved by specified dates. If every technique that is suggested is listed on this form, then every technique used will have been introduced in the service of one or more of the clients' stated goals.

Use of the Master Case Record form greatly facilitates record keeping. Long narrative histories are rarely useful or accurate. They also tend to be highly deficit-oriented. This record is short and oriented to process and outcome. It can be completed during the treatment session, and it can be reviewed in a minute or two prior to each succeeding session. In that way, the therapist is assured of following up on every instigation given. This is very important because the failure to follow through on any directives leads the clients to feel that the therapist does not take seriously all of the recommendations given for changes in their behavior, a belief that can seriously undermine their motivation to follow through, particularly on the more challenging directives that they receive. Finally, because these records are free of any negative labels, they can be freely shared with the couple in periodic reviews of the progress being made in treatment.

5. *To facilitate adherence to the natural progression of the stages of behavior change, the therapist should share with the clients some of the reactions that other couples have experienced in responding to each of the stages.* Miller *et al.* (1975) have

Figure 3. Treatment Planning Worksheet.

Client's name: Sheet ____ of ____

Therapist: Date: _____

I. Client's stated objectives

    A. H-W   D. H-W

    B. H-W   E. H-W

    C. H-W   F. H-W

II. Therapeutic goals, techniques, and results

Therapeutic goal	Corresp. cl. obj.	Techniques	Date start	Results, date
A.		1.		
		2.		
		3.		
B.		1.		
		2.		
		3.		
C.		1.		
		2.		
		3.		
D.		1.		
		2.		
		3.		
E.		1.		
		2.		
		3.		
F.		1.		
		2.		
		3.		

suggested that couples progressing through the stages of their program experience a sequence of four reactions. First, they undergo a "beginning awareness stage," in which they greet the challenge with a mixture of confusion and excitement. At this time they may have a tendency to make unrealistically heavy commitments, and it is the task of the therapist to keep their enthusiasm within the boundaries of their capacity. Next, they undergo the "awkwardness stage," in which they emit the new behavior with a noteworthy lack of finesse. If the partners are not equally committed to this specific step in the change process—that is, if both do not have an equal stake in accomplishing the targeted change because it is not especially meaningful to them—then one will find the performance of the other unconvincing and will have a tendency to use

Figure 4. Master Case Record.

Name	Address		Work phone	Hours	Home phone

Husband:

Wife:

Referral: (a) Date: (b) Source: (c) Acknowledgment date:

First session: (a) Date: (b) Who participated: (c) Fee:

(d) Date socialization tape used: (e) Date precounseling forms returned:

(f) Instigations given:

1.

2.

3.

4.

(g) General impressions:

Second session: (a) Date: (b) Who participated: (c) Fee:

(d) Progress on prior instigations:

1.

2.

3.

4.

(e) New instigations and repetition of former instigations numbers:

1.

2.

3.

4.

(f) Progress rated: excellent good fair poor worse

(g) General impressions:

this reaction as a basis for distancing from the treatment process. At this stage, it is incumbent upon the therapist to help the less-involved partner to enjoy the intent if not the outcome of the other's actions.

The "conscious skillful stage" comes next. At this time, both partners are more attentive to their own efforts to do what is expected than they are to enjoying the fruits of the other's efforts. The less-committed partner is likely to feel that the experience lacks authenticity and may use this feeling as a rationalization for hesitant follow-through. The therapist can deal with this reaction by assuring both partners that they are not expected either to perform the task naturally or to enjoy these early efforts, denying the less-involved spouse use of either the "it-

174   HELPING COUPLES CHANGE

```
Session number: _____ (a) Date:        (b) Who participated:              (c) Fee:
    (d) Progress on prior instigations:
        1.
        2.
        3.
        4.
    (e) New instigations and repetition of former instigations numbers:
        1.
        2.
        3.
        4.
    (f) Progress rated:    excellent    good    fair    poor    worse
    (g) General impressions:


Session number: _____ (a) Date:        (b) Who participated:              (c) Fee:
    (d) Progress on prior instigations:
        1.
        2.
        3.
        4.
    (e) New instigations and repetition of former instigations numbers:
        1.
        2.
        3.
        4.
    (f) Progress rated:    excellent    good    fair    poor    worse
    (g) General impressions:
```

doesn't-feel-right" or the "I'm-not-getting-enough-out-of-this" ploy. This tactic is somewhat similar to the use of paradoxical instigations advocated by Haley (1973), The Mental Research Institute group (Watzlawick *et al.*, 1974), and Raskin and Klein (1976). In a sense, it is an attempt to help the couple lose a symptom by telling them that they are expected to keep it. It differs from therapy by paradoxical intent, however, in that this experimental approach asks therapists to advocate that clients emit behaviors that the therapist would actually prefer they not make, thereby introducing into treatment a highly deceptive tactic. The risks inherent in this approach are that the client may not resist as the therapist expects and may behave in self-defeating ways as directed, that the client may sense the therapist's manipulation and generalize skepticism about all other instigations made by the therapist, or that the client may imitate this highly manipulative style of interpersonal behavior in interactions with others. In contrast, the present recommendation simply asks the clients to be modest in their expectations and does not involve any bold-faced manipulation, thereby avoiding the risks intrinsic in the use of paradoxical intent.

Finally, the couples who persist in treatment reach the "integrated stage," when their skills mature and the new behaviors pay off in more shared satisfaction. This, of course, is the essential goal of every treatment experience.

At each of these stages, a simple test-and-change strategy is useful. Awkwardness should vanish as skill begins to develop. Uneasiness about planning can be reduced by clarification of the positive value of the thoughtfulness that motivates such plans and by reminders of the unreasonableness of the expectation that one will always spontaneously fulfill the other's expectations. Resistance related to the failure of the partners to be fully committed to the goals can be avoided through full discussion of and contracting for goals and methods before attempts are made to elicit commitment to specific behavior changes. Finally, periodic checking to determine if the goals are still important can help to maintain if not to renew this commitment.

Two additional stages can also be identified as an aftermath of each successful instigation. Each spouse can be expected to engage in a bit of testing to assess the other's commitment to the new interaction as opposed to his or her willingness to revert to their old patterns. Testing can take the form of simply dusting off the former behaviors, of questioning the motivation of the other, or of sharing with the other a secret feeling that the entire treatment process generates superficial and artificial behavior changes. If this test is failed—that is, if the listener to these maneuvers indicates a willingness to slide back—then any gains of treatment are vitiated. Conversely, if this test is passed, the couple move into the final or consolidation stage, in which the new interaction becomes more or less firmly accepted in the rules of their relationship.

As with the earlier stages, the therapist can build the clients' resilience in the face of this testing by some anticipatory socialization. Telling the couple in advance that either or both will challenge the strength of what they have just worked so hard to accomplish and asking them to attempt to moderate the force of the test and their reaction to one another's probes can be helpful. Even more important is the skill of the therapist in assuming ownership of the very process of testing itself. This he or she does by telling the couple that not only is testing natural, but it is also a desirable means of consolidating change. This tactic stops short of paradoxical instigation (Haley, 1977), although it is a maneuver that certainly has parodoxical overtones and great potential benefit. Finally, the great weight of testing can also be lessened if the couple are trained in appropriate means of response to the urge to test and to the experience of being tested. Techniques for this purpose are discussed in Chapter 12 in the context of maintenance procedures.

ADAPTING THIS APPROACH TO SPECIAL GROUPS OF CLIENTS

The general approach that has been described thus far calls for weekly one-hour interviews with couples who are married, living together, and at least somewhat interested in strengthening their relationship. Marriage therapists are called upon to offer service to couples in other situations and with different therapeutic objectives. In this section is found suggestions for adapting this approach to several of the more commonly encountered situations.

Premarital Counseling. At least one member of each couple seeking premarital counseling has sufficient ambivalence about the impending marriage to feel that the commitment should not be made without the mediation of a third party. While younger, more naive couples tend to expect the therapist to be able to tell them either to go forward or to turn back, it is obvious that no therapist possesses the prescience that would justify such fateful advice. Therefore, the therapeutic tasks in this situation aim at helping the couple to experiment with identifying and/or changing varied dimensions of their interchange, using the data produced by these changes as a basis for their impending decision. It should be noted, too, that similar to the approach of others (e.g., Purcell, 1976), the techniques recommended here are intended for use whether or not the couple anticipating marriage are living together.

First, the couple need help in clearly describing each other's strengths and honest expectations about postmarital privileges and responsibilities. Stuart (1975) has developed an inventory that facilitates the collection of many of these data prior to the first treatment session, analogous to the form used in prestructuring marriage therapy. Unique to this form is an adaptation of the Role Construct Repertory Test (Kelly, 1955) that facilitates comparison of the dimensions that each person uses for evaluating self, partner, and others—a description of each person's "interpersonal space." Responses to this section of the form cue the therapist as to the vocabulary that each partner uses in assessing his or her reactions to the other as well as to people in general. With this information, the therapist can have some notion of the kinds of alternative relationships the clients value, offering leads as to ways in which they might wish to change their focal relationship. During the first few treatment sessions, these data can be fed back to the couple in constructive ways, with the goals being to help them to disclose aspects of the "secret contract" that may underly their thinking about the potential marriage (see Chapter 8) and to help them formulate change goals during their courtship.

During the first session the couple are told that the objectives of counseling are to help them to formulate goals for relationship change, to work toward achieving these goals, and to explore the implications of this experience for their long-term relationship. They are reassured that value judgments *per se* will not be made, but that the cognitive and affective effects of their interactive behavior will be carefully examined for leads toward the prediction of future outcomes. They should also be told that there is good reason to believe that relationships change dramatically after the marriage vows have been spoken (e.g., Bentler & Newcomb, 1978; Meck & Leunes, 1976; Stuart, in press), and that their premarital counseling is intended to help smooth the transition into marriage by making explicit some of the expectations that are often unspoken before marriage, only to become the seeds of mortal combat during the marital years.

It is then wise for each client to state the kinds of changes that the other could make in the service of resolving some of the uncertainties that elicit his or her hesitation about making a commitment to marry. These can then either be adapted to the stages of change that have been outlined for married couples, or they can be engineered to occur concurrently. For example, if the wife-to-be feels that her chosen tends not to follow through on promises, leading her to feel that she cannot trust him to behave in certain ways in the future, this problem can be addressed along with the introduction of caring days and communication change. For example, follow-through can be assessed by willingness to deliver on the promised number of small, positive behaviors called for in the caring-days list. During communication change, the man could be helped to differentiate between two levels of undertakings. (Promises should be written and always kept, while statements of positive desire might be verbal instead of written and might be understood to be desires as opposed to commitments.) In this way the couple can collect data pertaining to their specific change goals while passing through the stages of orderly relationship development.

Premarital counseling can be offered on an individual or group basis, as can any of the other services described here. Whether offered to the couple alone or as part of a group, it, like the other services, should be offered conjointly, for a fixed period of perhaps six sessions, and in a highly structured format. Unfortunately, there are no immediately available criteria for evaluating this treatment. Decisions to marry or not to marry are neither necessarily successes nor failures, and on this dimension, only the couple's happiness together or apart in future years can be the acid test of long-range outcome. On the shorter-range dimensions, the couple's compliance with instigations for behavior change and their capacity to describe new areas of their interaction in objective terms acceptable to both, and leading to change efforts, are reasonable outcome criteria. Unfortunately, most of the premarital counseling programs thus far described either include no evaluation or rely upon somewhat irrelevant standard measures of personality or uninformative probes of how much the clients liked the service they received.

Should the couple decide to marry, it is wise to ask them to agree to return for one or two sessions at the following critical times:

1. Just prior to the wedding ceremony, if it is three or more months hence.
2. When they begin to plan for their first child.
3. When either partner anticipates making a career or lifestyle change of major proportions.

Premarital counseling can thus be extended as a kind of marital well-being insurance, enabling the partners to use the assessment and change skills that helped them overcome their entry-level ambivalence to increase the success of their resulting union.

Separated Spouses. Couples who have separated and then request either marital treatment or "predivorce counseling" are experiencing the same level of ambivalence as the premarital counseling candidates. If they were certain about the desirability of marital termination, they would be unlikely to make any commitment to evaluation and/or change of their marital relationship. The fact that they choose counseling— even though one partner may be leaning far out of the marriage, with the other clinging to his or her coatttails in a restraining effort—is an indication that either the glue that keeps them in the relationship is strong or the barrier forces that inhibit marital dissolution are quite strong.

The therapeutic task with these couples is much the same as that chosen for premarital couples: they must develop a means of collecting data that will aid them in deciding whether to continue or end their union. Like those contemplating marriage, they must be told that the therapist is an expert in the process of decision making and not an expert on the content of the decisions that couples must make for themselves. The stages necessary to this process are comparable to those found in premarital and marital counseling: they begin with self-assessment through completion of the Marital Precounseling Inventory (Stuart & Stuart, 1973), build commitment through caring days, and so forth. Two differences do, however, require adaptation in the approach.

First, the couple generally need a rather tight time frame. Phillips and Toomin (1975) asked couples to make a commitment for a three-month period of structured separation therapy. Both Phillips and Too-min consider personal growth an important dimension of their program, and both feel that a period of less than 12 weeks would be insufficient for such growth. The goal of the present approach, on the other hand, is simply to aid the couple in making a decision about relationship maintenance or termination based upon data produced by their efforts to change their interaction. Moreover, the separated couple is considered, by definition, a couple facing a crisis. As Phillips has noted, the great stress placed on togetherness, with the implication that couples who separate for even a short period of time are inferior in some important way, is at least somewhat guilt inducing for the couple involved in the separation process. Separation also represents something of a state of suspended animation for them as partners, parents, and autonomous adults. Therefore, because the focus here is on relationship evaluation rather than personal change, because the couple are perceived to be in a crisis state, and because the party leaning out cannot be expected to make a long-term commitment, the present program asks the partners to agree to a *three-week* trial only. It is understood that at the end of this period the partners will be helped to assess their experience: should the results be discouraging, they will be offered help in structuring further separation, with only positive experiences justifying the instigation that they stay together longer. The fact that a commitment of a mere three weeks is called for often overcomes the reluctance of the less-committed spouse to become active in the treatment program.

Second, the caring days and related procedures must be adapted to the times that the couple agree specifically to spend together. Phillips asks couples in his structured separation program to have no contact, while Toomin does permit contact by mutual agreement. The approach here falls between these two, insofar as it recognizes the need to provide partners who have opted for some distance an opportunity to have designated periods apart and other times together. Rather than allowing either spouse to phone the other at will, or worse yet to drop in spontaneously at potentially embarrassing times, the couples are asked to agree to some *specified, inviolate, and unexpandable* times of contact. They must be specific so that both spouses can plan other activities in their lives. They must be inviolate so that neither spouse suffers the pain of rejection by the other if something (someone?) important comes up. They must be unexpandable so that neither spouse feels pressured to increase contact time and neither feels rejected by the other's hesitance to do so.

Phillips asks the couples he treats to have no contact with other partners during the time of their separation. He believes that trying to help the spouses to develop their relationship while either is dating is like "trying to get a person to learn to eat straw while feeding him/her champagne and caviar" (Phillips & Toomin, 1975, p. 5). Toomin, on the other hand, encourages her clients to actively explore other relationships in an effort to learn about options and to gain a better understanding of their primary relationship. The approach taken here is that partners may try to enlist the therapist as an ally in working their way out of what might be termed "collateral relationships" (Stuart, in press) with others; but that this is best done by the partners themselves. On the other hand, it is recognized that it is possible to generate great resistance to treatment if partners who are in important relationships with others are asked to terminate these contacts in the interests of counseling. Therefore, these relationships are not discussed in the present approach. Instead, each partner is asked to consider time not spent together as "private time," for which neither has any accountability to the other. They may have contact with others during these times but are responsible not to allow information about such contacts to intrude upon their marriage. It is expected that as the attraction of the marriage changes through suc-cessful intervention, interest in other partners will decline. In addition, it is often found that mutual respect between the mates often grows when one is in fact willing to agree to the other's private time and does not become defensive in the process.

With these structuring details fashioned into a formal or implicit treatment contract, the first treatment session should help them to agree to work out details about the way they will spend time together. They should be encouraged to plan some outside activity for their "dates" to protect them from endless discussion of "our relationship." Such discussions often degenerate into extended sessions of cross accu-sations and morbidly self-reproachful confessions. The couple should also be helped to agree on the level of intimacy they will share during their contacts. If one expects sex and the other doesn't, these conflicting expectations can become a new battleground. In this regard, it is essen-tial that the wishes of the person wanting the least level of contact should be honored, because this person is in the best position to thwart the progress of the partners' moving together; and this person can also inflict significant pain on the other. The first session can then conclude with the therapist's eliciting from the partners their description of the kinds of change each would like the other to make in the details of their interaction. These requests become the caring-days lists for what should be at least two structured contacts weekly.

In successive weeks the couple can be offered help in developing the expressive, negotiation, and problem-solving skills that underlie the behavior changes each hopes to see in the other. These changes are proposed in the same series offered routinely treated couples, because these stages follow the natural sequence of relationship development. Positive experiences can be expected to motivate the partners gradually to increase the level of their closeness. Conversely, when these rules are ignored or when they are followed but do not result in a more positive encounter, the couple can use this realization as a basis for more extended separation. Here therapeutic values come into play in very important ways. If the therapist is wedded to a model of marriage in which Bobby and Jo eat, sleep, and play together—indeed, do everything together but work—then anything less than total interpenetration would lead the therapist to recommend divorce. Conversely, if the therapist is more open and pragmatic in approach, it is realized that Bobby and Jo might undertake a permanent partial separation, remain married, and possibly prosper. In short, these are changing times and relationships are perhaps the leading edge of this change. Even lasting separation is not the kiss of death for attachment, and those who work with separated or separating couples would do well to dissociate themselves from dichotomous thinking, in which marriage with spouses involved in interpenetrating ways is conceived to be the only alternative to the spouses' going their separate ways.

Divorce Counseling. If measured by outcome, much of what is offered as marriage counseling might better be advertised as divorce counseling. With increasing frequency, couples are entering therapy with consideration of divorce as their prime concern. It is reasonable to assume that these couples can use either of two parallel services: they may benefit from training in relationship development that will draw them back from the brink of divorce as their interaction becomes more satisfying; or they may benefit from training in relationship development in order to build their skills in such a way as to improve their interaction as caring divorcees. In the first instance, they would be offered the same assessment and change program as the premarital and separating couples; in the second instance, they would be offered a chance to define the kind of relationship they would both like to have following divorce— ranging from absolutely no contact to a rich and meaningful series of mutually supportive exchanges—and then they would be helped to develop the skills either to let go gracefully or to redefine their mutual privileges and responsibilities in realistic and constructive ways.

There are times when the therapist will be asked to make Solomonic judgments about who should get the silver and who the Spode, or, more painfully, who should get Ginny and who Dan. If approached at all, these questions are best answered in cooperation with an attorney skilled in family law (Bernstein, 1976), although the equity issues in such disputes tend more often to be symbolic than real. During these discussions it is important for the therapist to clarify with each spouse any overlay of punitiveness in claims for greater than equitable control of money and children.

When divorce is the decision reached by clients, it is important for the therapist to help them separate relationship breakdown from personal failure in assessing their own situation. They can be helped to realize that marriage today tends to be more stressed than in bygone days, at least partly because of the greater complexity of our lives and because of the expectation that each spouse will be everything—and more—to the other. They should also be helped to learn what they can about their choice of mates and their contribution to the strengths and liabilities of their relationship. In addition, their needs can be well served if they can be helped to overcome any vestiges of irrational anger that would inhibit their gracefully letting go of each other and that would interfere with what for many couples is the possibility of a life-long friendship with one whom they know well and are well known by.

The outcome evaluation of divorce counseling is every bit as complicated as that of premarital counseling. It is never entirely clear that any pair are mismatched or that they could not change sufficiently to produce a satisfying relationship. They may stay together out of fear of separating, or they may separate because of falsely dire predictions. Their staying together or parting is therefore not a necessary criterion of either successful or unsuccessful therapy. Treatment can, however, be evaluated in terms of the quality of their interaction along either path. In this sense, the critical outcome questions are: Did the couple follow instigations to change selected aspects of their interaction? Did these changes help to improve their self-evaluations and their assessment of their mate? And of course the ultimate question is: Will the spouses believe in later years that they are happier apart than they would have been had they remained together? If there were a way to answer this question in advance of undergoing the travail of the route to its answer, the world would surely be a gentler place, and marriage counselors would have their hands firmly on its helm!

CONCLUSIONS

While services offered to each of these special client groups have their own distinguishing features, they also have two very important common themes. First, all such services must be undertaken with the guidance of pragmatic rather than absolute values; it is simply not necessarily better in any general sense for a given couple to marry or to stay married than for them to sever their ties either before or after they speak their vows. Also, in each instance, the services needed and provided deal with helping the spouses learn to assess the strengths in their relationship and to develop the skills to add to these strengths irrespective of whether they contribute to more successful matrimony or better friendship, albeit along separate paths.

This is an action-oriented approach that has its own unique rationale and service-delivery techniques. The structural model described in this chapter calls for a conjoint, short-term, and highly structured service in which the roles of therapist and client are highly specified, as is the sequence of stages of treatment. The model, as it has evolved in this chapter, is useful for services to married couples who are living together. The model may, however, be readily adapted to meet the needs of client couples who are unmarried but cohabiting, who are contemplating marriage, who are contemplating divorce, or who are, in fact, divorced.

Natural History of the Treatment Approach

Typically, the distressed couple begin by denying that problems exist. When stress overcomes denial, the partner who feels the most troubled may make requests for change in the other's bothersome behaviors, followed by gradually escalating confrontations over the failure of the other to comply with the requests. This aversive interaction generally becomes a negative experience for the noncomplying spouse, who, in turn, resorts to countercontrol measures. A negative interaction cycle is then established, leading each spouse to rely more heavily upon coercive as opposed to positive influence attempts.

Either or both spouses typically turn outside their marriage for support when the general tone of their relationship has turned from positive or neutral to negative. Whether they consult friends or relatives of like or opposite sex is determined by cultural bias and opportunity; but in any event, they seek support for their expressions of self-justification and frustration at the insensitivity or recalcitrance of the other. These outside contacts generally support the polarized position that each has taken, making matters worse.

As the stress level begins to mount, each partner assesses his or her potential gains or losses from maintaining the status quo or attempting to engineer change. As noted earlier, those who feel that they have the most to lose from termination of the relationship are likely to struggle to keep things as they are. In contrast, those who are aware of their ability to make successful independent choices are likely to insist upon change as a precondition for remaining in the relationship. Accordingly, those with the most to lose are the partners most likely to offer to make concessions, while those leaning out of the relationship are more likely to demand concessions.

Either of two configurations may motivate the partners' effort to make contact with a professional, following the breakdown of their informal efforts to evoke change. The partner with the most to lose may call upon a professional for help in mobilizing his or her skills to keep the other person tied into the relationship, seeking support for moving out of the marriage only if he or she feels that matters are utterly hopeless. The more powerful partner, on the other hand, is likely to ask for help in "cooling the other out." This implies either that help is sought in assisting the other to let go so that the more powerful mate is freer to leave, or that help is sought to neutralize the coercive tactics that are the last resort of the beleaguered mate.

The therapist can therefore receive an initial call from either the partner wishing to preserve the relationship or the partner who is inclined to think about ending it. The caller may ask for either individual counseling or conjoint services. If the caller asks for individual help with a marital problem, it is incumbent upon the therapist to make it clear that such help is likely to be hazardous to the health of the marriage for varied reasons. As noted earlier, one partner cannot offer an unbiased description of the relationship; efforts by one to change the behavior of the other often take the form of highly resented manipulations, and efforts by one partner to modify the behavior of the other can be greatly strengthened with the direct assistance of the therapist. Therefore, while individual counseling services can be offered to one spouse alone, there are strong contraindications for attempting to offer marriage therapy in this context. Accordingly, the client seeking individual sessions should be encouraged to invite the spouse to participate, at least in the first session, at which time the therapist can aid the couple in objectively determining who, if anyone, should be the client.

Marital conflicts can also be called to the therapist's attention when couples negotiate a different problem definition. For example, a husband might develop a problem of depression secondary to marital stress, or a wife may start abusing the use of barbiturates to quell the furies generated by her anxiety about her faltering marriage. In these instances the husband or the wife is likely to call for help with the personal problems of depression or substance abuse. An alert therapist with a relationship orientation will ask each caller if he or she is married and, if so, invite the client to come to the first session with his or her spouse. The caller can explain the therapist's wish for spousal participation on the basis of the possibility that the partner will have valuable insights to contribute and will have an important potential role to play in effecting change. With both partners present in the first session, the therapist is then in a good position to assess the role of marital stress in the creation of the personal problem as well as being able to evaluate the resources for the support of change that the "asymptomatic" partner presents.

If the case originates from the couple's definition of a marital crisis, the caring-days stage of treatment can be initiated immediately. Conversely, if the contact is initiated because of the personal complaints of one of the partners, the therapist first has to identify the marital interaction as an initial problem to be solved as a means of reducing the stress that may contribute to the personal difficulty. This can often be accomplished prior to the end of the first session, at which time the normal marriage-treatment routine can be established.

As noted earlier, it is wise for the therapist to begin the first session by reviewing the ahistorical, positive, conjoint, and time-limited characteristics of the treatment. This approach serves the multiple purposes of establishing his or her identity while the clients can relax a little in the new, therapeutic environment, of reinforcing the roles that the clients are expected to play in their successful therapy, and of establishing the therapist's authority in the direction of the treatment process. Clients are generally passive during these first few minutes, although one or another may occasionally challenge the ahistorical characteristic by wondering whether the therapist can understand the pair fully without a sense of their history. A statement that the present is a better predictor of the future normally quells this doubt initially, but therapists should be prepared for clients to reassert their preferred past orientations at varied times during the first few sessions. In each instance, the therapist is well advised either to ignore the statements or to respond by asking how the same issues are currently handled.

When the therapist asks the clients if they have any questions about the brief outline that has just been offered, and their questions have been answered, negotiation of the first stages of an informal therapeutic contract has been completed. The therapist next asks the partners to tell one another the things that each most appreciates in the other. Using the answers to the first question on the Marital Precounseling Inventory as a guide, the partner with the greatest number of most varied positive observations is asked to speak first as a positive model for the other. When the clients thus begin to be more active in treatment, they often take this first opportunity to speak as a time to vie with the therapist for control of the session and to make the hostile points that each has been storing up for the other. This maneuver will often take the form of qualifying positive remarks with negative barbs (e.g., "She is interested in my work, as long as she doesn't feel too competitive with me") or with allusions to painful history (e.g., "He talks to me about some important things now, although we have lived in silence for over five years"). To confront noncompliance or negativism at this early stage of treatment is to build considerable resistance in the client. Therefore, the therapist should reinforce the positive elements in each expression and either ignore or relabel the negative dimensions. For example, the therapist might reframe competition as the wife's desire to carry her end of the burden equally and can identify the change to greater expression now as a reflection of the husband's commitment to improve the quality of his interaction with his wife.

After some 10–15 minutes of discussion of these positives, the therapist is then ready to move on to a brief statement of the stages of treatment that are to follow: caring days are offered as a means of building commitments to the marriage by demonstrating that change is possible; communication change is offered as a means of building the skills needed to make, clarify, and acknowledge requests; behavior change is held out as a means of resolving the major issues that have troubled the couple. At this point it is essential that the therapist acknowledge the existence of major troubling issues in the relationship as reflected in the partners' evaluation of these trouble spots in Section H of the Marital Precounseling Inventory. To skip this step is to leave the clients with the feeling that the treatment will be superficial and will fail to address their more pressing concerns. The therapist then concludes by indicating that skills will be taught for making decisions, for resolving conflicts with minimal damage, and then for maintaining the changes that have been achieved.

The foregoing discussion should take about five minutes, with an additional few minutes allowed for the clients' questions. Agreement that the methods are understood constitutes a second element in the informal treatment contract. These informal negotiations are completed when the therapist points out that the goal of treatment is to change behavior so that each partner can base a personal decision about whether to continue or to abandon the marriage on the basis of the best level of interaction that each partner can achieve. The couple should be told that some partners choose not to make the negotiated changes and thereby deny themselves access to the data needed for sound decision making. Others do make the changes in behavior but remain dissatisfied with their marriage. When they have done the best that they are willing to do and still feel unfulfilled, the partners can decide for themselves whether to remain in a less than optimal relationship or to strike out in search of greater happiness in other relationships. The couple should be told that while behavior change can and often does lead to dramatic feeling change, this is not always the case, and one inherent risk in treatment is the realization that no achievable interaction change may yield the desired benefits for one or the other partner. Conversely, the hope should be extended that in light of the assets that each has just identified in the other's current repertoire, there is more than a reasonable chance that a change in the couple's behavior will lead to more positive feelings and a renewed commitment to their union.

The therapist should then ask the partner who has the least to lose—hence, the greatest power—how he or she would know that the other cared. Writing these prescriptions for small, positive, nonconflictual behaviors in the center of a sheet of paper establishes the basis of the "caring-days" procedure described in the next chapter. In helping both partners contribute to this list, the therapist has already begun the communication-change procedures and has helped the couple to understand how each person can help change the course of daily events at home. The session ends with the instigation that the couple plan to emit at least five of these behaviors daily, with two important cautions: each is instructed to meet a personal commitment to emit these caring behaviors irrespective of the other's actions; and each is alerted to the fact that it will feel unnatural to do these things at first. The first caution is important because in their effort to resist change, each partner is likely to scan the other's behavior carefully for some sign that would justify reluctance to change. The second caution is important because virtually all couples enter treatment with the erroneous belief that they must feel different before they act differently and will therefore use the nonoccurrence of impossible affective change to justify inaction.

The therapist is well advised to phone the couple after three days to reinforce the instigation to use caring-days behaviors; thus counteracting the couple's predictable reticence about adopting positive change techniques in place of their more practiced avoidance or coercion tactics. Even if the call is made, it is not unusual for clients to arrive at the second session with the disclosure that they did not follow through with the instigation. This lack of follow-through can be understood as their effort to force the therapist to deal with negative behaviors, consistent with most clients' expectations before beginning therapy. However, if an instigation was worth giving once, it is essential that it be repeated and fulfilled before moving on in treatment. Therefore, noncompliance is greeted by the therapist's asking; "What can we do a little differently to enable you to follow through on this most essential next step?" The answer may be found in clarification of the procedure, elaboration of more alternative caring behaviors, reestablishment of the principle that behaviors must be changed before feelings, etc.

When some success has been achieved with caring days, usually in either the second or the third session, the therapist should congratulate the couple on having so confidently taken the first step toward a better relationship and should then move on to establish the needed communication changes. For most couples, as suggested in Chapter 7, this step involves agreement about some communication norms, such as those governing the selection of things that will be prudently withheld from discussion as well as those governing the value of positive as opposed to negative expressions. For most couples in deteriorated relationships, two major steps are required at this time. First, they are encouraged to spend at least 10 minutes together daily to reestablish a habit of sharing some of the events of their respective days and to prestructure an opportunity for them to practice the other communication changes. Next, they are encouraged to make positive requests of one another and to provide each other with acknowledgment of the positives received. This procedure is intended to provide each spouse with some reinforcement for taking an active positive stance with regard to efforts to improve the marriage. At the conclusion of the second session—or the third, if two sessions were needed to gain compliance with the caring-days instigation—the couple is encouraged to continue the caring-days procedure, to identify specific times each day for some sharing of their daily experience, and to employ the request–clarification–acknowledgment techniques outlined in Chapter 7. They are also asked to give some thought to renovating their interaction.

The next session begins with a review of the couple's compliance with the last instigations. Strong reinforcement is given for positive achievements and help is offered in changing expectations, relabeling experience, or changing behaviors when things did not go smoothly. The couple are then asked to identify some of the major changes that they seek, with each partner assuming the responsibility for eliciting and clarifying the other's requests. These requests generally fall into two broad categories. Some are "lifestyle" issues, such as whether the wife will work and how spending versus saving decisions will be made. Others are specific concerns, like who has the responsibility for taking care of the children when they are sick or how much free time each spouse will have without the need to account for its use to the other. Using the negotiation techniques outlined in Chapter 8, the couple is helped to understand the process of formulating a "holistic contract," in which each lists his or her major requests and accepts the responsibility for granting some of the requests made by the other. Care is taken in this session *not* to complete the contracting procedure so that the couple can begin the next session with an opportunity to negotiate additions to the agreement with the therapist's participation in a coaching role.

During the next session the couple are also offered an opportunity to complete the "powergram" exercise as outlined in Chapter 9. In this connection, each identifies current and preferred areas of shared and independent decision making. Through a process that typically requires about half an hour, the couple develop a graphic display answering the questions who? will make decisions in which areas? with what degree of independence? The remainder of this session is used to help the couple determine when and how to invoke the powergram results, noting that the best exercise of power is the quietest. In addition, the couple are taught how to make use of a problem-solving tactic, also described in Chapter 9, as a means of resolving issues that might become conflicts before they reach the conflict stage. The couple are then encouraged to discuss the results of the power allocation at home and to look for opportunities to apply the problem-solving technique during the ensuing week, even if the issues at hand are comparatively minor.

During this phase of treatment it is common for one or both of the partners to test the other's willingness to follow through with the positive change process they have initiated. This testing typically takes the form of an expression of despair about the level of progress, an open threat to end the relationship, a regression to earlier coercive interaction patterns, or the generation of some new and unprecedented crisis, such as the threat that the male will quit his job to "find himself." Knowing that this kind of testing is likely, it is often helpful for the therapist to forewarn the couple about its occurrence. When the testing does take place, it should be so labeled and the therapist should lead the couple in an effort to apply to its solution those skills that have already been taught up to that point in therapy. For example, the partners can be reminded of the value of continuing to emit caring behaviors, to voice their desires for change in one another's behavior rather than identifying the crisis as an insurmountable barrier to their continued satisfaction, to negotiate ways in which changes in their respective behaviors can minimize the stress, and/or to apply the recently learned problem-solving strategies. In these ways the testing behavior is normalized and the couple can learn to treat each stress as an opportunity to refine their skills and to build relationship strength rather than reacting to crises as though they were major threats to the relationship.

During the final stages of therapy, the couple can be taught how to use the foregoing skills to minimize the frequency and intensity of conflict and then how to engage in issue-specific rather than intensely personally attacking conflicts, as outlined in Chapter 10. These discussions often have an academic quality if the earlier steps in treatment have been well taken and the ambient level of conflict between the spouses has substantially subsided. It is at this point, too, that the couple might be routed into sex counseling by the marriage therapist or into sex therapy by a sex therapist if, in the first instance, they wish to improve such details as the quality of their communication or decision making about intimacy or, in the second instance, they appear to have a primary sexual dysfunction. An overview of sex therapy techniques is found in Chapter 11.

Therapy ends with what might be termed a "graduation session," in which the partners are asked to recount what they have learned and the changes they feel they have accomplished. While the clients often feel compelled to tell the therapist how helpful he or she has been, it is essential that the therapist describe his or her role as that of facilitator of the release of their own positive relationship skills. The therapist should lead the clients in a review of the steps they have taken to meet each challenge that has arisen during the treatment, often writing down for them to take home a list of the steps they have found to be of greatest benefit. The final session can be continued with the couple's rehearsing the moves they will make when their new-found joy is challenged in the future, using as stimulus material some of the situations described in Chapter 12. As a final note, the couple can be strongly encouraged to return for a follow-up session between four and six months after this last session as a means of helping them view the therapist as a resource to catalyze future renewal and to alert them to the value of periodic review of their relationship. Typically, two or three of these sessions will be held over the next two years, with each being devoted to a review of how they have applied the treatment-mediated skills and to anticipation of how they will mobilize themselves to meet the challenges anticipated for the ensuing months or years.

It should be clear from this brief vignette that the skills taught in this approach are cumulative, and that once a technique is introduced, it is reapplied in each succeeding session. It should also be clear that the therapist must exercise great control over the early sessions in order to do the needed teaching and to protect the couple from the sabotaging effects of efforts to resort to traditionally ineffective coercive techniques. Later, as the partners demonstrate the willingness and ability to apply the positive relationship-management skills that are the core of this approach, the therapist fades the intensity of his or her control in favor of the opportunity to prompt and reinforce the clients' self-directive efforts. The therapist's early exercise of control also provides the opportunity to allocate time in the session to the spouse who has the greatest deficit in each skill area. It is always true that partners differ in their readiness to adopt each level of recommended behavior change, and the gatekeeper function of the therapist permits the allocation of time and attention to that partner who must reach the furthest to take each progressive step. In addition, it should be clear that the emotional tone of each session is quite even, on the supposition that learning will be more rapid when the partners are comparatively at rest and can concentrate their attention on the skill-building challenge at hand.

This overview has been necessarily sketchy. Each of the ensuing chapters provides much greater detail on the rationale and technique of each of the major stages of treatment.

C H A P T E R   6

Caring Days
A Technique
for Building
Commitment
to Faltering
Marriages

THE DECISION for couples to enter marriage therapy, in contrast to marriage enrichment programs, is typically prompted by the recognition by one or both that their interaction is essentially unfulfilling if not patently negative. Each spouse usually harbors an explanation of the trouble couched in terms of the other's shortcomings, although either or both may accept some measure of the negative responsibility in their recognition of the fact that everything that transpires in a marriage is a dance done by two. Typically, the couple have tried several self-selected remedies and have sought support, if not suggestions, from loved ones and friends before initiating the counseling process. Given this negative recent past, it is not uncommon for either or both spouses to begin treatment with limited if not negative expectations of the therapeutic outcome. Because the long-range effects of treatment are likely to be consistent with the couple's experience early on, it is essential for the therapist to offer clients an opportunity for measurable success very early in their treatment experience. The "caring-days" technique is an extremely effective means of offering this much needed experience.

On caring days couples are asked to act "as if" they cared for one another in an effort to elicit more frequent small, specific, and positive investments by both spouses in the process of building a sense of commitment to their marriage. This recommendation is consistent with many social-psychological principles of relationship management as reviewed in this chapter. It offers client couples an unprecedented opportunity for immediate change in the character of their relationship. The positive changes mediated by this approach provide the energy that fuels subsequent efforts to make more demanding changes in the pattern of the marital interaction.

Predictors of Attraction to Another Person

In Chapter 4 data were presented in support of the notion that if marital choices are not necessarily motivated by romance, neither are they the product of sheer chance. Couples who meet and mate tend to have a blend of complementary and similar characteristics sufficient to motivate them to move into a relationship expected to last many years, if not for the rest of their lives. For some couples, the music of their marriage is the voice of angels, while for others it is the cacophony of bent garbage can lids pounded with rusty spikes. Since most couples have at least a reasonable chance of catching the favor of the gods, their success or failure is as well explained by the way in which they play out the daily drama of their lives as by any other available calculus.

Since its inception, social psychology has been largely concerned with explaining the forces that motivate people to select one another from the bubbling multitudes, what leads them to seek to develop some relationships rather than others, how they manage the process of moving together, and what they do that either forms a bond between them or forces them apart. Writers like Newcomb (1956, 1961) and Byrne and his associates (Byrne & Nelson, 1965; Byrne & Rhamey, 1965) have suggested that after they have met and chosen to go forward with their relationship, one's attraction for the other is primarily under the influence of the relative balance of positive and negative experiences that each undergoes at the hands of the other. (In this regard, it is important to recall the role of the commitment value of behaviors as outlined in Chapter 4.) In general, it has been consistently found (e.g., Brewer & Brewer, 1968; Bramel, 1962, 1963; Eagly & Whitehead, 1972) that people tend to be more strongly attracted to others who have behaved toward them in ways that they define as positive. Accordingly, it can be assumed as a principle of human social interaction that:

POSITIVE ACTIONS ARE LIKELY TO INDUCE POSITIVE REAC-
TIONS, FIRST IN THE ATTITUDES OF OTHERS, AND THEN IN
THEIR BEHAVIORS.

Applications of this principle can be found in many diverse aspects of clinical practice. For example, researchers have found that the level of patients' depression can be predicted from the frequency of their positive social experiences (e.g., Ferster, 1973; Lewinsohn, 1974; MacPhillamy & Lewinsohn, 1973; Rehm, 1978). It may be that depressives emit few positive responses toward others, receive fewer positive responses as a result, and therefore miss the experiences that would support more positive feelings. As a partial test of this hypothesis, McLean (1976) has shown that when depressives are successfully prompted to act more positively, many experience more positive feedback and enjoy comparative relief from their depression.

Other social reactions are equally predictable consequences of social actions. For example, Stuart (1971a) found that interactions between parents and delinquent adolescents predicted the deviant status of the youths. Specifically, while parent-delinquent interactions were shown to be about equally balanced between positive and negative exchanges, parent–nondelinquent interactions were characterized by some seven times as many positive as negative exchanges. Presumably, these positive experiences built attachment to the family among the youths and led to their acceptance of the nondeviant social values of their parents.

Social experience seems equally able to predict marital performance. Weiss and Isaac (1976) addressed this issue and found that subjects' reports of the frequency of some 84 different behaviors during a 24-hour period correlated with their global ratings of marital satisfaction at the level of .57. In the same vein, Birchler et al. (1975) showed that during a period of self-reporting, nondistressed couples reported 541 shared activities with their spouses (58% of the reported activities), as opposed to the 344 shared activities reported by partners in distressed marriages (43% of the total). Others (e.g., Jacob et al., 1978; Marini, 1976; B. C. Miller, 1976; Robinson & Price, 1976) have also shown that time together reliably differentiates distressed from nondistressed couples. On the assumption that couples choose to spend more time together when they can anticipate experiencing more positive satisfactions during their shared time, these observations imply that nondistressed dyads enjoy a higher rate of shared time than do distressed partners.

In direct observation, Engel and Weiss (1976) found that coded videotapes of interactions revealed a rate of 1.85 helpful behaviors per minute among nondistressed pairs. Vincent et al. (1975) found that nondistressed couples made 25% more positive statements during a problem-solving interaction than did distressed partners. And Birchler et al.

(1975), observing that partners are more positive with strangers than with each other, speculated that "it appears that individuals learn to relate in an ineffective manner with their spouses while retaining social competence in their interaction with others" (p. 359).

While this finding of differential levels of positive reinforcement in association with varying levels of marital satisfaction has been noted in both clinical (e.g., Azrin *et al.*, 1973; Patterson *et al.*, 1976; Stuart, 1969) and laboratory observational (e.g., Stuart & Braver, 1973) studies, all researchers have not reached this same conclusion. For example, Robinson and Price (1976) and Olson and Sprenkle (1976) found that the presence of a high rate of positives is not a reliable characteristic of nonclinic couples. Moreover, Gottman *et al.* (1976b) found that while distressed couples were both less positive and more negative than nondistressed couples, it was not their intention to act in this manner. Therefore, while it is reasonable to hypothesize that the level of distress experienced by couples can be predicted by their differential rates of positive reinforcement, this association is not universally found.

One explanation for the failure of rates of positives to differentiate reliably between nondistressed and distressed couples may be that couples have very individual ways of assigning values to the behaviors they exchange.

Consistent with the concept of the commitment value of behaviors as explained in Chapter 4, it is also important to note that while some couples appear to place a high value on the range and rate of their positive exchanges, others assign greater value to the range and rate of negative experiences at one another's hands. In classic illustrations of seeing the cup half full, Marini (1976) and van der Veen (1971) found that members of couples and families, respectively, felt stronger attraction toward each other when the rates of their positive experiences were high. However, other researchers found that many couples look instead at the empty half of the cup and place greater weight upon the rate of their negative exchanges (Hawkins, 1968; Orden & Bradburn, 1968). For example, Wills *et al.* (1972, 1974) found that while the couples whom they studied experienced three times as many positives as negatives in their interaction, the positive events accounted for only 25% of the explained variance in marital satisfaction, while negative exchanges accounted for 65% of this variance. Moreover, they and others (e.g., Gottman *et al.*, 1977; Patterson & Reid, 1970; Raush, 1965; Weiss *et al.*, 1973) have noted that negative behaviors receive more prompt reciprocation than positive behaviors. In the light of the results of these studies, it can be concluded that the rates of both positive and negative behaviors play a role in determining the level of couples' satisfaction with their interactions. Therefore, relationships can be improved by increasing the rate of positives, which by implication would probably have a salutary effect upon the rate of negative exchanges by decreasing the rate of negatives, which would not necessarily have an impact upon the frequency of positive exchanges, or some combination of the two. The choice between these alternatives is the subject of the next section.

Formulating a Plan of Action

It has been shown that attraction in social relationships, mood level, and marital satisfaction are all strongly influenced by the course of social events. Unfortunately, while none of these data sets leads to an unambiguous conclusion, therapists are nevertheless faced with the necessity of planning clinical strategies based upon these as the best available data. This approach depends upon the acceleration of positive exchanges as a primary strategy for several important reasons.

To begin with, it will be recalled that evidence reviewed in Chapter 4 showed that reciprocation between spouses is better predicted by a lag Markov model than by a model positing immediate successive exchanges. That is, spouses may reciprocate positives gradually over time although their response in kind to negatives may be almost immediate. It is reasonable to suppose that trust in a continual flow of positives mediated by one's mate may have a lasting effect upon marital satisfaction, while the bite of negative events may have a more immediate but short-term effect. If this is true, the most fruitful way to promote lasting change in spousal interaction would appear to be an effort to increase positive exchanges. In this regard, Lott and Lott (1968) concluded that "learning to like another is essentially learning to anticipate rewards when the other person is present" (p. 200), a finding echoed in the research of other teams as well (e.g., Golightly & Byrne, 1964; Scodel, 1962; Wallace & Rothaus, 1969).

Beyond the fact that positive investments have been shown to have positive social effects and the fact that the most effective clinical programs are those built upon positive interventions, there are other important reasons for beginning marital treatment with an effort to increase the rate of positive exchanges. Most of the couples who enter treatment are either burned out or conflict-habituated. In either case, they seem to attend more closely to negative exchanges with each other and thereby often lose sight of the number and importance of those positives that still exist between them. An initial positive approach helps to recreate a more balanced appraisal of the behavioral dynamics of their relationship. In addition, the use of an incremental strategy at the start of treatment helps to foster the expectation that change throughout treatment will build strength and will be oriented toward positive goals. Presumably, couples are more comfortable continuing strategies that have met with early success than willing to change from negative to positive change programs. Finally, initiating treatment through a positive approach that is inconsistent with the nagging countercontrol interaction in which many clinic couples are well practiced helps to call attention to the fact that the treatment experience provides an opportunity for the couples to learn new relationship-management skills, which can help to weaken their attachment to their former, more destructive modes.

For these reasons, it is believed that a procedure that is ideal for the beginning of treatment is one that builds positive behavior, that produces a prompt positive effect, that trains the couple in using a new, change-oriented vocabulary, that demonstrates that gains are possible through planned behavior change, and that builds trust in the relationship in both spouses. The procedure should also be one that allows the couple to make changes in small steps. It is unwise to expect battle-weary clients to be willing to make concessions in the major conflictual issues of their relationship at the very start of their treatment experience. In the same vein, it is unwise to ask couples to give too much to each other too soon. Therefore, the present approach asks couples to make small positive concessions at the start of their treatment consistent with the thrust of many social-psychological studies, which have shown that small initial offers have a positive effect upon the long-term outcome of bargaining situations (e.g., Esser & Komorita, 1975; Oskamp, 1971; Pruitt, 1968; Pruitt & Johnson, 1970), the treatment situation being a special kind of negotiating setting. The program recommended here as the optimal strategy for phasing clients into treatment has been termed "caring days."

The Caring-Days Technique

As suggested in Chapter 2, acting "as if" couples care for each other may be the best technique available to them for building these sought-after feelings of mutual concern. Accordingly, couples are asked to begin the process of relationship change by acting as if they do in fact care for one another, while being forewarned that they will not in fact experience these feelings until they have changed their behavior.

Acts that are experienced as expressions of caring are naturally subject to very personal and individual selection. Rubin (1973) has attempted to operationalize the terms "loving" and "liking," each of which conveys an aspect of what is here meant by the word "caring." Caring, along with attachment and intimacy, are included in his love scale. Sample items in that scale are "If _____ were feeling bad, my first duty would be to cheer him (her) up"; "I find it easy to ignore _____'s faults"; and "It would be hard for me to get along without _____." In contrast, Rubin considers "liking" synonymous with favorably evaluating another person. The scale measuring liking, which Rubin (1973, p. 220) recognizes to be somewhat sex-biased, is illustrated by the following items: "I think that _____ is usually well adjusted"; "I would highly recommend _____ for a responsible job"; and "_____ is the sort of person whom I myself would like to be." As can be seen in these items, however, Rubin regards loving and liking as the effects of exchanges, the true nature of which is not studied in his scalar approach. The therapist must be concerned with promoting the emission of acts that elicit caring feelings, and only the spouses can indicate what those acts can be. Therefore, the effective use of the caring-days technique depends upon the therapist's ability to convince the couple that positive change early on is in their best interest, and that it will enable each to communicate to the other requests for small behavioral changes that would enable each to feel cared for by the other.

It is typical that couples entering marital treatment show a very low rate of caring behaviors toward one another, but some pairs entering treatment are found to have managed to maintain a reasonable rate of attentive behaviors despite their failure to rise to the challenge of other issues in their relationship. They are therefore less needful of the caring-days technique as a means of promoting commitment. However, they should still be offered the procedure because all couples benefit from some of the other gains resulting from the technique: for example, reinforcement of existing relationship strengths as a foundation for promoting interactional changes, learning to make positive requests and to acknowledge their fulfillment, and learning the power of small, specific behavior changes as a means of mediating change in the larger issues in the marriage. Therefore, all couples should be started with the caring-days technique, and those for whom commitment is already strong can be moved more swiftly to the succeeding stages of the intervention.

In introducing the caring-days procedure, it is important for the therapist to do three things. First, it is essential to recognize that the couple faces conflicts that must eventually be resolved. As enumerated in Scale H of the Marital Precounseling Inventory (Stuart & Stuart, 1973), the therapist should mention the challenges but should point out that change must be undertaken as an orderly process, and that the first step in the process must be the development of the request-and-acknowledgment skills and the simple behavior exchanges about to be described. Second, it is essential for the therapist to stress that the initiation of the change process depends upon the willingness of both spouses to make investments in relationship enhancement independently of the other. Each must act "as if" she or he cared for the other (see Chapter 2) if true caring is ever to be experienced. Generally, the spouse who has the most to lose if the relationship does not improve will be the one who is most willing to be committed to this change effort. It is therefore wise for the therapist to concentrate efforts on the other partner, who should be encouraged to view the caring-days process as a low-cost method of assessing the feasibility of relationship change. Treatment cannot proceed beyond this point without the concurrence of both spouses, but fortunately, factors such as the "halo" effect in the first session and the reasonableness of the request will lead to at least hesitant agreement by both partners for the one or two weeks needed for the couple to net some of the gains expected from this technique. Finally, it is essential for the therapist to use the word "caring" and not "love." "Caring" is a very positive word that does not have the complex mythical associations of "love." Couples are usually more willing to commit themselves to act as if they care for each other than to act as if they love one another. Love may or may not be the end point of treatment, but it can never be its start. Thus, delay of confrontation of conflict, adoption of an as-if strategy, and pursuit of caring and tenderness rather than love are a trio of antecedents, the absence of which is very likely to undermine any hope of success through the caring-days technique.

In caring days each spouse is asked to answer the question: Exactly what would you like your partner to do as a means of showing that he or she cares for you? Answers to the question are written in the center column of a sheet of paper specially ruled for the purpose[1] (see Figure 1). To be entered on the list, the behaviors should meet the following criteria:

1. They must be positive.
2. They must be specific.
3. They must be "small" behaviors that can be emitted at least once daily.
4. They must not have been the subject of recent sharp conflict.

A positive request aims for an increase in constructive behaviors, not a decrease in unwanted responses. "Please ask me how I spent my day" is a positive request that should be used in place of the negative request "Don't ignore me so much." A specific request is one that can be very easily understood. "Come home at 6 P.M. for dinner" is a specific request that might replace the vague "Show more consideration for the family." Small, potentially high-rate responses are needed at this stage of treat-

[1]Note that space is provided in Figure 1 for three weeks of recording.

Figure 1. Caring-days list.

Bill	Agreements	Jocelyn
9/3, 9/4, 9/6, 9/7, 9/8, 9/9 / 9/10, 9/11, 9/12, 9/14 / 9/17, 9/20, 9/21	Ask how I spent the day.	9/3, 9/4, 9/6, 9/7, 9/8, 9/9 / 9/10, 9/12, 9/14, 9/16 / 9/20, 9/21, 9/23
9/3, 9/4, 9/9 / 9/10, 9/14, 9/16 / 9/20, 9/21, 9/22, 9/23	Offer to get the cream or sugar for me.	9/4, 9/9 / 9/12, 9/15 / 9/23
9/3, 9/7, 9/9 / 9/15 / 9/21, 9/23	Listen to "mood music" when we set the clock radio to go to sleep.	9/3, 9/7, 9/9 / 9/15 / 9/21, 9/23
9/7, 9/8 / 9/11 / 9/19	Hold my hand when we go for walks.	9/7, 9/8 / 9/11, 9/16 / 9/19, 9/21, 9/23
9/9 / 9/14, 9/16 / 9/23	Put down the paper or your book and look at me when we converse.	9/4, 9/6, 9/7, 9/8 / 9/10, 9/13, 9/14, 9/16 / 9/18, 9/20, 9/21, 9/22, 9/24
9/4, 9/7 / 9/11, 9/12, 9/14, 9/16 / 9/21, 9/23	Rub my back.	9/5, 9/8 / 9/10, 9/14, 9/15 / 9/19
9/3, 9/4, 9/5, 9/7, 9/8 / 9/11, 9/16 / 9/19	Tuck in the sheets and blankets before we go to bed.	9/6, 9/9 / / 9/23
9/3, 9/8 / 9/15 / 9/17	Call me during the day.	9/5, 9/6, 9/7, 9/8, 9/9 / 9/11, 9/13, 9/14, 9/16 / 9/18, 9/20, 9/21, 9/22, 9/23
9/4, 9/6 / 9/13 /	Offer to play short games with the children when my friends drop in for a few minutes.	9/8 / 9/12, 9/15 / 9/21
9/7 / 9/11, 9/16 / 9/23	Offer to read the rough drafts of my reports and offer comments.	9/9 / / 9/20
9/5, 9/7, 9/8, 9/9 / 9/11, 9/14, 9/17 / 9/18, 9/21	Sit down with me when I have coffee even if you don't want any, just for the company.	9/7 / 9/10, 9/13 / 9/23
9/7 / 9/12 / 9/20, 9/23	Call my folks just to say "hello."	9/9 / / 9/23
9/6, 9/7 / 9/15 / 9/18, 9/20, 9/23	Fold the laundry.	9/9 / 9/10, 9/14 / 9/20
9/4, 9/7, 9/9 / 9/13 / 9/18	Buy me a $1 present.	9/8, 9/9 / 9/12, 9/14, 9/15 / 9/21, 9/23

ment if partners are to enjoy the immediate changes that they need in order to gain confidence in the treatment process. "Please line the children's bikes along the back wall of the garage when you come home" is a much more manageable request than "Please train the children to keep their bikes in the proper places." It is important to include relatively conflict-free requests on the caring-days list because neither spouse is likely to concede major points at this stage of treatment, that is, before both have made a durable commitment to maintaining their relationship. Conflict affords some immediate reinforcement in two forms: many enjoy the catharsis inherent in the expression of anger, and conflict sometimes succeeds in coercing immediate, if short-lived, change in the other's behavior. Neither partner is likely to forgo these gains before developing trust in the longer life of their relationship, a time during which they can expect longer-range reciprocation of the positives that they invest. Therefore, if the couple have been having arguments over when to turn off the television set and go to bed—one wishing to watch the late show through to the end, while the other wishes to retire much earlier—this would not be an acceptable item to include on the list.

It is typical for the clients to begin by making requests that are negative, vague, large, and conflict-embedded. It is the responsibility of the therapist to model desirable request lists, perhaps by showing clients acceptable models. It is also appropriate for the therapist to coach the partners' facilitative responses and to edit requests when writing them on the list. The couple should also be encouraged to add to the list during the week between sessions. The list should include *at least* 18 items for several important reasons. The items are contributed by both spouses, and some are of much greater significance to one spouse than to the other. Some of the items will seem much more relevant and feasible on some days as opposed to others. The actual opportunities to express caring and commitment are virtually limitless, and stimulating thinking about a range of these alternatives helps to overcome any stereotypical or monotonous tone in the daily exchange between spouses. Finally, interests shift over time, so keeping the list open-ended allows the list to keep pace with evolution in the partners' preferences. Coaching the couple to initially select 18 items and encouraging them to add several items to the list each week is an effective means of building a list with sufficient breadth and responsiveness.

When the list has been completed, each request should be discussed. The spouse making the request should state precisely what, when, and how he or she would like the other to respond. The spouse hearing the request should ask for clarification about any ambiguities during the treatment session. This process of making and clarifying requests prefigures the communication treatment that is the second stage of treatment.

Each spouse should be asked to make a commitment to emit *at least five of the behaviors on the caring-days list daily*. This number will provide frequent demonstrations of the couple's willingness to meet each other's expectations. Moreover, each should be asked to make these positive investments in improving their relationship *irrespective of whether or not the other has made similar gestures*. This condition is important because partners in distressed marriages tend to inhibit constructive interaction through their reliance upon what might be termed the "change-second principle." According to this principle, each decides that he or she will act positively only *after* the other has offered a positive. However, as each awaits a positive commitment from the other before acting, neither ever takes the constructive steps that are needed to improve their relationship. Therefore, the caring-days procedure asks each to abide by the "change-first principle," according to which each person is expected to change before the other, initiating that process of reciprocal change fundamental to the approach to relationship management based on social learning theory.

In addition to taking frequent, independent action, the spouses should also be encouraged to record on the sheet the date on which each has benefited from positive gestures by the other, the husband entering the date beside the behaviors emitted by the wife under the column headed "Husband," with the wife using the "Wife" column for the same purpose. These written records have several functions. Distressed couples tend to take for granted the positives that are offered to one another. Asking for written notation of these events helps to pinpoint their acknowledgment. Also, the written notations help each person to identify the behaviors that may have been overlooked. In addition, the record serves as a visual reminder of the amount of change that has taken place as a means of overcoming the pessimism that blights so many couples' belief in the possibility that they might improve their relationship. Finally, the record is also a source of data for use by the therapist in evaluating the willingness of each partner to take constructive, assertive action in response to therapeutic instigations.

The therapist is well advised to phone the couple two or three days after the first session to review with the clients any new items that they have added to the list and to prompt them to maintain a schedule of five or more caring behaviors daily. Apart from these focal benefits of the call, it also has the very important positive value of expressing the therapist's interest in the couple and his or her investment in their follow-through on therapeutic instigations. Their success with caring days as well as the expression of the therapist's interest and his or her expectation that instigations will be taken seriously will all contribute to an increase in the likelihood that the couple will follow through on future directives.

Barriers to the Success of Caring Days and
Why the Technique Works

The caring-days technique is intended to function as a low-cost means of initiating a much larger process of relationship change. Couples are asked to offer one another seemingly inconsequential, small, caring behaviors that serve to build their commitment to the therapeutic process and to their relationship. The procedure is analogous to the "foot-in-the-door" technique described by Freedman and Fraser (1966). They suggested that researchers might ask homemakers about detergents as a means of getting their foot in the door, ultimately to investigate in detail the items stored in their kitchens. They also suggested that drivers could be asked to place small "Drive Safely" cards in the windows of their cars as a means of building readiness to comply with later requests to place large "Drive Safely" signs on their front lawns. It is also similar to the process of "reinforcer sampling" described by Ayllon and Azrin (1968), in that the couple are prompted to make a small response designed to give them a foretaste of the potential reinforcement to follow larger changes later on.

Caring days can help the couple to enjoy some frequent, small, positive exchanges with each other. They are pleasant in themselves, often more so because they stand in sharp contrast to the conflict-bred pleasures that may have been the couple's pretreatment norm. They are also pleasant because they illustrate the ease with which change can be achieved, because they hold out the promise of more of the same in the future, and because they help to rebuild trust in the relationship. Pruitt (1968) has shown in laboratory studies that "the level of reward provided to another person is a positive function of the level of reward previously received from him" (p. 143). Therefore, nonrelated dyads have been shown to invest now to pay for rewards later. Gottman et al. (1976b) have observed a similar phenomenon in well-functioning married couples. They concluded that unlike distressed couples, whom they found more likely to engage in tit-for-tat exchanges, nondistressed couples seem to act positively toward one another now in order to be able to draw against their credit balances in the future. In this sense the caring-days procedure prompts nonreciprocated investments in the present, with the recording chart serving as a "receipt" for the investment, and with the very real possibility that reciprocal positives will be experienced in the future. In this sense the caring-days procedure also helps the partners build trust in one another.

Trust in relationships is very important because as Huesmann and Levinger (1972) have speculated:

> Irrespective of the depth of involvement, an individual often anticipates rewards in a dyadic interaction long before they occur. Yet even when the

future rewards are higher than the present rewards, a person does not always emphasize the future over the present. This occurs because of a discount on the future. One values future rewards less than present rewards, particularly if one is unsure about the continuance or the stability of that relationship. (p. 6)

By prestructuring the exchanges, both partners have an opportunity to develop some trust in the belief that their investments will be reciprocated, partly because of the formality of the exchange, including the recording; partly because of the therapist's involvement; and partly because the time frame for the exchange is brief and definite. They can then be helped to generalize from this isolated experience to the more expansive trust that they must have if they are to be confident and secure in their future exchanges with one another (Solomon, 1960). They will not make longer-range commitments without trust, and as trust must be earned through follow-through on commitments, long-range trust can be built only from a series of shorter-range trustworthy actions, such as those prompted during caring days.

Gains from caring days thus include an immediate change in the quality of the interaction—more positives—and an immediate opportunity to recapture a sense of trust in the other and in the relationship. But these changes are not an unmixed blessing. Stuart (1978) has elsewhere reviewed evidence suggesting that overweight persons who desperately wish to shed their extra pounds also harbor a fear of weight loss because all change is threatening. Change carries with it at least a temporary loss of predictability, and for some, the uncertainty brought on by change may be more painful than the unhappy relationship that it would replace.

Aronson (1969) has suggested that movement toward closeness in a relationship brings the potential for greater reward, but it also increases vulnerability to hurt. Fear of this potential pain is another source of the fear of change. In addition, when one accepts something from another, the acceptance carries with it an implicit obligation to reciprocate. For example, R. H. Turner (1970) has described a possible interaction between a dating couple. If he were to suggest the movies that they are to see for three weeks running, he would create a debt in the form of owing her the willingness to see movies of her choice. He may not wish to subject himself to this obliged reciprocation, so he may decline to make suggestions about ways in which they should spend their evenings. If she, too, were unwilling to accept this risk exposure, she would also pass up the opportunity to make the choice, and they would be at an impasse. The plight of distressed couples can be described in similar terms. Oftentimes, neither spouse is willing to make requests of the other for fear of having to grant reciprocal requests in the future. Thus, the fear of change may obstruct the efforts of couples who enter treatment in pursuit of change. When the fear of change is added to the distressed couple's pessimism about the possibility or even the desirability of rehabilitating their relationship, it is not difficult to understand why many marital treatment efforts fail to make even a worthy beginning.

The caring-days procedure helps to counteract this fear of change by specifying small, nonconflictual behavior exchanges that are likely to be reinforced promptly. Yet clients often resist this benign effort by reporting that they are "unable to think of things that I want my spouse to do," or by questioning whether they should be "dishonest in acting as if we care very much for each other when we are not certain what we do." The first resistance can be overcome by reviewing with clients caring behaviors that have been selected by other clients or that the therapist enjoys exchanging with his or her spouse. This resistance can also be weakened by taking care to ask the initial question in general rather than in specific terms: "What small, positive, and specific actions can one spouse take to express caring for the other?" is an easier question for many clients to relate to than the particular question, "What would you like Margaret to do to show that she cares for you, Bill?"

The second resistant maneuver is more of a challenge. The dissenting spouse can be asked if he or she has a better way to achieve the desired feeling state, and, if so, that person should be advised to follow the self-selected strategy because there will be little willingness to invest in the therapist's suggestions until this is done. The value of an "as-if" and "change-first" approach can also be reiterated, with the resister being told that the only way he or she can clearly meet an obligation to the other and to the treatment process is to take the prescribed steps for at least a week, during which time it is expected that the prevailing mood will be somewhat defensive and essentially neutral. At the following session the partners will have an opportunity to assess their feeling states, and neither will be asked to go further if they have not begun to experience a shift toward stronger emotions within a reasonable time.

To make caring days work, it is important that the therapist use a highly selective shaping strategy. For example, spouses may begin to make requests of one another by using what in the next chapter is termed "dirty positives." These are illustrated by responses like the following: "I like it when you ask how I spent my day, but I can't stand the fact that you read the paper while you do it!" or "I would like you to walk into the office with me from the parking lot, but only if you will wipe that pained expression off your face." The therapist may be tempted to attempt to split the negative "hooker" from the positive request, but to attempt to edit communication in this way before the clients have experienced some initial success is usually fruitless. Therefore, to give caring days a needed assist, the therapist must practice forbearance and reserve intervention maneuvers for their appropriate place in the treatment plan, exercising caution not to ask for too much change too early in the game.

Elements in the Success of Caring Days

Therapists who have used the caring-days procedure often express amazement at the speed with which their clients begin to show positive change. Clients, too, usually express surprise that the change process could begin before either or both underwent profound personality change or at least were "set straight" by the therapist. Rather than being a case of sleight of hand, these rapid and constructive changes can be explained by reference to several dimensions of the process of social influence unique to the treatment situation. An understanding of several of these phenomena can help to strengthen the therapist's confidence in the technique, certainly an aid to his or her making a convincing presentation of the technique to the clients.

First, it should be recalled that any couple entering marital therapy have some degree of ambivalence about the maintenance of their marriage, neither feeling clearly that either staying or leaving is necessarily the best move. Their entry into treatment is an expression of at least some optimism about the possibility of change in their relationship, and the therapist's reinforcement of this manifest positive pole of their dilemma with suggestions for positive changes that are nonaccusatory and quite inexpensive in a social sense can help greatly to reinforce this optimism.

The fact that the therapist attends to positive statements and positive requests made by each spouse in the presence of the other also helps each to feel more positive toward the other. In this connection, Rokeach and Kliejunas (1972) found that subjects' attitudes toward certain others could be influenced by pairing these others with individuals and/or situations that had strong positive or negative values. In this instance, any positive value attributed to the therapist redounds to the benefit of each spouse, as each is quite likely to be experienced as more positive by the other because of this association. (Parenthetically, it should be noted that this is one dimension of the power of the therapeutic relationship deemed to be an important facilitator of change by psychotherapists [e.g., Cox, 1978] and behavior therapists [e.g., Goldfried & Davison, 1976] alike.)

The effectiveness of the caring-days technique is also bolstered by the fact that the bargaining approach it embodies is prudent and provides an invaluable opportunity for social-skills building in the partners in the dysfunctional marriage. The coin of the realm for couples in conflict is usually bold-faced demands for massive change, but many researchers (e.g., Benton *et al.*, 1972; Chertkoff & Conley, 1967; Osgood, 1962) have shown that large demands at the start of bargaining often lead to large counterdemands and the breakdown of negotiations. Instead, this "incremental" approach prompts partners to make modest initial requests, with the explicit realization that the requests will broaden in demand as trust develops in a relationship to which both partners feel increasing commitment.

The fact that caring days is a positive strategy in which each person implicitly affirms his or her caring for the other is another source of its effectiveness. Working in social psychology laboratories, many researchers have found that interactors are likely to feel very positively toward one another when their initially negative exchanges undergo a positive transition (e.g., Aronson & Linder, 1965; Byrne *et al.*, 1969; Lombardo *et al.*, 1972; Stapert & Clore, 1969; Worchel & Schuster, 1966). As with most other social-psychological findings, some exceptions and contrary evidence can be adduced (e.g., Hewitt, 1972; McClintock & McNeel, 1967; Mettee, 1971; Sigall & Aronson, 1967). Nevertheless, these studies do suggest that when Bill starts to treat Amanda positively after weeks, months, or years of subtle put-downs, there is a more than reasonable chance that she will attribute sincerity and significance to this change and that she will respond accordingly.

In summary, the caring-days technique helps the couple to step aside from the weighty, negative interaction that occasioned their request for treatment. Without forced apologies for past wrongs done, without the assignment of blame, without the fruitless search for the first negative cause of chains of stressful events, caring days offer couples an opportunity for relatively risk-free change under the skillful guidance of a therapist whose perspective is valued. The caring-days-mediated interaction is consistent with evolving social-psychological principles of constructive relationship management, and the instigation of changes consistent with caring-days techniques helps to move the couple from an aberrant course back into the mainstream of constructive and facilitative social experience.

A Special Note on Noncompliance

As mentioned earlier, many couples can be expected to resist those very changes that they sought to make when entering therapy. Phrasing the instigation for caring days in the terms suggested in this text can increase the likelihood of compliance. So, too, can making the suggested phone call aimed at prompting follow-through. Despite great skill in these efforts, however, any given client couple may find what are for them compelling reasons to resist the instigation and maintain their stressful interactive ways. When this happens—that is, when couples come for the second interview without having followed through—it is essential that the therapist avoid the trap of trying to determine which partner was largely responsible for the failure or which tactic was effective in subverting the change effort. Instead, the therapist is well advised to recognize the couple's hesitance to make such simple changes when they feel that their problems are so complex in origin and dynamics, and should state her or his recognition of the need to deal with higher-order issues in the marriage. At this point, the therapist should reiterate that larger changes must grow from smaller shifts aimed at building commitment, trust, and other emotions that each would like to see strengthened in their marriage. A reiteration of the logic of the approach, an effort to add to and to refine items on the list, and strong encouragement to follow the instigation in the next seven days (avoiding encouragement that they "try" because this prefigures the expectation that they may fail) should then conclude the session, which might be shorter than sessions in which new steps are proposed. It is only through the therapist's reaffirmation of the value of this or any instigation that the clients will learn to take the instigations seriously, and their failure to follow through should be viewed as testing not only one another's motivation for change, but also the strength of the therapist's convictions about the value of the advice that has been offered. Therapeutic tenacity, when it is closely keyed to the clients' behavior, is one of the elements of therapeutic success, and at no time is it more important than in this first phase of treatment when the clients struggle hard to prove to themselves that improvement of their marital life is all but impossible, despite the sage advice they have sought.

C H A P T E R 7

Communication Change

COMMUNICATION IS perhaps the one process that is basic to the survival of all organisms. Without skill in a continuum of abilities ranging from the sending of information to the reception and interpretation of data, organisms can neither know about the resources and threats in their surroundings nor effectively control their environments. As essential as effective communication is, so, too, is it complex. This chapter begins with a review of the multilayered nature of communication, in which there is an ongoing juxtapositioning of explicit and latent meanings about specific ideas and the nature of the relationship between message sender and message receiver, using many dimensions of nonverbal and verbal channels to get the message across. Following this appreciation of the complexities of information exchange, the chapter then reviews some research relating to the acceptable goals of communication change in marriage therapy. While many writers assert that marital communication should be completely open, the preponderance of available evidence suggests that discretion rather than overexuberance is a better norm for a relationship-enhancing communication pattern. Therefore, modest goals are set for this phase of treatment: building clients' skills in making their desires known, in understanding the other's requests, and in bargaining toward a common understanding. The chapter concludes with a five-step treatment program aimed at making these goals a reality.

Communication certainly is important. It is axiomatic that all biological and all social life depends upon communication processes for its very survival. All single-celled organisms must reliably "communicate" with their environments if they are to obtain nutrients and monitor and protect themselves from predators and other dangers. Humans, too, whether acting singly, in tandem, or as members of small face-to-face groups, large social institutions, nations, or multinational organizations, depend upon their abilities to send and receive information to identify and maintain the basic requirements for their physical, psychological, and social survival (e.g., Goffman, 1959; Jourard, 1971; G. H. Mead, 1934; Malinowski, 1923; C. Rogers, 1961).

For Birdwhistell (1970), the social system goals of communication include keeping the system in operation, regulating the interaction process, cross-referencing individual messages as to comprehensibility in various contexts, and developing rules for decision making at all levels of the organization. At the level of social interaction in small groups, communication provides the basis for defining, communicating, accepting, refining, and changing expectations that each party holds of the other's behavior as well as being the vehicle through which each interactor assesses the quality of the other's compliance with these expectations (e.g., Bennis, et al., 1968; Gordon & Gergen, 1968). On the individual level, communication with others provides the data base for forming and maintaining a sense of social identity. In Hora's (1959) words, "To understand himself man needs to be understood by another. To be understood by another he needs to understand the other" (p. 237).

The communication process through which these life-, self-, and role-sustaining functions are accomplished is perhaps best characterized by the so-called Shannon–Weaver model (Shannon & Weaver, 1949). According to this model, (1) an information source (2) encodes a message, (3) which is transmitted (4) over a circuit that can be affected by irrelevant "noise" (5) to a decoding source, (6) where it is interpreted and received as a message. In this model it is clear that the message sent may not be the message received because of encoding, transmission, or decoding errors: we may not find the best means of expressing our intended message; our message may get lost or sullied as it is being expressed; and the other may reach an understanding of the message that is inconsistent with our intention.

The real hazards of communication lie in the fact that individuals always respond in part to their outer experience and in part to the stimulation of their own thoughts, feelings, and expectations. Thus, the expressed message is only one part—and perhaps a very small part, at that—of the experience that every person has at all times. It may take a very forceful and compelling message to claim and maintain the attention necessary to accurate understanding. Unfortunately, though, virtually every social communication is multidimensional: it has one or more explicit content layers and one or more implicit metacommunications that qualify the explicit message (Watzlawick et al., 1967). Both the content and the metacommunications can be either nonverbal and/or verbal, and more often than not, they are both. Factors such as posture, orientation in space, mannerisms, facial expression, and eye contact are among the nonverbal contents and/or qualifiers that are expressed. Factors such as the choice of words, syntax, timing, and vocal quality are the contents and/or qualifiers of explicit messages. In a sense, nonverbal communication is informationally more simple than spoken words because it contains multiple messages on only two levels: a content and a qualifier, both of which are nonverbal. In contrast, spoken communication always involves at least four levels of message: manifest and implicit information on both the verbal and nonverbal levels. Perhaps because of the greater simplicity of nonverbal communication, research has shown that it is often the more forceful of the two types of messages. This research will be reviewed first, to be followed by a selective review of research on spoken messages.

Nonverbal Communication

While reading the newspaper one evening, Dan told Alice that he loved her. Alice responded with an angry rejection. The "I love you" was the content of Dan's message—its report dimension. His reading the newspaper was the relationship-qualifying metacommunicational dimension of his message. It told Alice how to interpret his words, and she read the nonverbal message to mean that she was certainly—at that moment, at least—of secondary importance to Dan. Feeling patronized, she reacted with fury; when the content and relationship-qualifying dimensions of a communication are inconsistent, the nonverbal layer always has the greatest effect. Therefore, it is extremely important to understand the relationships among the spoken, paraverbal, and nonverbal aspects of any communication.

The redundancy in human communication is well expressed in the classic study of implicit word meanings through the use of the semantic differential by Osgood *et al.* (1957). They found that the evaluative, potency, and activity dimensions of words in common use account for approximately 65% of their referential meaning. In a series of classic studies, Mehrabian (1969) and others (e.g., E. T. Hall, 1966; Mehrabian & Williams, 1969; N. E. Miller, 1964; Scheflen, 1968, 1974) have shown that three dimensions also underlie much of the diversity in nonverbal expressions. A *like–dislike* dimension is expressed by maintaining closeness or distance, by looking at or away from the other, and by various vocal inflections. A *potency* dimension is expressed through expansiveness in expression, by standing straight as opposed to slumping, and by quickness of movement. *Responsiveness,* the third dimension, is often expressed facially, by vocal tone, and by speech volume. Thus, one would express liking, respect for the other's power, and responsiveness by, for example, standing close, maintaining eye contact, moving somewhat uncomfortably while speaking, and speaking rapidly and with considerable animation. If the other person disliked the speaker, considered the other a status inferior and somewhat dull at that, he or she might turn slightly away during the conversation, sit while the other stood, or speak softly and with little affect. These and other dimensions contribute to a taxonomy of propositions about interpersonal space with which Lett *et al.* (1969) summarized what might be termed the "golden decade of research in nonverbal communication."

The profound importance of the nonverbal dimension of communication is well expressed by Mehrabian (1972), who believes that of the total feeling conveyed in a spoken message, 7% is verbal feeling; 38% is vocal feeling; and 55% is facial feeling. Because we are more likely to censor our words than our actions in expressing our words, it is very common to find inconsistencies between these two levels of communication. We are more likely to use words to comment on the other's actions and more likely to use nonverbal messages to comment on the other as a person. It is the latter set of messages that appears to dictate both satisfaction with the encounter and attraction to the other person, as well as to qualify the ways in which the spoken words will be understood.

Ekman and Friesen (1969) would consider the newspaper reading accompanying the statements of Dan's love for Alice a much more persuasive expression than his words. So, too, will Alice—to Dan's lasting disadvantage. Ekman and Friesen believe that all people learn to decode nonverbal behaviors as a means of penetrating deception in all social encounters. They believe that the face, followed by the hands and the feet, are the most fertile sources of these valuable data. However, because the face is a recognized "giveaway," most people are more careful to control their facial expressions than to monitor the use of their hands and feet. Therefore, the latter often provide valuable cues to the relationship meaning of spoken words. For example, Alice might ask Dan if he loves her. His maintaining eye contact while saying "yes" would add greater strength to his words than almost anything else he could do. In the same vein, holding his hands palm up would say something very different than clenching his fists when he answers. And sitting with his knees tightly closed together would express a very different feeling than would his answering her question while reaching toward her with open, outstretched legs.

Sometimes nonverbal behaviors are used in place of words: they need not always provide the orchestration for the spoken word. Thus, they can express feelings of attraction or disdain. For example, when he pulls his chair at the breakfast table close to her, he expresses something very different than when he walls himself off from her with the morning paper. Couples develop what might be termed "local" meanings for a variety of these nonverbal expressions whether they do or do not accompany words. Because *any inconsistency between the nonverbal message and the spoken word will be resolved in favor of the former and at the expense of the latter, the clarity of communication and the maintenance of a high level of interpersonal regard demands training the couple in two sets of skills: maintaining consistency within the levels of their communication and finding ways to express feelings of interpersonal warmth nonverbally as well as verbally.*

To become aware of the nature of their nonverbal communication, couples can be helped to (1) categorize the ways in which they send messages nonverbally; (2) plan to send nonverbal messages that express commitment to the other; and (3) work on establishing consistency between the nonverbal and the spoken messages that they send. Several technical but excellent coding systems are available for classifying nonverbal communication (e.g., Birdwhistell, 1970; Mehrabian, 1972; Gottman *et al.*, 1977). Once familiar with these coding systems, therapists can utilize awareness-building exercises such as those developed by J. O. Stevens (1971) to help spouses learn how they sometimes rely on nonverbal messages entirely and how to help nonverbal messages work in support of their spoken intentions. This can be done, for example, by asking one spouse at a time to express interest in the other nonverbally, to express lack of intent, to express the desire for closeness, and to express the desire to be alone with his or her own thoughts. The partners can then be asked to couple these nonverbal messages with words, and to be aware, while speaking, of the tireless commentary that they nonverbally offer concerning the intent of their own verbal expressions. They can then be asked to discuss the communicational dimensions of such daily routines as the way they enter their home after work and the way they get ready for bed, reviewing which aspects of these wordless experiences reflect mutual concern and which reflect mutual distance. In this way, partners can be helped to "tune into the channel" that plays the nonverbal statements of the feelings of each for the other.

AS A GENERAL RULE, COUPLES SHOULD BE TAUGHT TO USE BOTH NONVERBAL AND VERBAL MESSAGES WHENEVER THEY WISH TO EXPRESS POSITIVE FEELINGS BUT TO RELY HEAVILY ON WORDS WHEN THEY WISH TO COMMUNICATE NEGATIVE FEELINGS.

This procedure is important because nonverbal messages permit one to avoid taking the responsibility for communications, even if they may be the most accurate glimpse into the black box of true emotions. When Alice comes home in the evening, mixes herself a martini, and slumps into an easy chair to read the evening paper and sort through the mail, she clearly communicates to Dan that she would rather be left to her own devices for the time being than to review the events of the day with him. If Dan asks her about what he experiences as her indifference, she can self-righteously respond that she meant nothing of the kind, that she was merely tired from a hard day and is, of course, interested in him. The sender of any nonverbal message always has this quick and ready escape from acceptance of the responsibility for the message sent, because it is always very easy to hide behind the cloak of misunderstanding. Therefore, in the interest of fair play, any negative messages should always be put into words so that the message sender has proper responsibility for the message sent.

Communication Chains

In the drama of human communication, every message that one sends to the other is (1) a response to a message from the other; (2) a reinforcement of the other's past action(s); and (3) a stimulus for his or her next actions (Adams & Romney, 1959; Bateson, 1963). Therefore, the only way to understand a communicational exchange is to realize that every event is stimulated by what has gone on before, affects the probability that past events will be repeated, and sets the occasion for future elements in the exchange.

To clarify the communicational process, it is helpful to think of information flow as a chain of events such as shown on the following page. In this sequence, information that reduces uncertainty is being exchanged directly and indirectly, through verbal and nonverbal means, concerning a manifest topic and the relationship between the speaker and the listener. The reaction of each person to the other is influenced by what is in fact happening between them and by the self-stimulating personal interpretation of these events. This situation is aptly summarized by Nierenberg and Calero (1973):

> Talk exists on at least three levels of meaning: (1) what the speaker is saying; (2) what the speaker thinks he is saying; and (3) what the listener thinks the speaker is saying. (p. 12)

The process of effective communication thus involves a struggle to make certain that the spoken or nonverbal communication accurately reflects the sender's intent, and that the message communicated is, in fact, the one that is registered and understood by the receiver.

Complicating this difficult process of information transmission is the fact that every communication relates to the social relationship between message sender and message receiver at least as importantly as it relates to the explicit content of the message. The social definition at issue in every message concerns the balance of control or influence

An inner message
generates an intention
to communicate.

      The message is
      encoded and set.

            The message is
            received . . .

                  subject to a personal
                  interpretation.

                  This outer + inner message
                  generates an intention to
                  respond.

            The new message is
            encoded and sent.

      The new message is
      received . . .

subject to personal
interpretation.

This outer + inner message
generates an intention to
respond.

---

between the two parties. In this context, Haley (1963b) asserted that social interactions can be classified as "symmetrical" if both parties have the option of doing the same things or as "complementary" if the actions of one narrow the options of the other. In symmetrical exchanges, one is "up" and the other "down" in a hierarchy of powers to shape the interaction. Most long-term relationships between intimates pass through phases of symmetry and complementarity, and inflexibility with regard to power adaptations can be regarded as a major threat to the stability of a marriage and to the abilities of the partners to adapt to the demands of a changing environment. What is most important is that these power negotiations are more often implied than openly nego-tiated in communication exchanges.

Writers such as Barnlund (1968) have recognized that everything that transpires between two interacting people qualifies their relation-ship along this power or control dimension. One exercises "one-way" communication when in a complementary relationship with another; this implies phrasing messages that communicate the speaker's intent without eliciting feedback from the listener. One exercises "two-way" communication when in a symmetrical relationship with another; this implies phrasing messages in such a way as to encourage feedback. In one-way communication, the speaker makes it clear that he or she will not be influenced by the listener: the army officer does not ask the enlisted man if he wishes to stand at attention, for example. In two-way communication, the speaker makes clear his or her intention to adjust what will be done in response to the wishes of the other: the wife who asks her husband if he would rather invite friends in for dinner or go to a movie operates this mode.

Life would be simple and spoken communication clean if we were always willing to acknowledge our definition of our relationship to oth-ers. But for many reasons we sometimes intentionally conceal our notion of the role of the other. Watzlawick *et al.* (1967) have offered a taxonomy of pathological control-manipulating maneuvers. One can reject the other's message by indicating an unwillingness to communi-cate. One can unwillingly accept the other's communication and allow resentment to build. One can disqualify the other's communication by acting as though something else was said, by sidetracking, or by speak-ing in self-contradictions, among other ploys. Rejection and acceptance imply recognition of the other's being, while disqualificating maneuvers imply that the other does not exist or at least does not matter.

Each of these ploys is a tactic designed to manipulate control of the exchange. Without unmasking the motives for attempting to exercise control in these ways, it is possible to limit their use and importance in the communication between spouses, using some rather simple and straightforward techniques. Before describing this program, however, it is important to discuss one common—and, unfortunately, misplaced—goal in many communication-change programs: the pursuit of "total openness."

The Goals of Communication Change: How Much Openness?

Open communication is synonymous with uncensored self-disclosure or the act of revealing personal information to others (Jourard & Jaffe, 1970). It has long been believed that open communication is also synonymous with happy marriage (Locke, 1951; Satir, 1964; Terman, 1938), and more recently scores of writers have touted efforts to open communication as the *sine qua non* of relationship therapy (e.g., Gottman et al., 1976a; S. Miller, 1975; Miller et al., 1975; Scoresby, 1977). So energetic are these exponents of free expression between spouses that Kursh (1971) observed:

> An ailment termed "lack of communication" has taken the place of original sin as an explanation for the ills of the world, while "better communication" is trotted out on every occasion as a universal panacea. (p. 189)

In order to prudently plan the communication phase of the present marriage therapy program, it is necessary to evaluate critically the validity of this commonly accepted goal of helping our clients to "let it all hang out."

Unfortunately, there is a wealth of information to suggest that uncensored, open communication may be more than any relationship can bear. Societies in general seem to have "a tacit agreement not to express or become aware of what may be dysfunctional" (R. Williams, 1951), and they seem to rely on lying as a safety valve for system maintenance (Brittan, 1973; Moore & Tumin, 1949). Societies, then, depend upon selective information flow. What happens when dyads and couples do not?

It appears that there are implicit boundaries of acceptable self-disclosure levels for stranger dyads (Fitzgerald, 1963; Jourard, 1959, 1971; Savicki, 1972). Actually, a curvilinear relationship exists between self-disclosure and attraction: some self-disclosure may be necessary for strangers to attract, but too much disclosure has a repellent effect (Cozby, 1973; Jourard, 1971; Taylor, 1968).

Total openness and its resulting more complete understanding also may have a curvilinear relationship with marital satisfaction. At the most global level, it is expected that husbands and wives will disclose more of themselves to each other through the successive years of their marriage. Merrill (1959), for example, believed that "Even the most obtuse husband who lives for a quarter century with a woman gains some understanding of her motives" (p. 208), while Blood and Wolfe (1960) believed that "sheer living together provides the basic condition for understanding another person" (p. 218). These and similar writers have thus predicted what might be termed a "joyful unfolding" as each comes to know the other thoroughly. There are, however, two flies in the ointment. First, many studies show that through the years, couples do not often increase in their ability to predict each other's behavior accurately (Budd, 1959; Goodman & Ofshe, 1968; E. L. Kelley, 1961; Udry et al., 1961), and when such understanding does exist, it is found to be associated as often with dissatisfaction (e.g., Clements, 1967; Corsini, 1956; Locke et al., 1956; Luckey, 1961) as with satisfaction (Dymond, 1954; Hobart & Klausner, 1959; Karlsson, 1963). Second, it has been shown that marital satisfaction tends to decline over the same years during which more spousal communication would be expected to aid its increase (e.g., Cimbalo et al., 1976; Mathews & Milhanovich, 1963; Pineo, 1961; Rutledge, 1966).

Writers like Simmel (1964) and Blau (1964) have attributed a negative relationship impact to high-level communicational expressiveness. Their beliefs have been substantiated in a number of different studies of spousal satisfaction. Cutler and Dyer (1965) and Goodrich et al. (1968) found that as early as the first year of marriage, couples begin to quarrel over things that would have been better left unsaid. Bienvenu (1970) found that the item from his inventory that best discriminated well-communicating couples from poorly communicating couples was a negative answer to the question: "Does your spouse have a tendency to say things which would be better left unsaid?" Levinger and Senn (1967) found that nondistressed couples differed from those with problems by their greater expression of positive sentiments in contrast to distressed couples' freer expression of negative feelings. Later, Sprenkle and Olson (1978) found that "the prevalence of negative support to put-downs rather than the absence of positive support typified the distressed couples" (p. 71). All of these researchers reached the conclusion that joining the bandwagon for fully uncensored communication is a ride that couples and therapist should be careful not to take.

There are a number of explanations for the negative impact of these expressive behaviors, although none has the strength of a causal hypothesis. First, witholding some displeasing revelation can help to sustain the attractiveness of the speaker. Kanouse and Hanson (1972) concluded an exhaustive review of research assaying the significance of positive and negative data. They found that "People are generally cost oriented in forming overall evaluations—they weigh negative aspects of an object more heavily than positive ones" (p. 1). While negative disclosures could have a certain commitment value (see Chapter 4), it is more likely that their inclusion in any message draws attention away from any counterbalancing positive elements in that communication (Gilbert & Horenstein, 1975), in much the same way that the princess focused on the pea and not on the feather beds on which she lay.

Several explanations have been offered for this ascendance of negative over positive information in impression formation (Wegner & Vallacher, 1977). One is based upon animal studies now over 30 years old (Brown, 1948; N. E. Miller, 1944). These have shown that when negative and positive elements exist in the stimulus, the force of the avoidance reaction is greater than the force of the approach reaction as the goal is approached. Thus, the force of negative cues outweighs the force of positive cues. Another explanation is based on the work of Jones and

Davis (1965). It asserts that because we expect most people and events in our lives to be positive, positive expectations become the "ground" of social perceptions and negative events become the "figure" that has stronger stimulus properties than the ground. In this sense, negative perceptions may have greater "cue salience." Finally, it may be that vigilance with regard to possible sources of threat to our health and well-being may simply be more phylogenetically adaptive than attention to positives. We may use this vigilance even though it may have the odious secondary effect of undermining our capacity to enjoy our lives quietly because of hypersensitivity to the negative dimensions of any mixed messages that we receive. Whatever the explanation, it is clear that the frank expression of negative messages can have a relationship-eroding effect no matter how well embedded they are in countervailing positives.

But there is some reason to believe that it is even wiser to censor somewhat the number of positive statements that are offered. In a laboratory study, J. D. Davis (1971) showed that positive messages often unexpectedly reduce the level of social interaction: giving too much too soon may be a more potent conversation killer then a strenuous challenge of the other's point of view. In this regard, Berscheid *et al.* (1977) found that subjects attend much more closely to others who are novel and who are believed to be important. When reassurance of one's power and importance comes too early or too often in an encounter, it is possible that the loss of challenge that this implies may bring with it a loss of interest. Unfortunately, it is not possible to discern how many positives are too many, or how few are sufficient to be enticing rather than extinguishing—even more of a problem because very frequently our desires doubtlessly change without notice.

Finally, it seems as though too much information about one's mate can pierce the illusions that help to foster feelings of love. Walster and Walster (1978) observed that "just falling in love is not enough for most of us. We start out wanting—and really expecting—an unrealistic degree of perfection in a partner" (p. 113), and we are painfully disillusioned when we are forced to accept the one we've chosen. If the Walsters are correct, we may be better able to live happily in our marriages if we can cling to some shreds of the illusion that our one-and-only is indeed just that. This possibility is supported by Newcomb's (1953) speculation that we may be able to live more easily with an illusion than with a grim reality. Moreover, several studies reached the conclusion that more happily married mates assume greater similarity to their spouses than actually exists, while those less satisfied seem to have paid the price of better understanding (Stuckert, 1963; Styker, 1957).

Taken together, the studies just reviewed offer scant if any support for the notion that open communication brings the reality of greater marital bliss. It is perhaps this kind of reasoning, along with the recognition that communication has virtually irreversible effects (Patton & Giffin, 1974, p. 9), that has led many thoughtful writers to endorse what might be termed the "norm of measured honesty" in place of the "let-it-all-hang-out" ethic. Clinician–researchers like Haley (1963a) and Watzlawick *et al.* (1967) have recognized that incomplete communication can have great adaptive value, with Kursh (1971), for one, considering these "errors" of communication a source of valued family glue. It should not be surprising to realize that even writers like the O'Neills and Fritz Perls—writers whose work, perhaps better than that of others, captures the sense of the humanist revolution of the 1960s—caution against free and open communication. The O'Neills (1972) wrote:

> Blunt or "brutal" honesty . . . is seldom a disclosure of intimacy. It is usually an indulgence in destructive and unnecessary criticism. The "brutal" or blunt truth is, in fact, more often an exaggeration. (p. 114)

In the same vein, Perls *et al.* (1965) offered praise for the value of "retroflection" or the weighing of the messages sent. They wrote:

> When retroflection is under aware control—that is, when a person in a current situation suppresses particular responses which, if expressed, would be to his disadvantage—no one can contest the soundness of such behavior. It is only when the retroflection is habitual, chronic, out of control, that it is pathological. (p. 147)

With these cautions in mind, it is possible to reach a mixed conclusion that sets the stage for efforts to change couples' communication. First, it can be concluded that some effort to improve communication between spouses may be absolutely necessary as a means of building skills for interaction change. Second, however, it must be recognized that the communication changes that are undertaken must be aimed specifically at facilitating the more basic behavioral change, and they should never be undertaken as ends in themselves.

UNDERSTANDING AS THE GOAL OF COMMUNICATION CHANGE

If unbridled self-expression leading to total understanding of the other is not the goal of therapeutic communication change, what is its objective? It is application of the norm of measured honesty to help couples to develop the listening, expressive, request-making, feedback, and clarifying skills that they need for achieving genuine agreements. To be able to live together satisfactorily, two people must be able to make their wishes known, must be able to understand the requests made by the other, and must be able to negotiate shared objectives on the basis of these reciprocal requests. Once an agreement is reached, the partners must also be able to understand its meaning in the same way. Therefore, selective expression and accurate understanding are the two clusters of abilities that couples must have.

The problem presented by Cora and Jim illustrates the first of these needs: Cora believed that if Jim really loved her, he would be able to anticipate her desires. Joining in the *folie à deux*, Jim heard every request for change as a criticism of his recent past behavior and as a demand. As a result, neither Cora nor Jim helped the other to know when and how to please, both felt uninterested in their mate and their marriage, and neither could explain their feeling of being "burned out." Al and Betty illustrate the other problem: They agree that they will be active in their church. For Al, "being active" means attending church on two or three special holidays and contributing a few dollars to the church building fund each year. Betty, on the other hand, interprets "active" as meaning the daily practice of her faith and sizable annual contributions to funding all phases of the church's programs. Al and Betty are further along than Cora and Jim because they do make requests of one another; but owing to their lack of understanding, they may as well be speaking different languages because they are little closer to effective agreements than are Cora and Jim. It should therefore be clear that "consensus" (Scheff, 1967), or what Skolnick (1973) termed a "self-correcting environment," is a skill basic to efforts to meet the challenge of problem solving in ongoing relationships. Therefore, the communication change program offered here seeks to promote judicious self-expression and understanding of these well-chosen messages.

Four Techniques for Communication Change

The argument presented above can be summarized as follows:

1. The process of exchanging information is complex because it is multilevel and invariably comes under the influence of the social dynamics of the communicating parties.
2. When conflict exists between the nonverbal and the verbal levels of any message, the former has greater impact than the latter.
3. While explicit messages should be honest, there is overwhelming support for the notion that it is adaptive to measure the amount that is communicated and that it is often interpersonally destructive not to do so.
4. Couples must develop the ability to express their offers and to hear and understand the mate's counterbids if they are ever to bring their relationship under reasonable, negotiated control.

With these assumptions in mind, the present program calls for training couples in five communication-change steps: listening; measured self-expression; selective request-making; provision of positive and corrective feedback; and clarification of intended meanings. These skills can be best understood as a modified Guttman scale: they are cumulative rather than discrete. Therefore, each of the first skills is a prerequisite for those that follow, and it is important for therapists to build systematic reviews of the earlier steps as the later ones are taught.

ABILITY TO LISTEN

From the Shannon–Weaver communication model presented above, accurate encoding and decoding are the basic skills necessary if effective communication is to take place. In the words of two popular authors, "For golden words to be of value, the sender and receiver are required to be equally proficient in totally different procedures and skills" (Nierenberg & Calero, 1973, p. 22). Because we send messages constantly, remembering that all socially relevant behavior is communication, it is the listener who actually determines whether or not communication will take place (Patton & Giffin, 1974). Therefore, without the ability to listen, we would be doomed to a life of monologue rather than dialogue, and we would be locked into a closed information system that would make adaptation to changing living conditions all but impossible. Despite its great significance, most people take listening for granted until it breaks down entirely, much as they take for granted, until times of crisis, their breathing and heartbeat.

A continuum of necessary listening skills has been described, with the points between the extremes of empathic and deliberative listening being differentiated mainly in terms of their goals (C. M. Kelly, 1970; Tubbs & Moss, 1974). The goal of *empathic listening* is to fully sense the other person and his or her message, while the goal of *deliberative listening* is to sort through the message to critically evaluate its components. Thus, while both types of listening aim at understanding, the active process in each is quite different.

We often believe that we are listening empathically when we are, in fact, hard at work sorting out the acceptable and the unacceptable elements of the other's message. Our empathic listening ability is hampered by the fact that we all tend to be listening specialists. Polster and Polster (1973) believe that some people listen for support, others for criticism; some listen for information, others for condescension; and some listen for statements, overlooking all questions, while others hear only statements when questions are asked. We are also all highly sensitive to certain key words, which signal us to tune the speaker in or out (Patton & Giffin, 1974). Virtually everyone has certain listening predilections about the communications that are received, and therefore, it is axiomatic that every message will be selectively perceived and substantially altered as it is decoded. Many of these biases work to support—indeed, may be the product of—stereotypes about others' behavior. Once stereotypes are formed—and they may be based upon leaping inferences from minimal cues—we tend to act in patterns consistent with our beliefs and force others to respond as though the stereotypes were valid (Harvey *et al.*, 1976). As one group of social psychologists has observed, "people are 'constructive thinkers' searching for the causes of behavior, drawing inferences about people and their circumstances, and acting upon this knowledge" (M. Snyder *et al.*, 1977). Motivated by our desire to maintain cognitive consistency, we may all tend to attend selectively to communications with others that support our beliefs about them, and we may fail to apprehend messages that would challenge our beliefs.

Aiding and abetting this selective and interpretive bias is the fact that while words are spoken at the rate of between 125 and 175 per minute, our ability to apprehend words is three or four times faster (Tubbs & Moss, 1974). Therefore, the thoughts of the listener are almost always sweeping past the words of the speaker, a fact that works significantly to hamper the sharing of meaning.

C. M. Kelly (1963) has shown that effective listening requires considerable effort, and this effort is expended only when it is reinforced. For example, he tested subjects' ability to answer questions about a 30-minute speech under two conditions: in one, they were told in advance about the test, while the test came as a surprise in the other. The results of this and other research (C. M. Kelly, 1967) clearly showed that those who were motivated to receive information, as through the awareness that they would be tested, were far more likely to be receptive to the information given.

The catalog of explanations for a failure to listen is long indeed. To name but three of many possible explanations, one may not listen because of simple lack of interest, because of a fear of having to change one's behavior in response to new information, or because of a desire to maintain a one-up position in a particular relationship. Unfortunately, listening for most people means "simply maintaining a polite silence while you are rehearsing in your mind the speech you are going to make the next time you can grab a conversational opening" (S. I. Hayakawa, cited in Addeo & Burger, 1973).

Nierenberg and Calero (1973) believe that good listeners are those who are able to separate their emotions from the other's words. They believe that poor listeners are those who (1) reject the other's words because they are uninteresting, already known, too simple, or too complicated; (2) attend to aspects of the speaker's appearance and manner instead of the words that are uttered; (3) stop attending as they concentrate on a single word or phrase; and (4) know in advance what they think they will hear. By implication, the benchmarks of poor listening are distracting behaviors, inattention to focal content, obsession with some aspect of the message, and undivided attention to inner messages in place of the spoken words. Conversely, good listeners do the following:

1. They are fully committed to listen.
2. They are physically and mentally ready to listen.
3. They wait for the other to complete the message before expressing their own ideas.
4. They use analytic skills to supplement, not to replace, listening (see C. M. Kelly, 1970; Nierenberg & Calero, 1973).

Combined, these skills build the ability to receive information in relatively undistorted form, and they give the listener the ability to help the speaker feel accepted and understood.

Commitment to listen involves making a decision that the words of the other have importance. Commitment to listen is behaviorally expressed by the listener's making the effort to relax, to clear all distractions (by, for example, turning off the radio or putting the newspaper out of sight), and to sit erect and maintain eye contact. Practicing waiting one's turn involves learning to refrain from jumping in to complete the other's sentence, not to ask for more information before the other has completed an expression, and to provide nonverbal signs of interest in what is being said (Duncan, 1972). Finally, the test of the use of supplementary analytic skills is the ability both to repeat and to acceptably and accurately rephrase the other's message.

Each of the four components of listening in the list above can be taught to clients through a series of very brief exercises during and between therapeutic sessions. A simple statement of the recommendations will help many clients make the desired changes. As a first step, it is helpful to assist clients in identifying some of their listener biases and hidden assumptions. What are some of the things that each expects the other to do quite often? Does Hal expect Midge to put him down frequently, and does Midge count on Hal to ignore her words entirely? If so, Hal will hear endless put-downs and Midge will forever feel discounted. Asking couples to write down for themselves the things that they think the other will say during a structured conversation can provide invaluable clues to these pernicious self-fulfilling prophesies. Helping clients learn to orient themselves toward one another as a sign of listening readiness, coaching them as to when and how long to speak and when to listen, and asking each to repeat and paraphrase selected messages of the other can all begin the process of skills building that can continue for a lifetime.

Self-expressive statements are believed to help partners orient
selves to each other and to help each person make sense of his
own experience by putting that experience into words (Miller ...,
1975). As has been suggested in the foregoing discussion of the fate of
total candor, however, some self-expressive statements can be expected
to have many more positive effects than others. Effective statements
should have at least seven important characteristics.

First, all self-statements should begin with the personal pronoun "I."
"I" statements are expressions of self-responsibility; they are clear, based
upon personal awareness, leave room for awareness of others, and
encourage the disclosure of differences (Miller *et al.*, 1976). Self-responsibility can be contrasted with "underresponsible statements," which
start with "it" and leave ownership of the statement in question, and with
"overresponsible statements," which speak for others because they begin
with "you," "we," "everybody," or "all" (Miller *et al.*, 1976). Statements
beginning with "it" externalize responsibility; the listener finds it difficult to respond because the speaker has not accepted ownership of what
is being said. Sentences that begin with "you" are almost always accusatory and lead to defensiveness, and they always involve an effort to
shift responsibility for the observation from the speaker to the listener
(Stevens, 1971). While "we" statements can sometimes bring people
together by pointing up similarities, they also mean by definition that
the speaker talks for both himself or herself and for the listener as well.

Just as most statements like "You make me angry" are actually
personal statements saying "I feel angry," so, too, are most questions
actually statements. Gestalt therapists believe that questions "represent
laziness and passivity" (Levitsky & Perls, 1970, p. 144), and that "very
few questions are honest requests for information" (Stevens, 1971, p.
105). They believe that questions are efforts to elicit a commitment
from the other person without the speaker's taking responsibility for a
position first. Moreover, when questions begin with "why" they almost
invariably are accusatory and put the other person on the defensive.
Thus, questions pose an important communication problem to the extent that they protect the speaker from responsibility for what is said
and to the extent that they reinforce the speaker in a "one-up" position,
holding the listener "one down."

With these considerations in mind, it is possible to generate two
additional dimensions of self-statements:

· Initially, they should be statements rather than questions whenever possible. (The use of statements that begin with "I" is not
likely to create a power imbalance between spouses and is likely to
keep the communication channels open.)

· When questions must be asked, however, the questions should be preceded by a self-statement; should begin with "how"; and should always be followed by a second question asking for amplification of the answer to the first.

Using the say–ask rule by preceding questions with self-statements is another way of increasing the level of responsibility that one takes for his or her utterances. For example, Ann might ask Harry if he would like to go to sleep now. A "yes" from Harry could bring on a tirade about his always withdrawing from her into bed, work, or through any other convenient door. Conversely, a "no" could lead her to accuse him of avoiding closeness, if not sex, by wanting to wait until she falls asleep before he climbs into bed. On the other hand, if Ann were to commit herself first (i.e., "I would like to go to bed now, Harry") and then ask her question (i.e., "Would you like to come to bed with me?"), she would give up the opportunity to set Harry up and would quite honorably accept responsibility for the message that she is communicating.

Using "how" to begin questions contributes to a problem-solving orientation in the exchange rather than the accusatorial set that is brought on by "why" questions. Following the "two-question rule," in which the speaker is always ready with a request for more information from the listener, has two advantages: it avoids using the answer as a "setup" for an immediate attack; and it expresses the asker's interest in the answerer's response to the question. In the following example only one question is asked, followed by a statement:

A: How are you feeling today?
B: I've been a bit under the weather lately.
A: I have not been up to snuff either. In fact, I went to the doctor just yesterday and . . .

It is clear from this exchange that A was using B's answer as a platform from which to launch a self-statement rather than having any genuine interest in B's state of health. Compare it with the following exchange:

A: What did you do today?
B: Nothing much, I guess.
A: Were you able to make some progress on the new project that you started last week?

Clearly, in this exchange, A's second question can be taken as an expression of genuine interest in the events of B's life. Use of the second question is likely to elicit a far more positive reaction in B than did the question–self-statement sequence described in the first illustration.

The sixth requirement of self-statements is that they must be present-oriented. Ben Jonson, in the prologue to *Irene* (III, ii, 33), urged that we "learn that the present hour alone is man's." This concept, which stresses the importance of sensations of the present, plays an important role in the theory of Gestalt therapy. Levitsky and Perls (1970) stated that "The idea of the new, of the immediate moment, of the content and structure of present experience is one of the most potent, most pregnant, and most elusive principles of Gestalt therapy" (pp. 140–141). Perls (1973), for one, believes that any effort to leave the present for the past or the future denies people the capacity to realize their potentials, for life can be mastered only in the present. And Nierenberg and Calero (1973) believe that use of any tense or voice other than the present creates a distance in verbal communication that helps the speaker escape at least part of the responsibility for the words that are uttered.

Finally, it is important for self-statements to be made directly, openly, and honestly—free of verbal excess. Nierenberg and Calero (1973) have offered an extensive catalog of phrases that are intended to manipulate the listener into the frame of mind desired by the speaker. Among them are "softeners" to create a positive reception ("You're going to like what I'm going to tell you"), foreboders that are intended to create anxiety in the listener ("Don't worry about me, but . . ."), and downers, which are intended to build the position of the speaker ("You couldn't have heard this yet, but . . ."). All of these ploys and a great many like them are word salad intended to maneuver the listener's attention and mood in such a manner as to increase the likelihood of his or her expressing the reaction that the speaker hoped for—despite the true impact of the spoken message itself.

Self-summarizing statements can be abused (Gottman *et al.*, 1976a), but they are also essential if both partners are to establish their identities for one another by expressing their convictions. When they are begun with "I," are made declaratively, are present focused, and are free of manipulative ploys, self-summarizing statements can be the essential building blocks of a social interaction, the basis of all verbal communication.

Clients can be taught to use self-statements successfully if they are taught the "I rule"; the "statement rule"; the "say–ask," "how," and "two-question" rules regarding questions; the "now rule"; and the "simplicity-speaks-the-truth" rule. Taught in this way, the rule statements have mnemonic value, and clients are more likely to put the rules into practice. A shaping program is best when training in self-statements is needed. The therapist can begin by commenting when each of the rules is put into practice by either spouse, followed by instructions to either or both to concentrate on using one or more of the rules during the session. Assignments can be given to the couple to spend 5–10 minutes daily in discussion of neutral topics such as items from the local newspapers—periods during which each person can either self-monitor or monitor the other's successful use of specific rules. When such an assignment is given it is important to provide the couple with 3″ X 5″ note cards on which are written the one or more rules they are asked to follow. When these cards are in the view of both during discussions, they will have considerable prompt value and will soon be unnecessary.

As an additional training tool, the therapist can help each partner learn both how to hold the floor and when the turn to take the floor is at hand. The analyses of interactions between spouses cited earlier have consistently shown that spouses are more likely to interrupt one another than to interrupt strangers with whom they converse. For example, Tim frequently rushes in to finish June's sentences if she pauses long enough to take even a very quick breath; this habit infuriates her because it is, in her eyes, an expression of Tim's lack of interest in her words and an excessive preoccupation with his own ideas. Another manifestation of this same problem occurs when one partner interrupts the other to challenge something that has been said without waiting to hear the complete thought and granting the possibility that subsequent qualification may change the meaning of the earlier statements. To deal with these problems, simple techniques for training spouses in how to respect one another's privilege of holding the floor may be in order. While Duncan's (1972) rather sophisticated coding system can be used to identify the speaker's willingness to yield the floor, simply asking each person to hold a pencil vertically when he or she wishes to hold the floor can help the other to learn when it is his or her partner's turn to speak. During treatment sessions, the coaching that this simple signal system can offer can go far both toward maintaining an orderly exchange of self-statements and toward training both partners in how to take their turns in conversation.

CONSTRUCTIVE REQUEST-MAKING

J. O. Stevens (1971) observed:

> Most demands are not expressed openly and directly. Usually I don't want to take responsibility for my demands, so I hide and disguise them in sweet requests, suggestions, questions, accusations, and countless other manipulations. I would like you to satisfy my desires without my having to ask you. If I demand directly, I run the risk that you might refuse. (p. 110)

Many people, then, have a tendency to be quite indirect in their attempts to garner from their spouses the favors they seek. While this approach reduces the likelihood that positive things will happen on the desired schedule, the loss of positives seems, for many, to be a less expensive price than the costs associated with openly making requests.

There are several possible explanations for the tendency to refrain from making requests. Many times people feel a desire but may not be aware of the way in which it can be satisfied. Another problem is that making a request of another implies valuing something that the other has to offer. In couples with balanced interaction, this acknowledgment poses no threat, but between spouses with a power imbalance—couples in which one partner is "socially bankrupt" because he or she wishes to have more from the other than he or she is asked to give to the other (Longabaugh *et al.*, 1966)—there may be a tendency to try to restore balance by requesting less. Also, conflict-habituated couples may wish to "disqualify" and/or "disconfirm" one another's very existence (Watzlawick *et al.*, 1967) through requesting less and thereby minimizing not only the power of the other but also recognition of her or his very being. Finally, one may hesitate to make requests of the other for fear of being asked to reciprocate the favors granted. Doubting one's capacity to satisfy the other's requests, one may prefer not to take the risk of failure or of expending commitment energy that is expected to be dissipated.

Successful experience in making structured requests through the caring-days exercise can help to overcome this request reticence. Training in making less-structured requests can be a further aid. The necessary skills fall into two categories: framing the request; and timing its delivery.

Request statements should meet all of the requirements of self-statements. For example, they must begin with "I," they must be present-oriented, and they must be made openly and directly. Thus, full responsibility is taken for the things one asks of another, a goal that is incompatible with the ideas of some that a "suggestion box" might be used to make requests (Gottman *et al.*, 1976a). The problem with this idea, while intriguing, is that it structures a mask behind which one can hide as if to escape at least part of the responsibility for having made a request. Self-statement requests should begin with "I want" rather than "I need." A want is something that "you want a lot but which is not necessary for your survival" (J. O. Stevens, 1971, p. 198). When one partner expresses a desire to the other, the listener is under no constraint to comply. However, when needs are expressed, an implicit obligation is created, a factor that often contributes significantly to a hesitance to comply; it's so much more pleasing to do things for one's spouse out of desire rather than out of compulsion!

Apart from choosing the proper words, it is also important to choose the proper time to make requests. Recognizing that the desires of two vital and alive adults are often dissynchronous, Polster and Polster (1973) believe that:

what is needed is the development of skill in managing these temporary but inevitable incompatibilities—through a process we call bracketing-off. In bracketing-off, the individual holds some of his own concerns in abeyance in favor of attending to what is going on in a communicative process. (p. 43)

Both partners must learn when their desires should be temporarily set aside in deference to the desires or needs of the other. It is obvious, for example, that Nate should not ask Sue to sit down with him for a few minutes to discuss his problems at work while she is studying for an important exam scheduled for that evening. It may be less obvious that Sue should delay talking about her need for a new car, or some very major repairs on the old one, until after Nate has decided how much responsibility he feels that he and Sue should take for the care of his recently stricken mother.

It is not difficult to help couples learn appropriate phrasing for their requests; it is more difficult to help them learn when to express their desires. While it may have been forgotten, we all learned the importance of saying "please," but somewhere along the line we may have failed to learn how to read the cues of the other's readiness to hear and to grant our requests, which requires the skills of a good empathic listener, as outlined above. Perhaps the surest way to have cue reading happen is for each spouse to assume the responsibility of telling the other when he or she is willing to put himself or herself at the disposal of the other. Bill might ask Judy if there is anything she would like him to do, or Judy might tell Bill that she would like to sit down with him for a few minutes to discuss what each might do to lighten the other's load or to bring new joy to the other's life.

SELECTIVE, SPECIFIC, AND TIMELY FEEDBACK

The fourth skill that helps to improve the quality of couples' communication concerns the way in which they express their reactions to one another's behavior. When Bill tells Joann how he feels when she wins a case in court, he is giving her information about the impact of her behavior on his feelings. Information is anything that reduces uncertainty, and feedback is a particular kind of information that reduces uncertainty about the effects of any individual or system action (Attneave, 1959). We all need feedback if we are to be able to perform any physical or social task successfully. The perils of driving with the eyes closed, or of jogging while wearing a headset radio that masks the sound of oncoming cars, or of trying to sell a vacuum cleaner to a customer who is unseen and who makes no response to the "pitch" all point up the extent of our dependency upon feedback. Unfortunately, in social interchange "direct and honest feedback is very rare" (Wegner & Vallacher,

1977, p. 234). We simply tend not to express to others the way we feel about their behavior—expressions that would enable them to know whether to offer more of the same or to change what they do to win our favor; instead, we sink into complaining withdrawal because of the other's insensitivity to our *unexpressed* reactions.

When feedback is given it is very often negative rather than positive. With those whom we love we have a great tendency to overstate our negative reactions at times of crisis. Several researchers have shown that husbands and wives are far more likely to give negative feedback to each other than are nonmarried men and women who are asked to solve similar laboratory-posed problems. This is as true of verbal behavior (e.g., Birchler *et al.*, 1975; Ryder, 1968; Stuart & Braver, 1973) as of nonverbal behavior (e.g., Baekel & Mehrabian, 1969; Gottman *et al.*, 1977). It has also been shown that parents and disturbed adolescents are more likely to exchange high rates of negative feedback (Mehrabian, 1969) and low rates of positive feedback (Stuart, 1971a). Thus, couples and families seem to expend their communicational energies on precisely those behaviors that are most likely to limit their shared satisfaction and to vitiate their growth potential.

This negative feedback functions principally to maintain stressful interactions, and it does little if anything to change them. Systems theorists (e.g., Laszlo *et al.*, 1974) have shown that negative information, such as data from a thermostat indicating that the temperature in a room has varied from set point, serves to activate a control system to restore the steady state. For example, if Max makes only negative comments on Pat's clothes, ignoring the days when he is pleased with her appearance, she will quickly learn to wear the very things he does not like in order to elicit some reaction from him. In contrast, studies have shown that when positive feedback is given, it is very likely that positive risk-taking, higher performance, and better outcomes will all result (e.g., Canavan-Gumpert, 1977). Therefore, feedback that is negative can generally be considered change-inhibiting, while positive feedback is change-stimulating.

Vague feedback and feedback that occurs long after the desired behavior are as likely to cause frustration as to have any beneficial effect, as has been shown in decades of psychophysical experimentation (Annett, 1969). Telling people that they are doing a good job without telling them how or telling them that they have done a poor job long after the task both undermine performance.

In addition to the recommendations that feedback be positive, specific, and timely, Filley (1975) has offered other guidelines for the giving of feedback; feedback should be descriptive rather than judgmental; it should concern things that can be changed; and it should be given when it is desired.

The first of these added recommendations may be the most difficult to achieve. All of those who have studied semantics (e.g., Osgood *et al.*, 1967) have recognized that all words have multidimensional meanings. It is equally true that our use of words in combination tends to be organized around a number of meanings that may be hidden not only from others but from ourselves as well. These hidden meanings and assumptions are shortcuts that help us to organize our impressions of ourselves and the world around us; but the price of this efficiency is often self-deception. Consider, for example, the ideas of Nierenberg and Calero (1973) concerning two everyday words: "'Sunrise' and 'sunset' contain a hidden assumption that for thousands of years may have prevented earthlings from ever considering that the earth might re- volve around the sun" (p. 85). Husbands and wives can bind themselves into interminable agonies when they use what Hurvitz (1970) termed "terminal language" in their exchanges, when the use of "process lan- guage" could so easily point the way to a resolution of their dilemmas. Terminal language involves the use of static labels such as "He is depressed" or "she is not interested," while process language describes what people do, such as "He spends several hours in bed every day" or "She seems to play tennis when she could be spending time with the family." Use of terminal language has three very obvious effects:

1. It creates negative affective reactions and blocks constructive thinking.
2. It leads to changes in behavior that, in turn, lead to reactions by the other that fulfill the prophecy implicit in the vocabulary.
3. When expressed, it is often experienced as an attack, against which the other mounts a personal defense.

Therefore, in giving feedback, it is important both to cleanse the lan- guage of self-statements to reduce the probability of negative self- cueing and to give feedback in process terms so that it can be con- structively received.

When feedback is offered in descriptive, process terms, it almost invariably addresses things that can be changed. Bob may not like the fact that Judy is short, but there is virtually nothing that she can do about her height other than perhaps donning a pair of dangerously high heels. Therefore, any comment that he makes about her height would by definition fall into the judgmental and terminal category. Con- versely, he may very much want her to be ready to leave for work with him in the morning on time so that her tardiness does not result in his lateness. He can give her feedback by observing that she has not been out the front door before 8:15 once in the last week, words that describe what she does in process terms that can result in change.

There are times when we are more and less ready to receive feed- back. For example, Jill was hard at work plastering a crack in the cellar wall when Glen came into the basement. He told her that he hoped dinner would be ready—an indirect way of giving her the feedback that she was taking too long on the job. It was clear from the intensity with which she was working that she was doing as well as she could, and his feedback to her fell on angry ears.

It is important to note that the true value of feedback is its feedforward effects; that is, the value of feedback lies in its influence upon future behavior. Jerry has felt that Pat has been quite aloof, and he would like to have a greater feeling of closeness to her. He could wait several weeks and tell her that he felt she had been distant for some time, in which case he will have gone on suffering with a gnawing sense of isolation. However, he could also tell her immediately that he would like to feel closer to her, moving into a request that she sit on the sofa with him for a while and talk about things they could do together to gain an opportunity for sharing and the closeness it could bring. In this way, feedback about Jerry's present feelings can be used to help Pat make changes that can have an immediate and positive effect.

It is now possible to formulate the skills enumerated above. Feedback statements should ideally have the following characteristics:

1. They should begin with "I."
2. They should refer to specific behaviors.
3. They should stress the positives in those behaviors, and if not positives, they should be phrased as requests for positive and specific changes.
4. They should use process versus terminal language.
5. They should be expressed as soon after the focal behaviors as possible—so that the feedback is present-oriented.
6. They should be offered at a proper time and in a way that is most likely to be received.

Training in giving feedback can begin in the therapeutic sessions and can be the target of instigations for changes between sessions. During sessions, couples can be asked to give nonverbal feedback by smiling, nodding, or pointing the index finger at the other in response to any preferred verbal or nonverbal behaviors. This procedure can then be coupled with verbal expressions about perceived positives in the interaction, with the therapist coaching improvements in the way in which the feedback expression is phrased. Couples can then be asked to provide feedback for one another at home. During the caring-days exercise, the spouses offer feedback by writing the date on which caring behaviors were received from the partner. A written feedback mechanism can be replaced with verbal expressions as skill develops.

At the same time that couples are trained in giving feedback, however, they should also receive training in receiving it. Unfortunately, the tendency to overreact to feedback seems to be inherent, for all feedback recipients, "whether mechanical or human, have in them a tendency to overreact to stimuli" (Scheidel, 1972). This tendency can be minimized by the verbal and nonverbal structure of the feedback that is given. For example, Tom can tell June that he didn't like her blue dress but does like the red one she now has on, and by pairing a negative and a positive message in the same sentence, he creates a defensive overreaction. Or he can tell her that he likes the way she looks without looking up from his book and totally undermine the value of his message. Keeping feedback messages univalent and maintaining consistency between the manifest and the metacommunicational dimensions of the messages greatly facilitate the listener's measured response. Training the listener to answer several silently asked questions can also result in further progress toward the goal of constructive response. Although these are difficult steps to take, the listener should ask:

1. Is the message positive?
2. Is the fact that it was offered an indication that the other is concerned about what I am doing?
3. Does the message help me see how I might perform well in the future?

If the answer to these questions is positive, chances are great that reaction to the feedback information will be positive as well.

CLARIFICATION

The fifth communication skill is clarifying the message that has been received. Whenever Stan asked Ellen a question, she jutted out her chin and tightened her lips. That was a red flag for Stan because he felt that this was a sneering rejection of the wisdom of his question, and it literally brought him to violence. When Ellen saw Stan in a rage, she felt that he was being insanely insensitive to her need to take a few minutes to think before she answered his thoughtful questions. Each one thus thought that he or she shared an understanding of the situation with the other, but both were cruelly off the mark. Habermas (1970) termed this illusion of understanding "pseudocommunication." Laing et al. (1972) believe that "people are aware of being in agreement more than they are aware of being in disagreement" (p. 104) and that both disturbed and nondisturbed couples "tend to assume that they agree when they disagree" (p. 107). As suggested earlier, these pseudounderstandings can lead to bitter fights, but fortunately, they can be avoided if couples are trained in the use of clarifying responses.

Katz (1947) long ago noted that "because language is symbolic in nature, it can only evoke meaning in the recipient if the recipient has experience corresponding to the symbol" (p. 21). Disjunctures between language and experience come about when no effort is made to trace the experiential referents of words, when the listener is unable or unwilling to transcend personal experience and stereotypes to apprehend the meaning of the spoken words, and when reification and personification lead to confusion between the precept and the concept. Unfortunately, interpersonal dynamics often disrupt the process through which two people negotiate their common language, because very often the listener confuses the speaker's intention with the message actually sent. For example, Maurine told Sander that she thought they should both vote progressively in the next election. Sander heard her telling him how he must vote—her inferred intention—and started a long harangue about that without ever clarifying whether she meant the Progressive Party or felt that one of the major parties was more progressive than the others. It is the confusion of the issue of the interpersonal mandates with questions of denotative and connotative meanings that can lead to many pseudounderstandings and unnecessary disagreements.

Virtually all communication-change programs include training in these clarifying responses. Gottman *et al.* (1976a) referred to the process as "validation" (p. 17). This is the same process that the Minnesota Couples Communication Program has termed "confirming/clarifying" (Miller *et al.*, 1976). In this approach, clarification is defined in terms of its objective: to check out the meaning of the other's message until it has consensual referents. Also, in this approach, it is as important to check out the meaning of nonverbal messages as it is necessary to arrive at a shared vocabulary.

The process of training clarifying responses begins in the treatment sessions. In his or her first response to ambiguous client utterances, the therapist begins to model the search for clarification. This search ideally takes place in a two-phase process. The therapist first says, "I am not sure that I grasp your meaning. Could you express that last thought in other words?" When the client does so, the therapist then restates the understood meaning of the spoken message and asks for verification. Typically, when spouses seek clarification they omit the first step. The original speaker then feels unfairly challenged and needlessly misunderstood when his or her words are fed back incorrectly. Asking the question first expresses the listener's interest in hearing what the other has to say rather than in making a projection and setting up a straw man.

When the communication-change phase of treatment begins, the therapist can ask the couple to practice the modeled two-phase clarification process, instigating them to ask for meaning and then to restate the message received. In each such cycle, the listener should probe the speaker for additional data until he or she can accurately paraphrase (rather than simply repeat in the same words) the speaker's message. It is important to stress that it is the speaker's responsibility to encode and send the message in the manner that is truest to the intended meaning, just as it is the listener's responsibility to use empathic receptive skills. It is the responsibility of both to avoid the tendency to become hypercritical of themselves or the other, in which case they can develop competitive exchanges and inadvertently turn the skill-building exercise into a contest. Therefore, feedback must be given constantly by the therapist as a model for the clients to follow in their effort to achieve these skills for genuine understanding.

As its method for helping couples to develop skill in expression, listening, and clarification, the Marriage Encounter movement (Genovese, 1975) makes use of written letters intended to serve as the basis of daily dialogue. Each spouse is asked to write a brief 10-minute letter to the other, with both partners answering the same question in their letter. The question may be couple-generated, or it may be chosen from a list prepared by the ME sponsors. The couple are then asked to "dialogue" about their letters for 10 minutes. During this exchange, each can ask the other for clarification of meaning. The positive aspects of the approach are that it allows each to communicate with the other without interruption as the letters are written; writing lends a seriousness to the selection of words; and by having both written and spoken messages, couples have an opportunity for multisensory inputs as aids in the challenging process of arriving at a truly reciprocal understanding.

Conclusion

Practice of the skills of purposefully using both nonverbal and verbal expression of feelings and ideas can help the spouses learn about one another's desires and the success of each in fulfilling these desires. This skill is a prerequisite to the next phase of therapeutic behavior change: the negotiation of a plan for making major behavioral changes. As attention shifts to subsequent therapeutic goals, however, communication skills should not be forgotten. Indeed, they should be taught as adjuncts to each of the succeeding stages of intervention. Rather than stressing specific techniques, communication skill building should stress the handling of larger relationship issues as treatment moves along. Because these larger issues call for greater accuracy and understanding, an analysis of the flow of information is never out of place. Indeed, it often provides a profitable change of pace when thorny issues arise as a function of therapeutic progress.

C H A P T E R 8

Structuring Behavior Exchanges

WE ALL SEEK predictability in our relationships with others, and we achieve this cognitive control through formulating norms, rules, and contracts in our relationships. Norms are shared, unstated expectations about how individuals will interact. Rules formalize these expectations in words, and contracts seek to establish reciprocal balance in rule-governed exchanges. Several different levels of contract are operative in every marriage, and violation of the provisions of one or more of these levels often lies at the core of the strife that the couple experiences. In this stage of treatment, the couple are helped to formulate a "therapeutic contract" with one another. This is a formal agreement to change some of the larger patterns of interaction in their relationship. To accomplish this negotiation, couples are taught to use a two-winner bargaining strategy—one in which shared rather than individual gain is sought. They are also taught to utilize holistic agreements in which each agrees to make any of several changes while the other is expected to do the same; but in holistic contracts neither is specifically required to do any one thing, and both have the obligation to grant at least some of the requests made by the other. A specific negotiation format is then presented, with the understanding that the couple will learn the skills basic to this format, which will enable them to renegotiate their contract at various times during the ensuing years, thus allowing it to remain responsive to the changing demands of their lives together.

Norms, Rules, and Contracts in Marital Interaction

Among animals (Latane *et al.*, 1972; Sloan & Latane, 1974) and humans (Insko & Wilson, 1977; Werner & Latane, 1976), it has been found that attraction grows as a function of predictability in the actions of the other. We seem to be drawn to others when we can make reasonably accurate guesstimates about how they will respond to our actions, and we tend to withdraw from others when we are taken aback by their response to us. Without predictability we cannot see our past experience to anticipate the consequences of our actions, and we give up an important measure of potential control over our social experience and the comfort that it can convey. Norms, rules, and contracts are three successively formalized means of achieving this sought-after predictability.

NORMS

According to Thibaut and Kelley (1959), a norm exists whenever two or more people share expectations about regularities in their interaction and about acceptable forms of recourse when these expectations are not met. A norm is thus a shared understanding about who? will do what? how? and under what circumstances? Some norms originate from cultural, subcultural, and socially mediated training that begins with the first breath and ends with the last. That is, we are shaped by our cultures in everything from the way we enter the world of the living to the way we make our peace when leaving it. Other norms develop through patterns of interaction in which the actions of one become precedents for the other's expectations about how they will relate in the future. For example, Pete first met Midge by approaching her during the intermission of a theatrical presentation in the auditorium of the local college. Midge had noticed Pete and thought it would be nice to meet him, but she felt restrained from approaching him by her culturally transmitted beliefs about behaviors that are not "ladylike." Pete, for his part, felt comfortable in taking the lead, because in the culture they shared it was not only acceptable but attractive for the man to take the risk associated with a first approach. When they went out for a snack after the show, Midge took the conversational lead with a pleasing flow of humorous, good-natured small talk. They had already begun to form norms for their relationship—expectations that they would share, although these expectations would never be voiced. According to their implied pact, Pete would take the lead in structuring their interaction, and Midge would take the responsibility for making a success of the exchanges Pete initiated. Later, for example, Pete would invite friends in for a social evening, and Midge would plan the meal and the evening's entertainment.

Norms like these have great value for every social group: they regulate interaction, making it more predictable, and they lend to relationships their feeling of comfort and familiarity, so long as the norms facilitate fulfillment of the desires of all concerned. Norms also reduce the need for power manipulations to the extent that they control behavior without recourse to direct coercive attempts.

When their relationship functions smoothly, Pete and Midge both stay up late after company leaves to wash the dishes and set the house in order. This is a norm, and neither has to prompt the other to follow through. The motivation to meet this expectation stems from their identification with each other, their mutual attractiveness, and their internalization of the norm through recognizing the legitimacy of the expectation. When they do resort to prompting one another to lend a hand, they put the norm into words and thereby make it a rule.

RULES

Rules are explicit expressions of relationship norms. Pete may tell Midge that he wants to be the jokester at parties because he has a quick wit and Midge takes so long to tell a story that all lose interest in her joke long before the punch line arrives. She may agree to Pete's "life-of-the-party role" and counter with the request that Peter hum silently in church because he's tone deaf, allowing her to take the singing lead. These are rules. They may develop because unspoken normative understandings do not function smoothly, or they may develop in anticipation of a problem in an effort to prestructure a way to facilitate its smooth resolution.

The expression of rules adds a cognitive dimension to an interaction, a dimension that builds the accountability of each for his or her behavior. Failing to comply with a norm—that is, violating a precedent that has been established—may or may not generate immediate conflict, although resentment may wordlessly build over time toward an unexpected explosion. Failing to comply with rules, on the other hand, often leads to immediate rule-enforcement efforts—quicker but often more manageable conflict because the issues can be clearly stated.

There are times when formalizing interactions as rules can be a source of embarrassment or even conflict. For example, it is expected that family members will do one another favors on the assumption that the favors will later be reciprocated (R. H. Turner, 1970); directly expressing this expectation can lead to hurt feelings. For example, Midge was pleased when Pete offered to type the report that she was struggling to finish before an important meeting; but she felt deflated when he added that he would like her to have the car serviced later in the week in exchange. The problem was that she felt by putting the agreement into words, Pete had denied her the opportunity to reciprocate spontaneously, and she also felt constrained by his bid for a rule. As another example, Midge and Pete have silently agreed that she will initiate sex, but if she were to suggest as a rule that only she should signal the start of their intimacy, both she and Pete would be likely to experience on uneasy recoil. However, if either she or Pete becomes dissatisfied with the normative arrangement, rule induction would be an effective means of initiating the process of negotiation toward a more satisfying style of sexual expression.

In addition to specifying desired behaviors, norms and rules also establish the tolerable levels of deviance (J. H. Davis, 1969). For example, Pete and Midge have a norm that each will talk about social experiences with their prior loves, but not about the intimacies shared with the men and women of bygone days. In so doing, they have accepted the principle of measured honesty (see Chapter 7), which establishes a rule spelling out how much self-disclosure is too much.

CONTRACTS

When both parties accept a set of norms that provide satisfactions each desire, they develop implicit contracts or wordless agreements governing some of the ways in which each will behave toward the other. When they put these agreements into words, they fashion their rule statements into formal contracts. Whether implicit or formal, all of these relationship contracts help to stabilize interactions and make them predictable. As Stuart (1971a) has noted, these contracts also tend to contain a standard form, although their content varies greatly. That is, relationship contracts always specify patterns of reciprocal behavior in terms of either rights or privileges and obligations or responsibilities, as well as provisions for sanctions for noncompliance and bonuses for efforts made above the call of duty. Formal contracts tend most often to use the language of rights and obligations, while therapeutic and informal contracts are concerned with specifying the responsibilities that each must fulfill in order to earn desired privileges. Sanctions allow each person to deviate from an obligation or responsibility without destroying the agreement. For example, if Midge would rather go to sleep immediately than clean up after company leaves, Pete could do the job alone or he could leave the work for Midge to do the following day. The contract remains in force so long as either of these take place. By the same token, Pete could tell Midge that he is so pleased with the effort she put into making the evening a success that he alone will do the cleaning up—clearly a bonus for his deserving wife.

Formal contracts in marriage are sanctified by the state, by religious institutions, or by the couple themselves through antenuptial or postmarital agreements. Many couples find the strictures of state and religious contracts, with their stress on rights and duties or on "loving, honoring, and obeying," to be too constraining, too incomplete, or too anachronistic. For example, the formal signing of a Jewish marriage contract, or *ketubbah de 'irchesa*, specifies the 10 obligations and 4 rights of husbands (Schneid, 1973). The obligations are (1) to provide sustenance and (2) maintenance for his wife; (3) to cohabitate with his wife and (4) to make a cash settlement with her in the event of divorce: (5) to meet his wife's medical and (6) burial expenses; (7) to provide for his wife's support (8) as well as that of his daughters; (9) to meet the cost of retrieval of his wife from captivity; and (10) to name his sons as heirs in his last will and testament. His rights include (1) access to the proceeds of her handiwork; (2) ownership of any property that she finds; (3) a portion of the interest from her dowry; and (4) the right to be named as the sole heir in her last will and testament.

Many Jewish couples who do take the trouble to read the document they are asked to sign find several of these terms unacceptable, while noting the omission of others that they consider essential. For example, many couples feel the need to agree before they marry to a division of responsibility for managing their home and caring for their children, for meeting their separate career needs, and for dividing up the financial pie. These are often fashioned into individually written antenuptial contracts that can have either very strong positive or very strong negative effects. On the positive side, contracts can greatly increase the predictability of the marriage for both parties. Their negotiation can require couples to think through and discuss the handling of issues that, if confronted at times of crisis, might not be so readily resolved. The contracts can also specify the terms that will govern dissolution of the relationship, should it occur, so that each person has the freedom to leave under specified conditions and neither need feel coerced to stay. On the negative side of the ledger, Wells (1976) found that many of the clauses of these agreements are contrary to statutory or common law; he found many to be overly rigid in the provisions that they did include; and he found them often to be lacking in provisions that proved essential as the relationship unfolded. In addition, if the negotiation is coercive—that is, done in the spirit of "Agree to do the following or wave good-bye to our happy potential!"—the contract can stand as a monument to the ambivalence and lack of trust with which the couple begin their relationship, and therefore, it can create a specter that casts an ominous shadow over all of their experiences ever after. Therefore, when the couples themselves try to improve upon the lack of reality in the marital contracts framed by governors and religious leaders, their efforts have the potential for compounding rather than relieving the stress they will eventually face.

At the start of this century, Sumner (1911) noted that formal wedding contracts had little hope of successfully structuring the marital interaction:

No laws can do more than specify ways of entering into wedlock, and the rights and duties which the society will enforce. These, however, are but indifferent externals. All the intimate daily play of interests, emotions, character, taste, etc., are beyond the reach of bystanders, and their play is what makes wedlock what it is for every pair. (p. 310)

It is the implicit contracts that govern these all-important prescriptions. For example, it is understood that Tony will flirt at parties, while Pat is free to have "one too many." So long as Tony keeps his flirting at the "hands-off" level, he can expect to be free to enjoy himself, and so long as Pat does not become too "loose-mouthed" she will not be chided for her drinking. Their contract thus creates the freedom they both desire; it even creates the freedom for them to go beyond their agreed-upon levels of indulgence. For example, Pat knows that she can protest Tony's flirting at the price of his denouncing her drinking publicly. Tony knows that he can ask Pat to drink less after he has been flirting only if he is willing to risk embarrassment. Thus, the sanctions in their contracts create the freedom to violate the agreement with predictable penalties, enabling them to keep their relationship on a steady if not too happy keel.

Berne (1961) referred to these implicit agreements as "relationship contracts." He also speculated that at a very subtle level, the couple may enter into a "secret contract" that establishes the boundaries of their evolving relationship-defining agreements. As an example of such a secret agreement, when Bill and Martha were married, he was setting out on a business career and she was prepared to be a dutiful housewife. This contract worked well for 20 years, during which time Bill became a successful executive and Martha kept a beautiful home. However, Bill became bored with the business world and quit his job without notice, deciding to live the life of a ski bum for a few years. A few months later, Martha, who had let the house run down, began having an affair with a much younger man; so long as Bill was not about to maintain his executive status, she saw no reason to hold to her commitment to sexual exclusiveness. To set matters straight, Bill would have to return to the executive suite, whereupon Martha would take up her place at hearth and home.

This secret contract is believed to spawn a series of relationship agreements with "the terms being successively revised as additional facets or possibilities of the relationship become exposed in the course of interaction" (Carson, 1969, p. 188). Unfortunately, these agreements are sometimes "fraudulent" in the sense that one spouse implicitly offers the other one type of relationship, an offer the other implicitly accepts, only to have the first alter his or her stance while the other is in the act of complying, justifying this switch in light of the other's exposed and vulnerable stance. In the language of Eric Berne (1964), the bid for a contract by the first person is a "setup," the switch in midstream is termed a "coup," and the entire transaction is termed a "game." For example, early in the evening the husband might make amorous suggestions about his desire for some "kinky sex." The wife, feeling uncomfortable about the invitation but having a strong desire to establish a new level of closeness, might make a few "sexy" innuendos of her own, only to have the husband turn on her and accuse her of being immodest and grossly seductive. Berne termed this game "RAPO," and it is one of the more vengeful of the games he described. Taken together over time, a series of these gaming actions can comprise a contract between the spouses. She might know that he will manipulate her sexually, but that she will get her revenge through engineering another of Berne's games, "Now I've Got You, You Son of a Bitch." In this game, she might complain about being overwhelmed with house-work at a time when she is also under great pressure at the office. Her husband might then be seduced into offering help, only to have her turn on him and say, "Why can't you show any respect for my ability to get things done? Why do you always undermine my sense of accomplishment by doing things I don't ask you to do and then hold it up to me later?"

Agreements to exchange games in this manner have been termed "disordered interpersonal contracts" by Carson (1969, p. 195). He noted that in well-functioning relationships, the existence of contracts facili-tates exchanges in an orderly fashion that helps each spouse to achieve expected levels of satisfaction with a minimum expenditure of energy. In troubled marriages, however, either the contracts can call for coordi-nated avoidance, in which each strives to minimize intrapersonal con-flict and ambivalence by maintaining maximal interpersonal distance, or they can allow each to secure desired relationship satisfactions through ignoble means at a very great cost to the other.

Improving Behavioral Contracts

Most of the norms, rules, and contracts that govern marital interaction are both effective and constructive, much as most of the behavior of those labeled "psychotic" is actually socially appropriate. For example, the couple who exchange manipulative games manage to help each other get to work on time, to keep food in the pantry and the house heated, and to get the children dressed and ready for school on time. They even handle themselves and each other well when they are with other people. Their interaction tends to break down when they are alone and otherwise carefree, or when one commits or omits some act that has symbolic importance to the couple.

Normally, at times of stress spouses perform for each other what Nye (1976) has termed a "therapeutic role," a service that accurately predicts their level of marital satisfaction and general role effectiveness

(Nye & McLaughlin, 1976). In the therapeutic role, one asks the other questions that highlight possible remedial actions in a climate of compassion and concern. As a result, the spouse who is under stress can often plan a course of action to resolve the problem. However, when both spouses are mired in a series of disordered relationship contracts, neither is likely to be able to have the perspective, the trust, or the courage to take the action necessary to improve the quality of their relationship. At these times, therapeutic contracts can offer several important advantages.

The very existence of a therapeutic contract can help to introduce an element of good faith into the ailing relationship because, as Lempert (1972) has observed, "there is a general norm in American society that valid agreements should be kept" (p. 10). The agreements also formalize a new understanding increasing the predictability of the exchange, and they serve as reference points for the resolution of any eventual misunderstandings. By making change more immediate, they expedite a return in expected levels of relationship-mediated satisfactions, and because they are explicit and open to review, they tend to be more equitable than less formalized agreements. Finally, the very fact that each partner is willing to make these commitments signals to the other that commitment to the maintenance of the relationship is at least tolerably strong.

Orientations to Contract Negotiation

These contracts can be negotiated through either of two strategies, and they can conform to either of two formal models. One negotiation strategy stresses a *"one-winner"* approach, in which both partners take hard positions and make few concessions (Siegel & Fouraker, 1960). Researchers like Komorita and Brenner (1968) have offered some support for this position with their data, which show that those who make early concessions tend to lose out in the bargaining process. Therefore, the one-winner bargainer starts with a hard position, concedes little, and strives for the greatest possible level of personal gain. The *"two-winner"* approach (Nierenberg, 1968) uses an "integrative bargaining" (Lewis & Pruitt, 1971) strategy, which often involves the "graduated reciprocation" recommended by Osgood (1959, 1962). This approach is based on the assumptions that both parties know in advance the nature of the ultimate agreement (Schelling, 1963; Stuart *et al.*, 1976), that this expected outcome is just (Homans, 1961) or equitable (Adams, 1965), and that both recognize the potential relationship costs of a personally damaging negotiation or an imbalanced outcome which could create a "relationship debt" that must be redressed at a later time. Thus, Hamner (1974) noted:

While the tougher bargainer has the potential of making a higher profit than his opponent, he runs the risk of extinguishing his opponent's conciliatory behavior and not reaching an agreement. It can then be argued that a strategy that is mutually rewarding proves superior in the long run to a strategy that has as its goal the maximization of individual profit. (p. 466)

While the two-winner negotiation model is most desirable, most distressed couples enter treatment with a highly practiced one-winner model foremost in their repertoire. Through weeks, months, or years of frustrated optimism, couples often turn from trust in reciprocated exchanges to the feeling that each must see to his or her personal desires first if they are to be fulfilled at all. Distressed couples also have a tendency to preface their requests for change with indictments for past wrongs: "You have always been self-centered and lazy; will you now try to demonstrate that you care for me by waking up and having coffee with me in the morning?" is the way in which distressed partners might request an affectionate moment. Phrasing a request this way is almost certain to guarantee its denial. Strangely, however, this background may not be all bad. Wilson (1969) has shown that when bargainers begin with hard demands and later soften their requests, they are more likely to achieve success than are those who begin with a soft-sell approach. Among distressed couples, the prior aversive ground may heighten the appeal of the present constructive request and thereby increase the probability that it will be granted. Finally, it should be kept in mind that even nonclinic couples have been shown to choose among three modes of interaction (Feldman & Rand, 1965). Sometimes each puts his or her needs first in an egocentric mode; sometimes each puts the other's needs first in an altercentric mode; and sometimes they seek shared gains from the start in a cocentric bargaining mode. Thus, the starting one-winner orientation of distressed couples is not their unique behavior; they differ from other couples primarily in the extent to which they operate in this mode.

Couples can be taught to identify their orientation through a pencil-and-paper exercise, and they can be taught to monitor their actual bargaining behavior through a personal editing process. To classify the orientation, each can be asked to draw three circles on a sheet of paper, labeling one "My Gain," another "My Mate's Gain," and the third "Our Gain." When they begin to negotiate change in a relationship pattern, each request should be noted in at least two circles. For example, Jane might want to buy symphony tickets (her gain) but may also be willing to go to Saturday afternoon football games with Sam (his gain). Her request would then be that they both attend symphonies and football games. Sam might want to buy a sports car and stresses the fact that they will both enjoy its use; but he knows Jane is a ski enthusiast and that she would find it impossible to pile ski buddies and equipment into a small two-seater. Sam would put the sports car in the "My Gain" circle and would have to find something to offer Jane to balance out his request. Through this method, which they can do privately or together, each person can gain an understanding of his or her negotiation orientation by estimating the probable payoffs of success.

Once the negotiation process begins, both partners will have to utilize the communication skills described in Chapter 7. To these should be added a "request–feedback–edit" function. Accordingly, after one spouse makes a request, he or she asks the other for feedback about the message that was received. Sam asks Jane to clean up the darkroom they both share and then asks her what she heard. She might have heard an indictment of her sloppiness, a criticism of the fact that they both share the darkroom that was originally Sam's private domain, or a statement that he's the photographer and she's the darkroom slave; or she might hear the simple request that she do her share of the work. She feeds back to Sam what she heard, and Sam can edit the exchange by restating his desire in the simple terms in which it was originally expressed, thus reassuring Jane, clearing the air, and preparing her to hear his request. Of course the dangers in this exchange are that Jane will not own up to what she thinks she heard but will react as though the expected words were spoken; or that if she does bite the bullet and express what she feels, Sam might feel called upon not merely to restate his request but rather to defend himself, or, worse yet, to counterattack because of Jane's response. Therefore, the feedback–edit clarification of request behavior should begin in the therapist's office—with strong coaching—before it is practiced in the riskier environment of the home.

Selecting a Suitable Contract Model

Just as there is a choice of negotiation strategies, so, too, is there a choice between contract models. A "partitive" agreement is a tit-for-tat or *quid pro quo* agreement in which the partners agree to exchange one specified behavior for another equally specified action. In contrast, a "holistic agreement" is one in which several behaviors by one are exchanged for several by the other, with no requirement that the offerings by one exactly match those of the other (Erickson *et al.*, 1974). There are advantages and disadvantages to both approaches. The partitive agreement offers a level of predictability and precise control not gained through holistic agreements. This predictability may be just what the doctor ordered for distressed couples who must work hard to regain this predictive power in order to renew their trust in their relationship. Moreover, there is good reason to believe that such exchanges are quite effective (e.g., Esser & Komorita, 1975; Turner *et al.*, 1971).

However, Jacobson (1978) found that this form of the contract did not predict treatment outcome as Weiss *et al.* (1974) suggested, and that tit-for-tat agreements give doomsday control to both partners, who can, through noncompliance with a specific obligation, seriously undermine the agreement. (Also see Tsoi-Hoshmand, 1975.) Moreover, some have argued that such agreements also weaken the marital commitment by creating inappropriate expectations. For example, Stapleton *et al.* (1973) believe that attraction to another is based upon attributing benevolent motives to that person. To the extent that one sees the other as acting for personal gain, attraction is weakened. This weakening might result from the utilization of a *quid pro quo* agreement, in which each believes that the other offers positive behaviors solely because of their expected return. Moreover, Heider (1958) also believed that one person will depreciate the value of the things received from another if it is believed that these things are one's due—a likely outcome in partitive contracts. In addition, the expectation of immediate reciprocation can also weigh heavily on interest in the marriage. Murstein *et al.* (1977) asked subjects to indicate their agreement with statements like "If I do dishes three times a week, I expect my spouse to do them three times a week." They found that agreement with items like these was negatively correlated with marital satisfaction, suggesting that a *quid pro quo* expectancy may be contraindicated with regard to marital success.

Holistic agreements, on the other hand, are less precise but do offer the advantages of preserving at least the illusion of altruism. They may also be more natural in that it may be more convenient for spouses to do certain things as opposed to others for each other at different times. Holistic agreements offer each person a range of constructive choices, any one of which can satisfy their reciprocal obligations. Finally, the use of holistic agreements also creates an expectation of less immediate reciprocation, which may increase the likelihood that reciprocation will occur.

Figures 1A and 1B provide illustrations of partitive and holistic marital contracts. Notice that there is no time sequence implied in the partitive agreement because neither person is expected to make a change until *after* the other has acted. In contrast, the holistic contract sets a time frame and asks each to act *before* the other. Notice, too, that in the partitive contract, either Sam or Jane can prevent relationship movement from getting started merely by not granting any of the other's requests. Because one or the other is likely to have more ambivalence about and less commitment to change in their marriage, the more reluctant spouse thus has doomsday control over the contract through simple noncompliance. With the holistic contract, on the other hand, either person can initiate the change process; because one is more likely to have confidence in and be committed to the relationship, one partner

Figure 1A. A partitive therapeutic marital contract.

Sam will wash the dishes . . .	when Jane has prepared dinner on time.
Sam will mow the lawn . . .	when Jane has weeded the rose garden.
Sam will initiate lovemaking . . .	if Jane takes a bath and comes to bed before 10:30 P.M.
Sam will visit Jane's parents with her . . .	if Jane accompanies him on a fishing trip.

Figure 1B. A holistic therapeutic marital contract.

It is understood that Jane would like Sam to:	It is also understood that Sam would like Jane to:
wash the dishes;	have dinner ready by 6:30 nightly;
mow the lawn;	weed the rose garden;
initiate lovemaking;	bathe every night and come to bed by 10:30;
take responsibility for balancing their checkbooks;	call him at the office daily;
invite his business partners for dinner once every six or eight weeks;	plan an evening out alone for both of them at least once every two weeks;
meet him at his store for lunch at least once a week.	offer to drive the children to their soccer practice and swim meets;
	accompany him on occasional fishing trips.

It is expected that Sam and Jane will each do as many of the things requested by the other as is comfortably manageable, ideally at least three or four times weekly.

will probably take this constructive, assertive action. Moreover, once either spouse has made a positive investment in the relationship, the quality of the interaction is likely to change, and the other may be drawn into the restorative routine. Finally, it is also important to note that partitive agreements tend to be narrow and holistic agreements more expansive; the former offer fewer change options, while the latter offer more such opportunities. Thus, Sam is permitted to demonstrate his commitment to change during weeks when he doesn't have the least inclination to mow the lawn, while Jane can do the same despite the fact that she is too busy with work even to think about laying a sumptuous spread before Sam's partners. As with the sanction clauses that permit partners to keep their agreements intact despite their temporary wish to not comply, the range of choices and the softer expectations of holistic contracts make these agreements a great deal more realistic and therefore more likely to achieve the expected result.

Helping Couples Negotiate Therapeutic Marital Contracts

Given the pairs of choices outlined above, it should be clear that the best therapeutic, marriage-enhancing contracts are those negotiated through the two-winner strategy and those that are holistic in form. Given the fact that every marriage is always a norm- and/or rule-governed relationship, and the fact that formal and implicit contracts give every relationship its unique, stable character as well as creating the freedom through predictability that every person needs, couples must be skilled in negotiating these agreements on their own. Indeed, marriage has been described as "a negotiation that never ends" (Karrass, 1970, p. 213).

The agreements described here have been labeled "therapeutic marital contracts" for a very important reason. Many couples hesitate to formalize their relationship through explicit contracts, some because they feel that these agreements take the spontaneity out of their marriage, others because they would prefer to avoid a situation in which they are formally expected to change. By terming these "therapeutic" agreements, the couple can be helped to view this as no more than a transitional step—a "behavioral prosthesis," as discussed in Chapter 5. Thus, they can be helped to approach this process as an exercise that will help them formalize now a process that will occur spontaneously after it has gained strength in their repertoires. In addition, formal identification of the role of the therapist in the agreement can help each to have a bit more trust that the other will follow through. Trust is fundamental to honest negotiation (Erickson et al., 1974), for neither person will make concessions without believing that the other will reciprocate. The fact that the therapist will help the partners monitor their evolving agreement may contribute enough to the aura of trust in the agreement to permit both to venture to reach agreement and then to make the desired changes.

It is important for the couple to view these therapeutic marital contracts as evolving agreements, much as they recognize that their lists of caring-days behaviors must continue to grow. In the context of family- and school-oriented services for delinquents, Stuart and his associates have found that about half of those served received only a single contract, 32.4% negotiated two contracts, and 17.6% negotiated three or more contracts during the course of their time-limited therapy (Stuart & Lott, 1972), with this contracting procedure alone contributing to a significant level of change in the behavior of both parents and their labeled adolescent children (Stuart et al., 1976).

To realize these gains, several steps should be followed.

1. *Each partner should be asked to list his or her positive and specific requests for change in the behavior of the other.* The key words in this requirement are "positive," "specific," and "behavior." The contracts seek action, not nonaction; therefore, only positive change is relevant. The contracts seek immediate change, which is possible only when instructions are clear and targets specified; and the contracts seek measurable change that can be found in actions, not attitudes. Finally, while the caring-days exchange list calls for small, high-frequency behaviors that are *not* the subject of conflict, the behaviors listed in therapeutic marital contracts can be larger, lower-rate actions over which the spouses may have had disagreements in the past. The justification for these changes is found in the fact that couples will have experienced an increased commitment to their marriage and will have learned that changed feelings can result from changed behavior through their success with caring days. They will also have learned how to frame and to clarify self-statements through successful completion of the communication-change exercises. Both of these sets of skills can be expected to aid them in rising to the challenge of the exchange of more complex behaviors through these therapeutic agreements.

2. *Both spouses should be asked to rephrase the other's request to clarify their meaning.* During this clarification process, couples can be trained in asking the "What do you mean?" "When do you want it to happen?" and "How would you like it done?" questions that can give them a true understanding of one another's wishes. In addition to the "feedback-edit" skill mentioned above, this is a second communication-change technique that is introduced during the process of building new behavioral exchanges.

3. *The couple should be asked to write their requests in the form of a holistic contract.* This procedure will give them the experience of building some accountability into their reciprocated requests for change.

4. *The couple should then be asked to put the contract into action, making note of their own and the other's efforts to abide by its terms.* Just as with the caring-days exercise, there are several ways in which the couple can be encouraged to act on their new agreement! They may be asked to take the agreement as a whole and to spontaneously offer each other as many of the items as they wish, or they may be asked to commit themselves at the start of each week to comply with at least a selected number of the other's requests. Then they can be asked to rely upon verbal or written acknowledgment.

Renegotiation of the contract can be an ongoing process; either person should feel free to add requests, and as neither is under any obligation to grant any of the requests already on the list, those that were made first need not be removed because they can provide valuable options later on.

Conclusions

We live in a contractual culture in which explicit agreements structure many different relationships. For example, we sign a contract when we borrow money through the use of our credit cards, when we order materials from book or record clubs, or when we pledge money to our favorite church or other charity. We enter informal contracts when we seek professional services, when we enter universities, or when we take our cars in for repairs. Normative contracts govern every interaction that we have with others, whether they are the drivers of the taxis in which we ride, strangers we meet at an elevator door, or friends we have known for years. We depend upon these contracts to clarify expectations in our relationships with others and to offer some guarantee that our investments will be reciprocated in some way at some time. Marriage is a multicontractual relationship: at least one of the contracts is formal, and implicit contracts exist at many different levels.

One way to understand relationship breakdown is to construe it as a consequence of violations of the expectations embodied in some of these many contracts. Therefore, therapeutic contracting is one means of restructuring relationships. When these contracts are negotiated through the use of a two-winner orientation, both spouses can be helped to restate and to reinforce their own investments in seeing the relationship improve. When the contracts are holistic in form, they can provide the foundation for a realistic exchange of new behaviors, a process of exchange that can grow with the relationship. And when the contracts are mediated by the therapist, their negotiation can be a skill-building process, and the activity of the therapist can help each to build the trust needed to make the promises explicit in the contracts a relationship reality.

Couples should be encouraged both to begin and to build upon a therapeutic marriage contract, living according to its terms for at least two weeks before moving on to the next stage of treatment—the development of a framework for allocating decision-making authority and development of the skills needed for problem solving. Once they have built commitment into their marriage through caring days, have acquired communication skills both as a focal effort and as an adjunct to contract negotiation, and have developed the capacity to negotiate changes in important marital behaviors, they will indeed be ready to negotiate the larger means through which they can plan and follow through on strategies for coping with challenges as they arise within their marriage or in their dealings with the outside world.

C H A P T E R 9

Allocating the Authority to Make Decisions

T HE CHANGING situational demands of daily living, the evolution of our bodies and ourselves, and the shifts in cultural patterns and values all call for kaleidoscopic adaptations by partners in successful marriages. It is simply not possible to sustain on their 10th anniversary the same strategies for coping with most areas of their functioning that the couple negotiated during their honeymoon. Therefore, every couple must have in their kit of survival skills the ability to make decisions constructively and efficiently. This chapter offers a framework for helping couples determine how to allocate the authority for decision making in important individual and shared areas and then how to negotiate means of meeting challenges that arise within that framework. This is one major technique introduced during intervention in order to help couples sustain gains when treatment ends; for in learning how to make decisions, they are helped to acquire the skills to process issues alone, but as though they had the aid of a sensitive therapist.

This chapter begins with the recognition that the marriage and family literature has yet to produce a generally accepted measure of social power. However, while social scientists may still be struggling to find measures with adequate reliability and validity, families must continue to apply power in their efforts to achieve satisfactory outcomes to the problems they face. It is suggested here that power is a process rather than a static property, and that it has varied bases and changes over time. The "powergram" procedure suggested herein is one means of helping the partners identify how their power is currently distributed, how each would like the distribution to be changed, and, most importantly, how they agree that it will be changed. While the literature touts the virtue of equal power distribution, many couples in fact operate with an equitable but by no means equal allocation of their decision-making influence. The chapter then concludes with an analysis of the requisites for effective problem-solving discussion, a taxonomy of the techniques used to subvert this discussion, and a method for establishing better techniques for managing these frequent and quintessential exchanges.

Barbara and Alan both work. Their son, Billy, cut his knee in a gym accident at school and must go to the hospital to get the knee stitched. Should Barbara or Alan leave work to get Billy the care he needs?

Barbara has been offered a job in another city and she would like to move; but Alan is two years away from finishing graduate school, and a move would undermine his new career goals. Should they move or stay where they are?

Alan's rich uncle just died and left the couple $5000. Barbara would like to use the money to buy a new car, while Alan would like to invest in common stock. How will they decide how to use the money?

These are some of the larger decisions that couples may face in any year of their lives together. They also face dozens of smaller decisions, like who should shop for food? take out the garbage? decide whether the TV should be left on or turned off when one is interested in the program and the other is tired? Literally scores of decisions like these are made every day by every couple, sometimes with greater friction and sometimes with the smoothness of a well-oiled machine.

Conflict arises from decision making when both parties seek maximum personal gain and when the partners lack rules for resolving these major and lesser issues of their shared lives. Broderick (1975) believes that every family must have rules for distributing resources—from money to closet space. He believes that two other and more far-reaching sets of rules are also necessary: a set of rules for allocating decision-making authority and a set of rules for the use of equity- or coercion-oriented bargaining strategies when conflicts of interest arise. Virtually all distressed couples have much to gain from developing a set of rules for allocating the authority to make decisions and by identifying a mutually acceptable strategy for decision making. After a review of the nature of power in couples, this chapter presents methods for helping couples to allocate authority and make decisions effectively.

The Nature, Measurement, Sources, Constraints, and Uses of Power

Many social scientists agree with Veroff and Feld (1970) in their observation that "power problems in decision making are an essential element in all interpersonal interactions [and] they seem particularly unavoidable in American marriages" (p. 302). While some of the sources of power are beyond therapeutic influence, others can be strongly influenced by treatment-induced interaction change. An understanding of the nature, measurement, sources, constraints, and uses of power is basic to the planning of treatment aimed at redirecting the influence process within the marriages of distressed couples.

DEFINITION OF "POWER"

Most reviews of the concept of social power generally agree (e.g., W. D. Jacobson, 1972; Rollins & Bahr, 1976; Smith, 1970) that "power" refers to the ability of one person to change the probability of another person's behavior (e.g., Bannester, 1969; Cartwright, 1959; Emerson, 1962; Nagel, 1968; M. F. Rogers, 1974). Power in this sense is a property of a dyadic relationship and not a static characteristic of one of the actors; when no relationship exists, no power is possible. Thus, an understanding of power requires an assessment of the control efforts of one and the supportive responses or countercontrol efforts of the other (Schuham, 1970; Straus, 1964).

Because every social interaction can be viewed as the coordination of efforts by two or more people to influence the attainment of their goals, and because the "clout" that underlies each influence attempt is social power, the study of social power is as basic to social science as the study of energy is basic to physical science (Russell, 1938) and the study of force to the science of motion (March, 1955).

Whenever social groups form, people inevitably seek to channel the course of the interaction along personally selected lines (Mills, 1953). To avoid chaos, every social system, including the family, must develop rules for channeling the direction and manner of these influence attempts (Scanzoni, 1970). Indeed, every effectively functioning social organization has a definite power structure (Gilman, 1962; Smith & Tannenbaum, 1963; Williams et al., 1959). In families, the centralization and legitimation of authority is a necessary precursor to successful problem solving (Tallman, 1970), to maintaining an adequate definition of spousal (Parsons, 1949) and parental (Smith, 1970) roles, and to the containment of conflict (see Chapter 10). In every subcultural community, norms for balancing power between spouses and within families are widely understood. Between any pair of family members, however, these norms may serve as the starting point for a negotiation of influence patterns, with the outcome being an agreement that is unique to the couple. Where there is inconsistency, the normative standard always gives way to the idiographic standards developed by family members (Bott, 1957; Tallman, 1970), but when the influence patterns have not been established, both marital (e.g., Jacob *et al.*, 1978; Veroff & Feld, 1970) and family (e.g., Murrell & Stachowiak, 1967; Ferreira & Winter, 1965, 1966) functioning can be adversely affected.

MEASUREMENT OF POWER

Before going on to analyze the use, constraints, and distribution of power in couples, it is important to note the many problems that remain unsolved in the measurement of power. Whether it is because of the vast complexity of the social influence process or because many people have a tendency to deny their exercise of power as if out of embarrassment (Sampson, 1968), most of the conclusions reached about power operation and distribution are based upon very tenuous data bases.

Most studies of family power are based upon self-report, although some researchers make inferences about power from observation of the process and outcome of decision making. Among the self-report measures are the efforts of Blood and Wolfe (1960) to obtain answers to the question "Who usually makes the decisions in . . ." eight different areas of decision making; Heer's (1962) effort to learn from spouses who usually wins arguments; and Kenkel's (1957) attempt to learn how spouses think they should spend $300. Among the process measures, Mishler and Waxler (1968) inferred relative power from the number of times that each spouse interrupted the other; Straus and Tallman (1971) inferred power from couples' influence attempts during their "SINFAM" game; and Olson (1969) inferred power from observation of the outcome of couples' efforts to reach decisions in which their gains were unequal.

Unfortunately, there is little agreement between these two clusters of measures (e.g., Hadley & Jacob, 1973; Kenkel, 1957; Olson & Cromwell, 1975; Rollins & Bahr, 1976; Turk & Bell, 1972). For example, in one series of studies (Olson, 1972; Olson & Rabunsky, 1972), when couples were asked who should prevail in a decision (normative power), who would prevail (predictive power), and who did prevail (retrospective power), their answers correlated quite weakly with the actual result of their bargaining (outcome power). Earlier, Hill (1965) had asked some 300 families spanning three generations to classify their bases of decision making as husband-centered, egalitarian, or wife-centered. While some 16% of the couples felt that the husbands dominated their decision making, observers felt that over 32% fell into that category. For egalitarian and wife-dominated patterns, the pair of spousal and observer scores were 77% versus 46% and 7% versus 28%, respectively. Thus, while most couples believed their interaction to be egalitarian, many behaved otherwise.

Because of these common patterns of inconsistency, the multitrait-multimethod (Campbell & Fiske, 1959) is the only acceptable approach to measuring spousal or family power (Cromwell *et al.*, 1975; Douglas & Wind, 1978). This method approaches the assessment of power from various perspectives, such as the outcome of decision making and the partners' beliefs about who holds decision-making power, at the same time taking into account generalized patterns of power allocation and the way in which these general patterns can be affected by special situations. The measurement package should include some self-report measures, both because what couples think they are doing may have a greater impact on their marital satisfaction than what they actually do (see Chapter 4) and because self-report measures are comparatively inexpensive and highly flexible. When they are used, it should be remembered that couples can be more reliable in discussing specific tasks like taking out the trash than more general interactions like their discussion of who decided who would take out the trash (Burchinal & Bauder, 1965; Douglas & Wind, 1978; Granbois & Willet, 1970; Larson, 1974; Olson & Rabunsky, 1972). The reliability of self-report measures can also be improved by clustering related items (Douglas & Wind, 1978) and possibly by allowing couples to weigh items according to their perceived importance (Price-Bonham, 1976). For example, the wife may not consider the number of hours that her husband works nearly as important as her own choice of jobs. Therefore, she might assign a "significance level" of only 2 on a scale of 10 to his work hours, while assigning an 8 to her own job choice. Presumably, she will then be more willing to concede authority on his working hours than on her job choice. The measurement package should also include observational items, because what the couple is seen actually to do assures a certain level of validity to inferences about their relative power. Indeed, all therapists observe clients' interactions during sessions and use these data to construct models of the couple's interaction. These observations may, however, be subject to observer bias, and couples may adjust their normal patterns in response to their beliefs about the observer's expectations (see Chapter 4). The interests of reliable and valid judgments can perhaps best be served by averaging over a combination of self-report and observational data. Any conclusions that are reached, however, must be tempered by a realization that our knowledge about marital and family power is at best in a "Preparadigmatic stage of development" (Sprey, 1975, p. 61) and may remain so for many years because of the vast complexity of the questions: Who decides? Who decides each issue? For what reasons? (See Haley, 1963a; Sprey, 1972.)

Several different bases of power have been identified in the social-psychological literature (Centers *et al.,* 1971; French & Raven, 1959; Gillespie, 1971; Harsanyi, 1962; W. D. Jacobson, 1972). Among the various sources of power that have been identified are the following:

1. Legitimate power, which derives from laws or norms that suggest a status of role occupant should have greater decision-making influence.
2. Expert power, which derives from agreement among others that one person has greater skill in a given area and is likely to guide the group to the wisest decision.
3. Referent power, which derives from the feeling that two or more people are members of the same social group and should be influenced by one another.
4. Coercive power, which stems from the belief by one that the other will punish noncompliance.
5. Reward power, which stems from the belief by one that the other will reward compliance.

A critical dimension in each of these power bases is acceptance by one of the other's status, in the case of legitimate, expert, and referent power; or the other's willingness to use the punishment and reward resources that are available. The latter factor has been termed the "subjective expected utility" (Pollard & Mitchell, 1972; Tedeschi *et al.,* 1972) associated with punishment and reward, that is, the belief by one concerning the other's estimate of the potential gains and losses from using either punishment or reward strategies. All of these sources of power are thus dependent upon acceptance of the definitional power of the person in the one-up position by the person who is then one down.

Three other sources of power should also be mentioned. One person can gain power in decision making by managing the flow of information. Open influence through the persuasive use of warnings and mendacious and manipulative influence through managing cues for action and feedback about action outcomes are highly effective ways of building one's power through the control of information (Tedeschi *et al.,* 1972). One can also gain power through simply talking more than anyone else. Several researchers (e.g., Feldman & Rand, 1965; French & Snyder, 1959; Mack, 1974; Strodtbeck, 1954) have found that group decisions tend to accord with the thrust of the person who dominates the discussion. Finally, power can also be gained in a relationship simply by virtue of one person's being more and the other less committed to the maintenance of the relationship. This is the effect of the operation of the "principle of least loss" discussed in Chapter 4. Power in this sense stems from the fact that one person is in a position to mediate greater rewards than the other, and therefore, the former exercises greater resource control than the latter. However, it is the balance of the potential reward capacity rather than the absolute value of the rewards themselves that accounts for this eighth source of influence within marriages.

The strength of power deriving from each of these sources—that is, its ability to overcome resistance and obtain compliance—is naturally variable among couples, areas of decision making, and stages of the relationship. When commitment levels are high, referent power can be expected to be strong. When the problem at issue is one of adjusting to some external demand, the ability to supply information builds the power of its possessor. When the principle of least loss operates to build the power of one person, coercive strategies are more likely to be effective; but when power is equally balanced, reward power is likely to be more potent. Finally, in settings in which ties to extended families and norm-setting reference groups are strong, legitimate power is likely to hold sway.

Independent of source and setting, researchers have developed a set of axioms about the use of power (see, for example, Emerson, 1962; W. D. Jacobson, 1972; Nagel, 1968; Pollard & Mitchell, 1972; Tedeschi, 1972):

1. *Power is the property of social relationships, not of people.*
2. *One will accede to the power of the other only if the former believes that his or her goals will be better served by accession than by resistance.*
3. *Power is always relative.* Because the exercise of power by one requires the compliance of the other, each has some measure of reciprocal control over the other; therefore, power is always relative and never absolute.
4. Because power is relative, *it is always transitory.* Situations change, and the weaker of the pair can later become the stronger. For example, parents have greater control over their young children than they will have when those children grow to become adults. As the parents age, their adult children often gain the more powerful position.
5. *Power is usable only to the extent that its use does not penalize its possessor.* For example, Sam is much stronger than Alice. He does not want her to flirt at parties. He has the ability to carry her bodily out of the house if he believes she is flirting, but the social cost to him of so doing can be exorbitant.

There are two corollaries to this fifth axiom. First, that power is always greatest which requires the least effort to exercise. For example, if Sam does try to carry Alice from the party, one can question whether he or she has exercised greater power. He has removed her from the party, but she has set the occasion for his displaying violence in public. Second, it is clear that the exercise of power is never without its costs. Every influence attempt elicits in the other at least a small measure of resistance, and when resistance is strong enough, countercontrol and/ or counteraggression is likely to result. The urge to resist is likely to be smaller when the influence strategy is through positive reinforcement (Cartwright, 1959; Kelley, 1965; Komorita et al., 1968). But even positive reinforcements may have costs reflected in diminished attraction for the relationship experienced by the other (Aronson & Linder, 1965; Gergen, 1969) and loss of the opportunity to use the same reinforcer as a consequence for other target behaviors.

The use of negative influence strategies generally incurs costs greater than those following from mediating reinforcements, although Tinker (1973) found:

> High attempted dominance caused negative–hostile interaction, irrespective of the sex of the dominating spouse. Moderate attempted dominance, on the other hand, did not cause an increase in negative–hostile interaction. (p. 418)

The use of negative influence strategies was found by Raven et al. (1975) to be half as effective as the use of positive methods of influence, with 10% as opposed to 20% of the subjects reporting that they complied with negative and positive maneuvers, respectively; but both of these lagged far behind the 47% who responded to legitimate power, 54% to expert power, and 55% to referent power. This finding suggests that any time the exercise of power requires additional interactional behaviors, it may be less successful than the effortless power that inheres in the relationship between the two parties—that which results from respect for the role of the other, his or her competence, and commitment to the relationship unit.

The use of coercive power has additional costs as well. First, it is rather poor modeling for children, likely to weaken their attraction to the family, and may give rise to their reflexive and operant aggressive reactions (Bandura & Walters, 1963; M. L. Hoffman, 1960). Next, it requires close monitoring of the other's behaviors, which is a great relationship cost (Baldwin, 1971). When positive influence is used, the other is likely to report relevant behavior in order to receive reinforcement. However, when negative influence is used, the other is likely to hide relevant behavior in order to avoid punishment. The detection of relevant events is thus far more effortless in reward as opposed to coercion conditions. Finally, exercise of negative power can undermine enjoyment of the relationship by the person in the one-up position just as readily as it can adversely affect the commitment of the person who is one down. Kipnis (1972) suggested the following probable chain of reactions:

(a) With the control of power goes increased temptations to influence the other's behavior. (b) As actual influence attempts increase, there arises the belief that the behavior of others is not self-controlled, but is caused by the power-holder, (c) hence, a devaluation in their performance. In addition, with increased influence attempts, forces are generated with the more powerful to (d) increase psychological distance from the less powerful and view them as objects of manipulation. (p. 40)

In other words, the deference shown by the less powerful person can be viewed as a sign of weakness by the more powerful (Sampson, 1965), and therefore, the successful exercise of coercive power can actually weaken the appeal of the relationship to both parties—a very great cost.

In summary, it is clear that just as one cannot not communicate, and one cannot not behave, one cannot interact with another and not exercise some measure of power in an unavoidable effort to manage the flow of events. The power that results naturally from the appeal of the relationship is both stronger and involves less cost than power that requires the exercise of specific maneuvers. The former power, which grows from norms, competence, and attraction to the relationship, may be termed "ascribed" power, while the latter, which results from specific actions, may be termed "active" power. It is clear that the use of ascribed power is more efficient and cost-free than the use of active power. Following a description of the ways in which power seems to be distributed in contemporary marriages, a program will be presented for building legitimate power bases within the marriage and for applying this power to successful problem-solving.

The Balance of Power in Modern Marriages

While many commentators (e.g., Bell, 1963; Blood, 1969; Corrales, 1975; Kolb & Straus, 1974; Mack, 1974; Udry, 1974) have stressed the belief that most American families subscribe to the egalitarian ideal, others have argued that egalitarianism in marriage is far more a goal than a reality. For example, Gillespie (1971) believes:

The egalitarian marriage as a norm is a myth. Under some conditions, individual women can gain power vis-à-vis their husbands, but more power is not equal power. Equal power women will not get as long as the present socioeconomic system remains. (p. 147)

Goode (1970) also believes that an "unequivocally egalitarian family is rarely to be found [because] when the husband tries to dominate he can still do so" (p. 70). While some important strides have been made toward building women's power, cultural attitudes still favor male dominance in many situations.

Egalitarianism is a desirable goal for couples. It is an arrangement in which partners agree on how decisions should be made so that the exercise of power is unnecessary (Sprey, 1975). Therefore, both those who would wield and those who would be influenced by power are spared its ill effects. For example, Veroff and Feld (1970) believe that the wives in egalitarian marriages "have the possibility of influence 'without stimulating fear of weakness'" (p. 109), while husbands have the freedom to yield power without feeling compromised.

Concern about egalitarianism or its absence has generated considerable rhetoric, much of which may be unnecessary. If egalitarianism is taken to mean "absolute equality," then husbands and wives must open every decision to negotiation and possible dispute. Every decision, no matter how minor, would then be a potential stimulus for conflict, and it would be all but impossible to complete smoothly the business of daily living. On the other hand, if egalitarianism is understood to mean "relative equality" or "equitable parity" in decision making, then each spouse could claim authority in areas of his or her particular interest or expertise, while sharing those of common concern in an effort to facilitate the flow of events in marital life. Indeed, as was stressed in Chapter 4, the major issue in marital satisfaction may be less the objective facts of the matter than the comfort with which both spouses adjust to the reality of their lives together, such as they are.

In point of fact, couples have developed many of the options for the distribution of power that theorists like Emerson (1962) and Wrong (1968) have deemed possible. The husband may be vested with the independent authority to make some decisions, or he may be vested with the authority to make decisions in one or more areas after consulting his wife. The couple may agree to share in some decisions equally; they may vest the wife with the authority to make certain decisions with or without consultation with her husband. When couples believe that the husband or wife acts with relative independence of the other, they classify their decision-making basis as either husband- or wife-centered. However, if consultation or mutual decision making is their norm, their power balance can be classified as more-or-less egalitarian.

Table 1 summarizes the data on couples' self-reports of their decision-making patterns as observed in six different studies. In four of the studies, the couples believed themselves to be strongly committed to egalitarianism. Included in this group are two subsets of couples that Blood and Wolfe (1960) and Centers et al. (1971) termed "syncretic" because they shared power about equally and "autonomic" because they had approximately equal power in nonoverlapping areas.

Several factors may have contributed to the different conclusions reached in these six studies. Data were collected by different means, in different places, and at different moments during a time of rapidly

Table 1. Balance of decision-making power in selected studies

	Husband-controlled decision making	More-or-less egalitarian decision making	Wife-controlled decision making
Blood & Wolfe (1960) (modified according to Centers et al., 1971)	9	84	5
Komarovsky (1961)	45	27	21
Hill (1965) ("married-child" self-report data only)	15	80	5
Safilios-Rothschild (1969)	41	27	32
Centers et al. (1971)	25	72	3
Osmond & Martin (1978)	27	61	12

changing social values; any of these factors could explain the range of findings that were reported. These studies also drew upon populations with differing characteristics, and a number of different demographic factors have been found to predict differential power. Males, as has been said, have been found to have greater influence in marital decision-making than females (Kenkel, 1957), perhaps because they are more likely than females to be accorded expert power (Raven *et al.*, 1975). Males are also more likely to have higher levels of education, which build marital influence (Johannis & Rollins, 1959), and higher-status jobs, which have the same effect (Blood & Wolfe, 1960; Komarovsky, 1961). Perhaps because of the operation of the principle of least loss (see Chapter 4), husbands also become vested with greater power as the number of children increases. On the other hand, employment by the wife often increases her power (Blood & Hamblin, 1958; Heer, 1958; M. L. Hoffman, 1960; Middleton & Putney, 1960; Scanzoni, 1970), which seems to rise consistently over the longer term of the marriage (Hill, 1965). Finally, all of these sources of influence are tempered by social class (Blood & Wolfe, 1960; Komarovsky, 1961; Mack, 1974; Olson, 1969; Udry, 1974), with the importance of the wife's work as a source of power being different among lower- and middle-class families as but one example.

Note that in every set of comparisons more couples reported husband-centered than wife-centered decision-making patterns. Lewis (1972) found that many wives in the group he studied wished to have more authority, and at the same time, many husbands wished to have *less*. One factor that may lock wives out of areas of influence that they would like to have, while locking husbands into these same areas, is the traditional support for husbands' rather than wives' having the major role in making these decisions. Indeed, it has been found that couples tend to make decisions in culturally prescribed areas (e.g., Jacob *et al.*, 1978; Lovejoy, 1961). For example, a recent study by Douglas and Wind (1978) identified clusters of decisions in which either men or women appear to dominate. Some 74% of the decisions about which car to buy, 72% of the decisions about the amount of life insurance to buy, 92% of the decisions about car servicing, and 74% of the decisions about liquor purchases were made by men. In contrast, women made 86% of the decisions about how much money to spend on food each week and 81%–92% of the decisions about house cleaning, while the couples reported sharing equally in 89% of the decisions about inviting friends for dinner, 84% of the decisions about household furnishings, 66% of the decisions about which brand of television to buy, and 56% of the decisions about which bank to use. Clearly, these allocations of authority fall within broad cultural stereotypes. Another study (Henshel, 1973), this one conducted in Toronto, found that the initial decision to "swing" was made by husbands in 59% of the swinging couples, by wives in 12%, and by both partners in 28%. Even this pattern is not inconsistent with traditional norms. Indeed, surmounting these norms may in itself require realignments of duties and expectations that have been reinforced by decades of socialization, and for the present generation, at least, it may be more a source of anxiety than a source of egalitarian joy.

Lu (1952) did find many years ago that satisfaction was greater in marriages in which decisions were made on an egalitarian basis. This finding set the patterns of expectation for many later studies. The research by Centers et al. (1971) cited earlier showed little difference in the likelihood that couples would report satisfaction with husband-dominated, syncretic, or autonomic decision-making patterns (73%, 70%, and 79%, respectively), with only 20% of the spouses in marriages in which decision making was wife-centered reporting comparable levels of satisfaction. In a later study, these same social scientists (Raven et al., 1975) found that among couples reporting higher levels of marital satisfaction, those relying upon referent, expert, or legitimate power (49%, 27%, or 20%, respectively) were far more satisfied than those using reward or coercive power (3% versus 2%). Taken together, these studies suggest that egalitarian decision making, in which the power is based upon ascription rather than action, would seem to contribute significantly to marital satisfaction. Osmond and Martin (1978) also see egalitarianism as a major contributor to marital stability as well as satisfaction. At least 72% of the couples in egalitarian marriages were still married at the time of the study, in contrast to some 27% of those in which one spouse or the other had significantly less power.

When power is imbalanced, it is evident that husband dominance is more conducive to marital satisfaction than ascendance by the wife. Corrales (1975) noted:

> The wife-dominated context may be indicative of the situation where the husband is most uninvolved and where he is receiving most of his satisfaction from sources outside the family. Not only is he personally "absent" but the wife is then saddled with most of the family load. (p. 213)

Udry (1974) suggested that the least involved husbands attend to economic duties and possibly participate in social activities. Those with moderate involvement attend to husband household duties and may share in child care. And those who are most involved may share in common, even traditionally wife household duties. In contrast, the least involved wives still attend to wife household duties, child care, and social activities. As they are more involved, they take on common household duties, economic duties, and husband household duties. When wives "dominate" their relationships, it is often because the husbands reduce their family involvement, leaving the wives saddled with extra duties because they must assume full responsibility for home and child care. This finding may explain why past studies have shown that when the power balance tips slightly in the husband's favor, both marital (Hurvitz, 1965; Kolb & Straus, 1974) and family (Alkire, 1969) functioning appear to be better than when the reverse is true.

It is possible that wife dominance in decision making may occur by default: wives may wield the power that husbands are incapable of handling. In that case, the wife's dominance may be just a concomitant of the husband's inability to provide for the family or to function effectively within it, and the lower level of satisfaction could then result from the situational stresses induced by the husband's inadequacy. It is also possible that the lower level of satisfaction in wife-dominated families might be a result of the wife's feeling that she has more authority than her husband, but still not enough influence over the couple's decision-making processes. As a third possibility, husbands might have yielded power grudgingly and feel at a loss both because they have come out second best in a power struggle and because of the difficulty they face in accepting a normatively typical position vis-à-vis their wives.

It can be concluded that egalitarianism is a generally accepted ideal. Sensitively operationalized egalitarianism does not call for equality in all matters; rather, it would suggest that couples should develop an equitable means of allocating decision-making authority between the spouses according to their sanctioned roles, expertise, or interest in the various areas in which decisions must be made. If the resulting balance is imperfect, however, the available evidence suggests that slightly more husband influence may be more conducive to marital and family happiness than greater influence by the wife.

Allocating Decision-Making Authority

The effect of normative influences that support the power imbalances that strain marital satisfaction can be at least partially weakened through the development of decision-making rules such as those suggested by Broderick (1975). Such rules also serve as guidelines in advance of the need to make decisions, so that when these challenges arise, all available energy can be channeled into organizing the needed data and selecting from among the available options rather than being dissipated in unnecessary negotiation with the spouse.

Stuart (1976) has elsewhere suggested that any of a number of different points along the continuum of power balance might suffice for any given couple:

1. The husband and wife might each make most of the decisions independently, with little consultation and no overlap in areas of decision making.
2. Most decisions might be made jointly, with few made independently.

3. Some decisions might be made separately by each spouse; some might be made by each spouse upon consultation with the other; and some might be joint efforts.

None of these options is necessarily better than the other two, just as none is a fail-safe guarantee of effective decision making. Because shared decision making is time-intensive, younger couples tend to reserve it for major issues, while older couples, who perhaps have less time pressure, increase the range of their shared decision-making areas (Wilkening & Bharadwaj, 1967; Wolgast, 1958). Overall, the couples studied by Johannis and Rollins (1959) made only 7 of 43 decisions mutually, and those dealing with child care and major purchases were the ones most likely to be shared (Geiken, 1964; Wolgast, 1958). The two dimensions of a system of rules for allocating power in decision making are thus designation of authority and area.

Stuart (1976; Stuart & Lederer, in press) has developed a system termed the "powergram" for helping couples to make these allocations. A powergram is a graphic way in which clients can be helped to visualize the way in which they currently feel decisions are made, the way in which they would like them to be made, and finally, the way in which they agree to apportion decision-making authority between themselves.

Scale G of the Marital Precounseling Inventory (Stuart & Stuart, 1973) is the basis for powergram construction. This scale lists 16 areas in which couples commonly make decisions:

a. Where couple lives.
b. What job husband takes.
c. How many hours husband works.
d. Whether wife works.
e. What job wife takes.
f. How many hours wife works.
g. Number of children in the family.
h. When to praise or punish children.
i. How much time to spend with children.
j. When to have social contacts with friends.
k. When to have social contacts with in-laws and relatives.
l. When to have sex.
m. How to have sex.
n. How to spend money.
o. How and when to pursue personal interests.
p. Whether to attend church, and if so, which church to attend.

Couples are asked to read over this list and to add to it any areas of decision making that are important in their lives but are not included in the standard list. They are also asked to cross off items that do not apply. Couples have added items like "Decide on where to go for vacations," "Decide how to make investments," and "Decide how much money to donate to charity or to the church." Couples in which either the husband or the wife is not employed outside the home or in which there are no children naturally delete the clusters of items that are irrelevant to their marriage.

Next, spouses are asked to reread the final list of items, rank ordering their importance according to their individual evaluations. They are asked to indicate the most important items by designating them with a "1," and the items of secondary and tertiary importance by indicating each with a "2" or a "3", respectively. They are, however, asked to limit to *five* the items to which they assign highest priority.

When the list has been refined and prioritized, the couples are ready to complete Powergram A by answering the following question:

Please read the list of items that we have just developed. *At this time* in your marriage, who *usually* has responsibility for making decisions in each area?
1. Almost always husband.
2. Husband, after consulting wife.
3. Both share equally.
4. Wife, after consulting husband.
5. Almost always wife.

The couples are asked to write their answers in Powergram A in the following manner:

Please note that the powergram is divided into five sections corresponding to each of the possible ways of allocating authority for making decisions in the area. The wife should indicate her answer to each question by writing the capital letter (e.g., "A," "B," etc.) corresponding to each item (e.g., "A" for "Where couple lives," etc.) in the area of the form corresponding to her answer. The husband is asked to do the same using lower-case letters.

As seen in Figure 1, Boris and Marta both felt that they now share alike in the decision about where they live; therefore, they wrote "a" and "A" in section 3 of the powergram. Boris felt that he and Marta also share equally in deciding what job he takes, so he wrote "b" in section 3 of the form. Marta, however, believes that Boris alone makes this decision, so she wrote "B" in section 1 of the form. When this situation exists, Boris is said to have "pseudojuniority" because he believes that he has less power than his wife feels that he now exercises. A different situation exists in regard to item h, when to praise or punish the children. Boris sees this too as an area of shared decision making and entered an "h" in section 3, while Marta considered this to be mainly her domain and entered an "H" in area 4. In this case, she has "pseudostrength" because she believes that she exercises more authority than Boris has ceded. Pseudojuniority and pseudostrength are both potential sources of con-

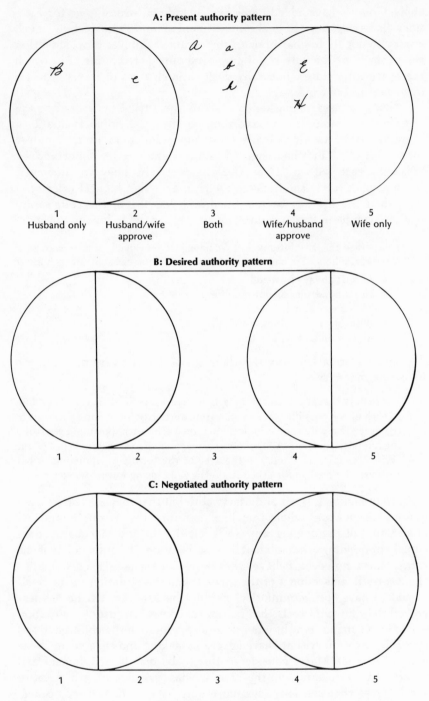

Figure 1. Powergram.

flict. When fights are spawned by such misunderstandings, they are often more virulent than those that are an outgrowth of straightforward disagreements. An illustration of the latter situation is seen in Figure 1, where Boris thinks he has major influence on the kind of job Marta takes (he wrote "e" in section 2 of the form), while Marta feels that she merely consults Boris but essentially makes the decision herself (she wrote "E" in section 4 of the form).

Couples are asked next to answer the following question:

> Now please use Powergram B to indicate the way you think decision-making authority *should now be* distributed in each of the areas under consideration. Wives should do this by entering capital letters corresponding to each area in the section of the form indicating the pattern they would like to follow in making each decision. Husbands should do the same but should use lower-case letters.

In completing Powergram B, couples often unmask latent conflicts—disagreements of two or more scalar points between the way in which they think decisions are now made (Powergram A) and the way in which they would like to have authority distributed. It is important to realize that not all of these conflicts revolve around the desire of either or both spouses to have greater authority in a particular area. Often spouses wish to have *less* influence in one or more areas, a desire that the other may view with considerable apprehension. The desire for less authority might simply indicate that one partner wishes to simplify his or her life by avoiding the necessity to collect data and weigh options in a variety of different areas of family concern. It may also reflect the desire of one to accord greater autonomy to the other. However, it can also reflect a wish to avoid potential conflict or the desire to cut one's investment in a relationship that is seen as offering diminishing returns. Meanwhile, the desire to have *more* influence may be an expression of the belief by one that he or she has more expert power or a legitimate right to autonomy in a particular area rather than necessarily suggesting that one wishes merely to overwhelm the authority of the other.

When both spouses have indicated their views of the present balance of power and their desired balance of power in each area, they are ready for the therapist to help them negotiate their new decision-making rules. This is done through the use of Powergram C, which will indicate the way that they agree to distribute authority in each area. The therapist's role is that of facilitator and mediator (see Chapter 5), while the couples are encouraged to adopt the two-winner bargaining strategy described in Chapter 8. The therapist should make three separate lists for each spouse: the first list should itemize all of the areas to which each spouse has assigned first priority; the second and third lists should itemize the areas that each has assigned to secondary and tertiary importance. While these rank orderings may not contribute significantly to the conclusions drawn from research on the balance of power between spouses (Price-Bonham, 1976), they do play a major role in helping clients to renegotiate the balance of their marital power.

If Powergram B indicates few areas of disagreement, the negotiation of Powergram C may be quite easy. If the spouses have numerous disagreements about how they should distribute power, however, the therapist's use of the three pairs of lists just described can help in the development of a pattern of decision making acceptable to both. In this effort, a holistic rather than a partitive strategy should be used (see Chapter 8). That is, rather than matching item for item—a process that seriously narrows options toward the bottom of the lists—the therapist should try to help the partners accommodate one another by clustering their exchanges. Boris might be willing to yield authority in a first-priority item for him (how to spend money, area n) in exchange for increased authority in the areas of their social interactions with others (areas j and k, which he accorded secondary importance). These kinds of trade-offs can be quite straightforward and often result in highly effective agreements about the balance of decision-making authority.

Three soft criteria can be used in evaluating these agreements. First, it is important to be certain that the couples express satisfaction with the accord. Without their verbal consent, there is little likelihood of their behavioral compliance. Next, the therapist should feel that the agreements approach equity. This is important because if the therapist feels that the agreement is inequitable, this feeling will surely be communicated to the clients, whose commitment to the agreement can be adversely affected. Finally, the couple should make a two-week trial of the pattern so that they can make certain they are both comfortable with it.

By making this agreement, the couple are able to establish formal relationship rules that build the basis for legitimate power in their decision making. Many, if not most, of the decisions that couples make are based upon value rather than factual considerations. For example, deciding when to make love, how many children to have, which church to attend, or which job to take are all choices guided by values, not facts. Other decisions—like which car to buy, how to spend their investment dollars, or whether or not to go forward with elective surgery for a member of the family—are all decisions that should be based upon the kinds of facts that require expertise. Legitimate power is a suitable basis for the first set of decisions, although legitimacy should yield to expertise in areas like those in the second set. When the patterns of authority are legitimated prior to the rendering of decisions, energy can be directed toward weighing the alternatives and will not be dissipated in jockeying for position. Moreover, after the decision has been made, the partners will not experience a postdecision dissonance (Festinger, 1957) that has been augmented by a feeling of having been ill-used in the relationship.

As a final note, it is important for couples to realize that the agreement they fashion through Powergram C is not cast in iron. It is only a working agreement, one that should be reviewed periodically in search of opportunities to make changes that will help both partners feel that they are enjoying the authority and support they desire.

Problem-Solving Skills

Couples need two somewhat distinct sets of skills to solve problems successfully. They need the information-gathering, organizing, and analytic skills basic to formal decision making. In addition, and of at least equal importance, they need the ability to work together throughout the often demanding and sometimes frustrating process of trying to find solutions to their dilemmas. Failure to have command of the basic logic can naturally sabotage their effort to rise to the problem-solving challenge. Because the logic of decision making is familiar to most professionals, it is reviewed here only briefly before consideration of the interactional aspects of problem solving.

FORMAL DECISION-MAKING PROCESS

Over half a century ago, John Dewey (1910) outlined five steps in problem solving: (1) definition of the problem; (2) collection of relevant information; (3) innovative listing of alternative options; (4) selection of one of these options; and (5) evaluation of the resulting action. Young *et al.* (1970) have correctly placed great stress upon the importance of problem definition, for they see in it the real key to problem resolution. They wrote:

> A statement of the unknown is actually a partial description of the solution. As such, it serves two functions: (1) It acts as a guide to inquiry, since it describes what you are looking for; and (2) it enables you to know when you have found your solution, since the solution will match the description. (p. 92)

Defining the problem incorrectly, therefore, introduces a biasing factor into every subsequent stage of decision making. For example, no amount of reasoning can answer the question, "*How* can one build a house with four southern exposures?" However, the question, "Where can one build a house with four southern exposures?" can very quickly be answered when it is realized that only the geographic north pole could meet the four-southern-exposure stipulation.

Stressing the importance of the internal logic of the problem-solving process, Young *et al.* (1970) described a four-stage process. They began with "preparation," in which one becomes initially aware of the difficulty, formulates the difficulty as a problem to be solved, and explores the problem by formulating the pressing question. This stage is followed by a "subconscious incubation stage," which forms the basis for the third stage, "illumination," when a hypothesis is formulated. In their view, a sound hypothesis (1) is consistent with actual experience, (2) is consistent with the generally accepted fund of knowledge, and (3) offers practical guidelines to the problem-solving process. To fulfill the latter requirement, the hypothesis must pass the test of Occam's razor: it must be as parsimonious as possible, including unverified assumptions only when they are unavoidable. Finally, the hypothesis must be verified through reasoning and subsequently through direct experimentation. Verification requires sufficient flexibility to permit management of the conditions that could modify the outcome and the willingness to accept the data whether they support or deny the hypothesis.

THE REALITIES OF FAMILY PROBLEM SOLVING

While this general formulation of the logic of problem solving has been accepted by a variety of authors concerned with solving the problems of daily living (e.g, Demars, 1972; D'Zurilla & Goldfried, 1971; Jacobson, 1977), for a variety of different reasons, families rarely approach this ideal. First, there is tendency to shrink from assertion in problem definition:

> In ordinary affairs we usually muddle ahead, doing what is habitual and customary, being slightly puzzled when it sometimes fails to give the intended outcome, but not stopping to worry much about the failures because there are too many other things still to do. (Miller *et al.*, 1960, p. 171)

Second, while it is difficult enough for individuals to come to the conclusion that "something has to be done," this conclusion is even more difficult for groups and families to reach because they must agree both that something is amiss and that group effort can lead to a solution (Lindley, 1971). Third, when consensus is reached that a problem exists, families tend to be more inclined to rush working out solutions than to concentrate first on a prudent formulation of the problem at hand (Aldous, 1971). Moreover, couples tend to turn to problem solving at the end of the day, when their energy level is low; they tend to pursue these efforts in the worst physical surroundings, where distractions are at a maximum; and they generally seal themselves off from outside inputs when new information is most needed (Weick, 1971). Couples also have a notorious tendency to "hitchhike" many unrelated issues onto their problem-solving efforts, so that crossed agendas hamper almost all of their efforts (Weick, 1971).

Perhaps the greatest difficulty of all in marital problem solving is its inevitable confusion of relationship and specific task-oriented issues. Bales and Strodtbeck (1951) found that groups composed of unrelated members tended to pass through three stages in their problem-solving efforts. During the "orientation" phrase, the members learned about the interests and capacities of each other, and they discussed the dimensions of the problem; during the "evaluation" phase, they developed their hypotheses and alternatives for action; and during the "control" phase, they sought to influence one another to accept a preferred action alternative. Across all three phases, they gradually increased the rate at which they exchanged both positive and negative feedback. Turner (1970), however, has noted that for families, orientation and evaluation are often truncated because each member thinks that he or she knows where the others stand, and each has argued in the past over the standard options that the family considers. Therefore, much more of the time that couples spend in decision making is passed in the control stage, and it may be this fact that accounts for the strikingly negative spousal interactions as compared with those of unrelated strangers (e.g., Stuart & Braver, 1973; Birchler et al., 1975; Gottman et al., 1976; Gottman et al., 1977). Thus, Cromwell and Olson (1975) believe that couple decision-making is more oriented to "power outcomes" than to successful change in the flow of external events. With so much energy being diverted into relationship management, it is small wonder that little is left for task accomplishment, often leaving the couple embroiled in conflict and still facing the original dilemma at the end of their efforts to arrive at a sound decision.

Prerequisites for Marital Decision Making

Effective decision making by couples requires at least six prerequisites, all of which are teachable and learnable skills.

BASIC COMMUNICATION SKILLS

The spouses must have basic communication skills at their disposal. They must be able to express their ideas, listen to and understand the other's expressions, ask for clarification, give feedback, and negotiate unambiguous agreement (see Chapter 7). Couples who do not speak the same connotative and denotative language have no basis for fruitful, shared, problem-solving efforts, because effective discourse can occur only across a bridge of shared meanings. Without such a base, neither can understand the other's intentions, suggestions, and willingness to compromise, so skills must be built to overcome the broad array of communication deficits described by Thomas (1977), ranging from acknowledgment deficits to undertalk.

OPEN LINES OF COMMUNICATION

Communication between spouses must be open to a free exchange of information and ideas. They must have a selective openness to outside inputs. Thomas (1977) has observed that "The family, being nuclear and relatively isolated, tends to be detached from most external corrective influences" (p. 18). At the same time, however, it is always open to the intrusion of the concerns in the extrafamilial lives of all of its members. Thus, it tends to function as a "closed system" in the sense that novel ideas from outside are limited (Bower, 1965), and there is little to help win the battle of "bounded rationality" that confronts all decision makers working in closed systems (Simon, 1955). However, if one family member has been frustrated at work or at school, the tension that this frustration creates will be readily injected into problem-solving deliberations with adverse effect. Thus, each couple must develop a filter system that draws relevant data into discussions while screening out unrelated issues.

ESTABLISHED LINES OF AUTHORITY

Each couple must have a flexible yet defined power structure. As noted above, this structure can facilitate problem-solving deliberations in task groups (Hall & Williams, 1966) as well as in family groups (Mulder, 1960). Ferreira and Winter (1965; 1966), for example, found that in normal families with defined power structures, decisions were made quickly, and provision was made for the opportunity for all to express their views, so that the decisions made were likely to be more equitable than those made in distressed families that lacked an authority structure. Beyond the existence of this defined power distribution, the basis of the power is also an important consideration. Weick (1971) lamented that the basis of decision-making power in families is more likely to be legitimacy than expertise, but some measure of both is conducive to negotiation toward solutions that are acceptable by all. Because families are also motivated to make decisions so that they can move on to the next issue in a manner that offers at least partial satisfaction to all concerned, referent power is the third important dimension of the ideal authority base.

Families should also have the capacity not only to tolerate but to encourage conflict in ideas. Moore and Anderson (1971) call this the "autotelic" principle of problem solving. They believe that "the best way to learn really difficult things is to be placed in an environment in which you can try things out, make a fool of yourself, guess outrageously, or play it close to the vest—all without serious consequences" (p. 107). If the couple are easily threatened by the exchange of opposing views, they lose the major advantage of shared as opposed to individual decision making. When this is true, it is often useful for the therapist to help the clients to relabel what they might see as the *threat* of disagreement as the *opportunity* that disagreement provides for growth. Groups make decisions more slowly than individuals, but they use this time to consider alternative solutions. Fear of conflict, however, can lead to a reticence about alternative approaches, to the point where the decision is the work of one individual to the dismay of the other. Unfortunately, there is a strong tendency for family members to confuse substantive issues with relationship issues; that is, for one to interpret rejection of his or her suggestion as a rejection of him or her as a person. Strangers are much better able to take the proper distance and thereby keep their disagreements on a factual level separate from their interpersonal dealings. Thus, Tallman (1970) recognizes that both partners must approach the decision-making arena with a set of flexible templates; they must be willing to focus their energies on the best possible solution rather than on gaining acceptance for their personally selected avenue of approach.

BALANCED TRUST

Both partners must also have a certain level of trust in each other if they are to take the risks needed for the development of an effective problem-solving strategy. Without trust, neither partner is likely to believe the other's communication (Young *et al.,* 1970). For example, knowing that Loren wants to buy a new car, Gail will accept his statement that the old one would cost too much to repair only if she trusts; otherwise, she will discount his argument as merely motivated by Loren's wish to achieve his own goals. In addition, trust is needed for the orderly flow of exchanges that is required by problem-solving discussion. For Turner (1970), "bargaining is simply a general term for any interaction in which the concessions that one member makes to another are expected to be reciprocated in some manner" (p. 106). Trust is the basis of good-faith bargaining (Blau, 1964) and of the integrative orientation (Lewis & Pruitt, 1971) that was seen as the basis of negotiation in Chapter 7. All collective problem solving requires some level of willingness to act, to submit to the judgment of others, and to share the risks and benefits of a pooled outcome; and bargaining based upon trust is the means through which these decisions are made.

CONSENSUS ON CRITERIA OF EFFECTIVE SOLUTIONS

Finally, the couple also need to agree on suitable criteria for deciding that problems have been solved. Simon (1955) made the differentiation between "optimal" outcomes in which a near-perfect solution is achieved and "satisficing" outcomes in which the outcome is at least minimally acceptable to all concerned. Unfortunately, too many family members seek optimization when a satisfactory decision is a far more realistic goal.

For family members, adoption of an attainable problem-solving goal requires adoption of an approach in which "everyone wins." In this approach, the objective is agreement rather than total victory; if one person wins "big," the other is likely to feel shut out, only to undermine the agreement later through direct or indirect means. One-sided decisions are therefore worse than no decision, because not only will they not succeed in solving the problem, but they also carry with them the likelihood that commitment to the relationship will be weakened.

In choosing goals for the problem-solving process, couples should realize that achievement of consensus is as close as a couple can come to an optimal solution unless they have spontaneous agreement about how to solve a problem. In consensus, either or both may (1) introduce a new alternative on which both spontaneously agree; (2) make a genuine shift in opinion; (3) change frames of reference through discussion of the other's values; or (4) change images of the dispute outcome. When these alternatives are related to those discussed in Chapter 3, the first corresponds to behavior change, the second to relabeling, and the third to change in expectations. Accommodation or an "agreement to disagree" (Turner, 1970, p. 98) is the other possible criterion for decision making. It involves a willingness by one to accede to a suggestion by the other, although it is not believed to be the best possible outcome. Accommodation is always actively pursued through bargaining, and one will be willing to concede only with the expectation that the gesture will be reciprocated at a later time (Edwards, 1961; Kirkpatrick, 1955). Finally, Turner (1970) has indicated that *de facto* decisions—allowing events to take their course without any active intervention—is the extreme of decision-making outcomes that is the opposite of spontaneous agreement. In *de facto* decisions, the couple, in effect, decide not to decide; these decisions are, then, "nondecisions" or acts of acquiescence to the spouses' fundamental differences. While fewer than the 12 outcomes discussed by Thomas (1977), the 4 discussed above do represent major points on an outcome continuum that can be depicted as follows:

Type of outcome

Spontaneous‑‑‑‑‑‑‑Consensus‑‑‑‑‑‑‑Accommodation‑‑‑‑‑‑‑*De facto*
Agreement   outcome

Optimal   Satisficing   Unsatisfactory
                                      Quality of outcome

Decision-Making Interaction

With the conception of the goals firmly in mind, couples can plan the strategy that they will use in negotiating toward consensus or accommodation. The nature of the interaction needed for effective decision-making is influenced by the nature of the problem at hand. Some problems require creative solutions; for example, if the breadwinner of the family suffers a loss of job, the whole family may get together to see if they can come up with suggestions for alternative sources of income, or all may contribute to a decision about what to give the grandparents for Christmas. In these situations, communication should be open and flexible, with each member of the family having an opportunity to make contributions (Bass, 1963; Hoffman, 1965). It should be remembered, however, that while this free-and-easy communication is desirable, limits should be placed because the expression of too many ideas can be confusing and therefore counterproductive (Dunnette *et al.*, 1963; Taylor *et al.*, 1958). On the other hand, challenges that require the coordination of the activities of all family members require centralized authority (Bavelas, 1950; Leavitt, 1951; Tallman, 1970). For example, the flooding of the basement during a spring runoff requires some quick decisions about how to contain the damage, followed by some prompt and willing action. Solving the problem therefore requires one person to take the lead in soliciting suggestions, making a quick decision, and delegating responsibility to all concerned.

All couples thus need at least two modes for problem solving, and it is helpful if both spouses have the vocabulary for calling signals indicating the need for "creative" or "coordinated" problem-solving efforts. When one thinks that the interaction is in the creative mode, while the other barks out commands as if in the coordinated mode, conflict is the almost certain outcome; one feels that his or her contribution is not valued, while the other feels that his or her authority is discounted.

Whichever mode is established, the couple must then proceed through the steps in the problem-solving process: identifying the challenge, posing alternative solutions, selecting one of these, putting it into practice, evaluating its effectiveness, and reconsolidating the relationship following problem solution. Each of these steps is accomplished through discussion, which has a double function: first, it weakens uniformity and helps both realize that a difference of opinion exists; and second, it develops a new norm, which gives the couple's stamp of approval to the decision (Moscovici & Doise, 1974). Without discussion, it would be impossible to generate alternative solutions. For example, Straus (1971) found that middle-class couples outperformed working-class couples in Bombay, Minneapolis, and San Juan in their abilities to solve problems. In all three cultures, those with middle-class backgrounds were more willing to suggest and to entertain alternative solutions; they had greater "ideational fluency and flexibility" (p. 253). In addition, when solutions are imposed rather than derived from discussion, the person who is "one down" in the process is hardly likely to accept the solution gracefully. Discussion is thus the key to accommodation to the solution that is reached. In this regard, Maier (1963) long ago recognized that reaching the solution is only half of the problem; convincing the other to go along with the solution is the larger challenge for many couples, one that is facilitated by the use of fair discussion technique.

Unfortunately, discussion during decision making is complicated by many factors. As noted above, couples sometimes confuse disagreement about a discussion point with rejection of them as people or role occupants. Discussion also stresses the creative capacities of the spouses, and they may tend to turn to conflict to mask their inadequacies. The formality of the decision-making process also tends to heighten the specter of forming precedents for all future decisions. This specter, in turn, leads both partners to strive for maximum gain now to avoid defeat later. Finally, the emotion that is mobilized during problem-solving discussion can sometimes trigger associations with other emotionally charged issues that filter into the problem-solving efforts, with serious ill effects.

These latter factors may account for the observations of Vincent et al. (1975), which were partially confirmed by Gottman et al. (1976b), who showed that distressed couples were more negative and less positive than nondistressed couples, even during laboratory-based efforts to solve artificial and somewhat isolated problems that should have posed little challenge to the couples. The achievement of consensus must be "actively pursued and does not usually just happen" (Turner, 1970, p. 104), and the maintenance of close emotional ties during problem-solving discussions is also the result of planful effort and not just a happy accident. These two dimensions—the hammering out of a workable solution and the strengthening of relationship bonds—can be achieved if couples follow decision-making rules such as those promulgated by Thomas (1977). He suggested three rules relating to partner interaction during problem solving: (1) both partners should be allowed to have their say so long as their contributions are relevant to the problem at hand; (2) communication rules such as those outlined in Chapter 7 (e.g., self-statements beginning with "I" and the use of good listening and clarification skills) should be followed throughout the discussion (also see Thomas, 1977, pp. 88–89); and (3) one partner's good decision-making contribution should be praised even if the other disagrees with its content.

Nierenberg (1968) suggested a series of questions that can be asked to determine the likelihood that these good discussion rules will be followed. For example, he would ask whether there are any penalties in the discussion, such as costs for expressing a dissident point of view; for offering false information; for failing to agree; or for trying to maintain the status quo while appearing to try to solve the problem. One would also be well advised to know whether either or both partners are attempting to use the problem-solving discussion to try to strengthen or to modify the balance of power in the relationship. Karrass (1970) has noted several different levels of "brotherhood" that may characterize the starting positions of both parties. They may be "equal brothers," based on equal status. One may be a "big brother," while the other is a "little brother"; the former may attempt to exercise benevolent control based upon higher status, while the latter may seek charity based upon inferior status. They may also be "long-lost brothers" who are searching for a relationship definition through the negotiation, or they may exercise "brinksmanship," in which they take high joint risks, allowing the relationship chips to fall where they may. Long-lost brothers interact with no clear allocation of authority; both jockey for control, and every maneuver can be understood as a tactic of position enhancement. Finally, those in a brinksmanship interaction set relationship issues aside and work toward the greatest possible level of outcome without regard to who directs the negotiation process.

Just as there is no particular balance of power that offers greater benefits than any other, so, too, is no one of these relationship patterns necessarily better than any other. In fact, successful couples have all five of these options in their repertoires and move from one to the other according to the nature of the challenge or the stage of its solution. For example, solutions to the problem of where to go for a vacation are best achieved by equal brothers, while decisions about whether to repair the failing oil burner or install solar heating is best made by the person with expertise, who should fill the big-brother role.

The role that each person takes is clearly reflected in the nature of the questions that each asks and the types of answers that are offered. Questions determine the direction of the discussion. As a starting point, it should be recognized that:

Communications between individuals clearly involve more than mere exchanges of information regarding respective positions. The purpose and goal of the communications is to induce change, to make a choice between two alternatives. Thus group discussion and communication cause involvement of the individuals and commit them to each other. (Moscovici & Doise, 1974, p. 252)

That is, all communication must be recognized as representing an effort to influence another person, and any time an influence attempt meets with success or failure, the relationship between the speaker and the listener is either strengthened or weakened. Therefore, questions asked during problem-solving discussions must be construed as efforts to influence the proceedings. These influence attempts are positive if they are an expression of commitment to a solution that is genuinely believed to offer the best mutual payoff, and they are negative to the extent that they are ploys designed to gain or maintain a challenged position of power.

Questions that seek factual information or that solicit the views of the other are the "meat and potatoes" of problem-solving discussions. General questions like "What do you think?" and direct questions like "Who has the know-how to solve this problem?" and fact-finding questions beginning with "where," "when," "what," and "how" can all facilitate the discussion, although the context in which they are asked can define the power balance and limit the risk of sidetracking. For example, Julia and Salvador are trying to decide whether to send their daughter to parochial school. Compare the following two exchanges:

JULIA: Sal, do you think we should send Anne to Saint Elizabeth's school this year?

SAL: It costs a lot and money's tight now. Maybe we should leave her in public school for another year to see how well she does.

JULIA: Why do you always look at everything in terms of money?

JULIA: Sal, I know that it's expensive but I think we should send Anne to Saint Elizabeth's this year because she really isn't getting the special help she needs in public school. And if I volunteer a few mornings each week at the school, we can even get a tuition rebate.

SAL: What do you know about class size and tutorial help at Saint Elizabeth's? Would it really be better than public school?

JULIA: That's a good question. I'll go and spend a few hours in class there next week to see just how individualized their program is.

In the first exchange, Julia made no commitment and Sal fell into a trap. Had he agreed to send Anne to parochial school, Julia would have been as likely to attack him for extravagance as to accuse him of being stingy in the present interaction. Moreover, the first exchange resulted in the couple's moving off onto a side track that carried them far away from an effort to collect the data needed for solving their problem. On the other hand, Julia took a position in the second exchange and initiated a well-focused discussion without asking a question. The first exchange was a "cat-and-mouse" dialogue; the second was a problem-solving discussion between equals.

Karrass (1970) would classify the first exchange between Julia and Sal as a "decoy," one that was aimed at snaring Sal into a one-down, defensive position. Karrass also offered several other classifications of negotiation diversions. "Denial" is withdrawing a statement after it has met with resistance. In the first exchange above, Sal might have denied that he was concerned with the expense in an effort to confuse Julia and thereby regain some of his lost stature. Either person might camouflage his or her intentions with a "sugar-and-spice" role play—seeming to be interested in negotiating a true bargain while actually waiting for the proper moment to strike. The "scrambled-eggs" ploy is one in which irrelevant side issues are swept into the discussion to keep the couple from reaching a conclusion. Julia's accusation that Sal is a tightwad is such a diversion. To the extent that it works, the couple will not reach a decision, and thus Julia will later be able to accuse Sal of being defensive and/or indecisive. "Low-balling," or adding on additional costs, is the traditional maneuver of the auto sales of business and of manipulative spouses as well. After the deal is apparently struck, the salesperson might then tell of the extra costs of dealer preparation, sales tax, and other "forgotten" charges. After Julia gets Sal to agree to parochial school for Anne for, say, $800 per year tuition, she might tell him about the mandatory contribution of $1000 yearly to the building fund and the $450 annual cost of uniforms and bus transportation. Finally, "scoundrel" is a maneuver in which one person lures the other into a never-ending negotiation, with the goal of building his or her position while preventing the other from ever reaching closure on the issue and gaining peace of mind. Finally, a ploy first described by Strodtbeck (1958) is termed "word screen." In this maneuver, one person maintains a constant stream of words that do not necessarily make sense but that do block out the other's efforts to influence the exchange, with disastrous effects upon the problem-solving process.

Description of these manipulations can be as extensive as the imagination is vast. Each is analogous to Eric Berne's (1964) "games." While it is helpful for spouses to be able to identify their own use of these ploys, self-confrontation is at best an often-suggested but rarely successful effort. To refocus these problem-causing maneuvers, the other spouse should be coached in the technique of "redirection." This means that the "victim" of the maneuver should take the responsibility of redirecting the exchange in a nonaccusatory manner, short-circuiting his or her natural but unproductive tendency first to right the wrong before getting back to constructive problem-solving. Indeed, it is the goal of every manipulator to provoke a response in kind, which guarantees the diversion of the constructive effort.

Use of the redirection technique has four very important requirements. First, it must be done without a labeling of the behavior of the other. If Sal were to tell Julia that she is belittling him as a diversion, she would quite spontaneously defend herself and escalate the attack, creating even greater obstacles to their problem-solving efforts. Second, the redirection should be offered without defense or apology. If Sal were to say, "I'm sorry Julia, but we have to stick to the issue at hand," he would again stimulate Julia's defensiveness. Third, redirection must seek positive change only; it must be aimed at keeping the couple on the track rather than at manipulating a confession from the other. "Let's concentrate on getting the facts" is far more constructive than "Let's stop trying to sabotage the discussion." Finally, the redirection effort must be repeated until it is successful. If Sal attempted once to redirect Julia and she came up with a second allegation, Sal must simply stick to his redirection guns and try to move the discussion along, avoiding the inclination to figuratively throw his hands up in disgust and then join the fray. Rarely is it necessary to repeat redirection efforts more than two or at most three times if the earlier stages of treatment have been successfully completed.

For example, if Sal were to introduce the "scrambled-eggs" ploy by accusing Julia of always trying to go beyond their budget, as shown by her buying a winter coat last year when it was *not* on sale, Julia could respond, "That may have been a mistake, but let's concentrate now on deciding how we can help Anne." If Julia were to start a round of "scoundrel" by also throwing into the hopper her feeling that Sal does not adequately support her efforts to bring Anne up in the faith, Sal should offer that perhaps he could do more, but that now they had best concentrate on putting together the facts relating to the problem of Anne's schooling. In each instance, the implicit attack is recognized but without counterattack, and the "victim," who thereby gains control, makes an attempt to refocus the discussion along problem-solving lines.

In optimal therapeutic situations, each spouse can be trained as the other's benevolent coach. The benevolence stems from the fact that each is prepared to "slip the punches" of the other, that is, to sidestep any assault without allowing it to interfere with the objective of the exchange. This procedure takes a definite amount of self-assurance and feeling of commitment to the relationship, both of which are the probable outcomes of the earlier stages of treatment. Also necessary are the willingness to lay idle pride to rest, the willingness to be forbearing in the interest of strengthening the relationship, and the willingness to resist the tendency to close all negative cycles, as described in Chapter 6.

Training in these corrective coaching skills begins in the treatment session with the therapist as model. Once the role has been demonstrated, the therapist can "put words into the mouths" of both spouses by telling them what to say to the other to redirect the discussion and then can later reinforce each for spontaneously assuming the mature and effective role of coach. These skills can then be reinforced through guided practice between sessions as couples perhaps tape-record their problem-solving discussions at home and discuss their tapes during therapeutic sessions, where positive feedback and constructive redirection are repeatedly modeled by the therapist.

C H A P T E R   1 0

Conflict
Containment

ONFLICT HAS BEEN variously described as the key to constructive change in marriage and as the bane of marital existence. It is suggested in this chapter that conflict can best be understood as an emotionally charged effort to coerce relationship changes from another person. The intensity of the emotions that are expressed as well as the focal request are the potentially facilitative communications inherent in conflict. However, the personal and relationship attacks that are part and parcel of these communications are the even more potent and potentially destructive dimensions of the communication.

This chapter traces some of the more familiar sources of conflict, contending that some form of conflict is virtually unavoidable in any long-term and complex human interaction. After a review of the research literature on the form and content of conflict between spouses, it is argued here that conflict is a second-best means of promoting relationship change and that efforts should be made to prevent conflict when possible, to contain it when it does occur, and to depend upon the communication and negotiation skills described in earlier chapters as the preferred means of facilitating relationship growth. A set of techniques for containing conflict, based upon an analysis of the six phases of the natural history of conflictual experiences, is presented at the end of this chapter. As an overall orientation, it is suggested that couples maintain a present orientation during conflicts, that they adopt conciliatory "two-winner" strategies, and that they approach problem solving during conflict one step at a time. Within this rubric, they can then be helped to select among issues that might serve as conflict triggers, find the least potentially damaging means of expressing anger reflexively, engage in some potentially humorous self-analysis during the commitment stage, and shift into a problem-solving mode during the reconsolidation stage so that a rapprochement can solidify whatever gains and minimize any relationship stresses that result from conflict.

The failure to deal with conflict constructively has been viewed as the single most powerful force in dampening marital satisfaction (Cuber & Harroff, 1965) if not the most prominent cause of marital failure (Mace, 1976). Sociologists, like Coser (1969), who study conflict in group settings have noted that it can sometimes function to unfreeze interaction, stimulate innovative solutions to problems, and build group cohesion. While it may have some of these effects upon couples, it is more likely to evoke rigidification, ritualism, and withdrawal between spouses (Rosenstock & Kutner, 1967).

Once conflict has occurred, it tends to be repeated. Contrary to the views of some that conflict has both a cathartic and a self-stimulating effect that dissipates the urge to fight (e.g., Casriel, 1974; Perls, 1969), this respite from battle is brief, and those who have engaged in violence can be expected to be at least as violent again in the not-too-distant future (e.g., Bandura & Walters, 1963; Hicks, 1965; Kenney, 1952). Moreover, negative interactions have a higher probability of reciprocation than positive exchanges (Doehrman, 1968; Deutsch, 1969; Gottman et al., 1977; Rausch et al., 1974; Wills et al., 1974). Therefore, coercive experiences develop an inertial force that makes them more difficult to change than to maintain. For these reasons and others, Ellis (1976) has wisely suggested that counselors "stop helping people 'sublimate,' 'control,' or express' their feelings of anger, and that instead they show them how to eliminate or dissipate it" (p. 305).

Sources of Conflict

Ethologists like Lorenz (1966) and Rochlin (1973) believe that the propensity for violence is inherent in all humans, while observers of the social scene believe that it is endemic in all social institutions (e.g., Barry, 1970; Lewin, 1948). The inevitability of conflict in marriage and the difficulty in keeping conflict within safe bounds are reflected in the following observation by the sociologist Goode (1970):

> We are all exhorted to talk out [our] programs, to be wise in presenting our grievances, and [in] listening to those of others. Most of us are not wise, however, and in any event the underlying problem is that both sides may honestly feel that they are being cheated in the flow of family transactions. If both believe they are already paying more than they should be, it is difficult to alter the terms without perpetuating more injustice. At the same time, since both are already emotionally close, they know the other's weaknesses, and have acquired great skill at neatly hurting the other. . . . Moreover, they cannot easily retreat to the masks and formulas that mere acquaintances or business friends can use to pass over the conflict. (p. 630)

As if to validate this pronouncement, Birchler et al. (1972) found that nondistressed couples experienced conflict weekly, while arguments were the daily experience of those who were classified as distressed. Given the everyday observation that conflict is a high-probability event, couples can be helped to avoid some disagreements if they understand and take steps to control at least some of the sources.

One source of conflict derives from some general assumptions about what "should" occur in married life. Some writers believe that an idealized picture of family life is set forth in order to encourage people to marry and to stay married despite the strains of married life (Steinmetz & Straus, 1974). Partly as a result of this myth, couples expect to grow ever closer over time (Kimmel & Wavens, 1966). Failure to achieve this mystical state leads to bitter disappointments that often translate into conflict. A second source of conflict is related to the observation that "precedents are always turning into rights" (Homans, 1961, p. 73). Thus, spouses often gird for battle when present misdeeds or omissions of expected positives are believed to portend more grief in the years to come. Third, married couples interact with each other over more facets of their lives than do any other pairs; this interdependency in so many areas creates a myriad of opportunities for conflict (Lewin, 1948). This multifaceted interaction complicates, for example, efforts to establish and maintain a personal identity (Brittan, 1973), and it has been shown that spouses whose sense of identity is weak are more likely than those with strong personal identities to engage in conflict with their mates (Barry, 1968). Related to this problem is the fact that a marital relationship typically lasts for many years, and each partner is certain to undergo changes that may not be well synchronized with those of the other partner. Finally, conflict can also result from faulty communication leading to misunderstandings (Chapter 7).

Couples are less fortunate than those in many other business, local, or personal relationships because couples tend to fall victim to many of these stresses, while parties to other important relationships often escape these social perils. This conclusion is reflected in the comparisons of interaction patterns between spouses and between spouses and strangers. As shown in Chapters 4 and 8, various researchers (e.g., Birchler, 1972; Birchler et al., 1975; Stuart & Braver, 1973) have shown that when interacting with one another, spouses show less consideration and tact than they show in their routine exchanges with others.

Why are we kinder to strangers than to mates? Several explanations are available, partly found in culturally mediated values and the situational dimensions of spouse–spouse versus spouse–stranger encounters. On the value side, while it is recognized that strangers may disagree, considerable pressure builds up on spouses who are expected always to arrive at consensus. These and other norms lead married couples into upwardly spiraling conflicts that unmarried pairs can readily avoid (Blood, 1960). Moreover, while interactions between unmarried dyads often take place in the public eye, spouses interact in the privacy of their own homes and beyond the reach of social forces that would help them keep their anger within bounds (Gelles, 1974). In addition, because marital conflict is most likely to take place at home, at night, as opposed to less intimate relationships, married dyads have far less opportunity to separate to lick their wounds and obtain relief from tension (Gelles, 1977). Compared with other pairs, spouses have more sources of conflict, live by norms that lead to more intense conflict, and play out their conflicts in settings in which intense conflict is most likely to occur.

Content and Form of Marital Conflict

Tolstoy observed in *Anna Karenina,* "Happy families resemble one another; each unhappy family is unhappy in its own way." The themes that recur in conflict between couples, nevertheless, vary over time in predictable ways. For example, Gurin *et al.* (1960) found that 42% of complaining couples were concerned about their interaction, 12% addressed issues of child management, and 5% were concerned with managing interaction with in-laws and others in their extended families. Thus, their own relationship is obviously the prime concern of conflicted couples. During the first year of marriage, Sternberg and Beier (1972) found:

> The topics which most often seem to disturb the young couples are sex, money, and generally speaking, concern for each other. It seems that in the first year of marriage couples shed illusions and focus on hard-core problems. (p. 4)

Women are most likely to be the complainants in early requests for psychological help (e.g., Gurin *et al.*, 1960), perhaps because it is they who are required to make the greatest adjustment during the first years of married life (Bernard, 1964; Burgess & Wallin, 1953), and with little preparation for the role (Rossi, 1968). Later conflicts are likely to center on readjustment to shifting role responsibilities as the partners become parents and attempt to balance intrafamilial responsibilities with extrafamilial roles and opportunities. For example, in their study of lower-income families, Osmond and Martin (1978) found that among the 561 couples they studied, 235 and 171, respectively, reported fighting often about money and children, while 85 had frequent conflict about relatives, 53 conflicted often about recreation, and only 6 reported frequent disagreement about sex.

The content of spousal conflict is less important than its form. The form of conflict, in turn, can be analyzed from two perspectives: the orientation that each spouse takes toward disagreement with the other and the intensity with which the battle is fought.

Mouton and Blake (1971) have presented a unique way to conceptualize conflict orientation. They pointed out that every human encounter can be viewed from the perspective of the extent to which each person seeks personal gain and the extent to which each seeks maintenance of the relationship. They scaled both motivations from one to nine, higher scores indicating strength in each objective. When both motivations are high, they believe, partners are apt to adopt a "problem-solving" orientation. At the opposite extreme, one at which couples see no hope of gain from continuation of the relationship and are content to see it die, Mouton and Blake predicted that a "lose–leave" strategy will come to the fore. When one's goal is personal gain with little regard for the other, the "tough-bargainer" strategy will be used. Finally, for those who are willing to sign off on personal gain and have a strong desire to see the relationship persist, a "friendly-helper" orientation is likely to be chosen. If we recognize that conflict orientations rarely exist in the extremes and that the strategy chosen by one will be influenced by the choice made by the other, the Mouton and Blake classification can help couples and therapists alike to classify the orientation that partners adopt in approaching disagreements with each other.

In a slight variation of the same theme, Filley (1975) has offered a means of classifying not orientation but the fight tactics used by each partner. In a "win–lose" approach, either spouse may resort to the use of coercion to achieve gains at the expense of the other. This approach can lead to a Pyrrhic victory: the city can be taken but not without its being burned to the ground in the process. In a "lose–lose" approach, either spouse may give up any hope of gain and try, instead, to prevent the other from gaining any advantage. Both of these sets or tactics are fueled by dichotomous "you-versus-me" language in place of the co-centric "we." Both proceed from egocentric assumptions about right and wrong in the other's behavior, with comparatively little effort to evaluate one's own role in conflict elicitation. Moreover, both tactics seek an immediate remedy for the perceived wrong without regard to the impact that this solution might have upon the relationship and with virtually no ploys excluded from the conflictual situation. In contrast, the "win–win" tactic is one in which the spouses look for the greatest possible mutual gain reflecting the greatest possible return for their relationship. As an indication of the general frequency of these various strategies among lower-income couples, the number of spouses who saw their mates as never, seldom, sometimes, or often willing to give in during conflict was, respectively, 84, 103, 228, and 132 (Osmond & Martin, 1978).

Conflicts are more likely to produce positive change when both spouses employ win–win tactics. When they do so, the disagreement tends to be issue-focused. Rausch *et al.* (1974) found that 67% of the conflicts in which the issue was clearly stated were successfully resolved, in contrast to 18% of the conflicts in which the issue remained vague because of nonspecificity. They noted that:

> Specificity and directness optimize information exchange. When each partner knows what the other is talking about and how the other feels about it, each has the possibility of modulating his own reactions toward the other. The goal may be attainment of his own wishes, achievement of a joint solution, or simply increased differentiation and refinement of information about the issue. (p. 99)

Specific issues tend to be of a lesser magnitude than global concerns, and this, too, tends to aid their resolution (R. Fisher, 1964).

When conflicts are issue-focused, stress tends to be placed on defeating the problem, not the other person (J. Hall, 1971). When attention shifts from the issue at hand, it tends to focus first on the alleged inadequacies of the other person and then on the relationship itself. Person-focused conflicts can be termed "*second-degree*" arguments in contrast to the "*first-degree*" arguments that stress a specific issue. These second-degree arguments always involve "issue expansion" (Rausch *et al.*, 1974) that moves toward *ad hominum* attacks upon the other person, as well as the "hitchhiking" that was seen to be a dimension of complicated problem-solving efforts. The words "never" and "always" punctuate exchanges in these conflicts. So, too, do efforts to steamroll the other through a barrage of forcing dialogue, expansion to other issues in the past or beyond the scope of the specific problem, and what Rausch *et al.* (1974) term "crucializing" with statements like "If you really loved me. . . ."

Through the operation of negative cycles in which wrong begets wrong, these personal attacks are likely to escalate. The more one attacks the other and becomes committed to the truth of the attack, the more difficult it is to maintain the necessary level of regard for the other. When the value of the other is sufficiently disparaged, it is but a small step to attacking the relationship itself: Why would one wish to maintain a relationship with another who has so little worth? Rausch *et al.* (1974) believe that "for some couples almost any discrepancy in viewpoint seems to impinge on core issues" (p. 202). Thus, disagreements about how to celebrate the first anniversary can quickly be translated into evidence that the other "is always selfish," which, in turn, lead to threats like "If that's the way you want it, then you can just leave me out of the picture entirely." Once divorce threats begin, both partners are freed from the necessity to think constructively about each other, and conflict tactics tend to become progressively more destructive and eventually reach the *"third degree"* of intensity.

Because issue-specific conflicts are far more likely than second- or third-degree arguments to produce constructive change, distressed couples need help in learning how to keep their disagreements on the issue-focused plane. This learning is facilitated by an increase in commitment, effective communication, negotiation skills, and problem-solving abilities, all of which can make conflict less likely to occur or more mild when it does take place.

Techniques for Avoiding Conflict

Conflict can be managed in a number of different ways. Of course, the best way to manage conflict is to prevent it. It has been suggested that wise mate selection can help to reduce conflict (e.g., Blood, 1960); unfortunately, it is not clear whether "wise" means marrying someone like or different from oneself. It has also been suggested that conflict is less likely between mature partners for whom "a problem, in retrospect, may appear not to have been a problem at all" (Gurin *et al.*, 1960, p. 102). Here, too, however, it is not practical to expect the spouses to age a little so that the storm can pass innocently by. Having a set of relationship rules such as those developed through the powergram procedure suggested in Chapter 9 is another means of conflict avoidance. Blood (1960) raised the possibility that conflict may have been a less common marital experience in cultures in which family power was centralized in the hands of one person rather than presumably distributed equally as in companionate marriages. He noted that "When two or more family members believe that they ought to share in making a certain decision, they have added another potential conflict to their portfolio" (p. 214). In addition to developing an authority-allocating strategy, couples can also reduce their conflict potential by having effective communication skills. Pondy (1967), for example, found that the antecedents to conflict are often imagined and not real. Effective communication can serve as a guard against these misunderstandings and "pseudounderstandings" described in Chapter 7. Nierenberg and Calero (1973) phrased this belief nicely with the words: "The spouse who listens to one word and hears two, and knows the many things conveyed without talk, has the basic ingredients for understanding" (p. 92). Unfortunately, as we suggested earlier, this interpretive dimension of communication is likely to be as much a source of marital strain as a means of conflict avoidance.

Couples can also avoid conflict by having at their disposal an effective early reaction to would-be conflict triggers. Cutler and Dyer (1965) found in their analysis of marital interaction that negative exchanges do not always lead to fights because spouses sometimes react to provocations with an adjustive response. This may be a neurotic reaction, as would be true in exchanges like those that Rausch *et al.* (1974) found to be indications of avoidance, externalization, and/or denial through a "mutually agreed on defensive contract" (p. 73). But they can also be efforts toward compromise and concession. Naturally, if one spouse is the constant compromiser and conceder, that person's desires are likely to be unfulfilled, possibly constituting a domestic powder keg. When conciliatory behaviors are equally practiced by both spouses, however, the ends of marital satisfaction can be very well served. Therefore, while the presence of conflict does not necessarily signal relationship distress, neither does its absence necessarily indicate that the potential for marital stress is low.

Guidelines for Controlling Conflict

Given the realization that some conflict must inevitably occur in every relationship, it is important for each couple to have at their disposal a set of well-rehearsed strategies for dealing with disagreements when they do arise. We have found it helpful to base these strategies on a series of guidelines for conflict containment.

PRESENT ORIENTATION

It is important to focus the issue in the present, not in the past. As Scoresby (1977) has observed, "Most of our society believes that the best way to solve a problem is to find out what causes it and eliminate the cause" (p. 151). At the best of times, this may not be a wise strategy because it directs attention away from the challenges at hand and because the past is rarely if ever repeated in the future; therefore, past-oriented solutions may offer little benefit for the future. In marital encounters, this approach has even more pitfalls. First, when the partners search through the sifting sands of their past, they are unlikely to agree upon which actions, by whom, lead to what consequences. There were no observers, and their recall is subject to marked denial, distortion, and therefore disagreement. Second, because neither spouse wishes to be cast in the role of the villain (which would require concessions in the future), both are likely to respond to accusations of culpability with counteraccusations, intensifying the level of conflict through succeeding thrusts and parries. Therefore, the search for the roots of conflict in the past should be abandoned in favor of the quest for solutions in the present. In this, as in all areas of marital interaction, "why" questions should be replaced with "how" questions, and past orientations should be exchanged for orientation to the present and future.

Impulse leads most spouses into what Shepard (1961) has termed the "win–lose trap" and to the use of "primitive methods" in which one seeks gain at the other's expense. Indeed, there can be some gain from the use of strategies such as violence, but the gains are far more often short-term, with the longer-term consequences very negative with regard to the satisfaction of the aggressor (Steinmetz & Straus, 1974). For example, Kimmel and Wavens (1966) have observed:

> As long as the players look at the outcomes from their separate perspectives and attempt to maximize individual utilities, they will think in terms of winning and losing and their *feelings of conflict* will not be resolved by any decision, no matter how rationally optimum it might be. Thus, an outcome that both parties *perceive to be* equitable is impossible. In marital conflicts, both the "winner" and the "loser" of any game are losers, because the conflict issues are seldom resolved and the relationship becomes less and less unified, more individuated. (p. 462)

Thus, adoption of a win–lose strategy not only affects the tactics that one adopts in conflict, it even affects the way in which one sizes up the outcome of the disagreement. "Winners" are losers because they can hardly savor their ill-gotten gains, and "losers" are bitter and steeled for later battles in which they can balance the books. It has long been recognized that one can win or lose a dispute, but the loser can accept or reject the defeat (Maier, 1963). When the loser does not accept defeat—commonplace in marital disagreements—the victory is only an illusion, safe for a time but sure to be overthrown. Therefore, a cooperative rather than a competitive model of conflict resolution is what is strongly needed. Elsewhere (Chapter 8), this concept has been expressed as a "one-winner" as opposed to a "two-winner" tactic, the former based on the incorrect assumption that marriage is a zero-sum game, the latter based on the much more correct and humanistic assumption that marriage is the essential non-zero-sum game.

Adoption of a two-winner model requires two important skills: one must truly label the behavior of the other in the most positive possible light, and one must plan moves that can "resolve the issue equitably" rather than moves that are intended to "win the battle."

Perhaps more than any other writer, Ellis (1976) has championed recognition of the fact that the way in which we label other people's behavior greatly influences the way in which we respond to it. He suggested that an activating event triggers a belief system that, in turn, mediates a reaction. For example, Margaret arrives home for dinner an hour late (activating event). Burt decides that she has no regard for his feelings at all (belief system), so he becomes angry (reaction) and rages at her about her selfishness (another reaction). According to Ellis, Burt's anger and raging are under *his, not Margaret's* control. He could have construed her behavior in any of dozens of other ways—for example, "She has difficulty managing time," "She really gets involved in her work," or "She tries to be prompt but she hates to cut conversations short for fear of offending others"—any one of which would have enabled him to have different emotional and behavioral reactions. The effort to train oneself to relabel, to shift perspectives, or to "decenter" (Stuart, 1967) can be greatly rewarded by the avoidance of unnecessary stress and by the adoption of socially constructive actions that are conducive to much greater social effectiveness.

One way to do this is to ask couples, as Scoresby (1977) has suggested, to concentrate on their similarities during times of anger rather than indulging in a fruitless feeding of their anger by dwelling on differences. A simple exercise for accomplishing this result is to ask each person to practice preceding every critical statement about the other's behavior with a positive observation about other things that are positively valued. This procedure can be learned through such simple mnemonic devices as asking each spouse to cross his or her fingers when he or she is about to criticize the other and to keep the criticism locked within the crossed fingers until a positive observation has first been made.

Adoption of a win–win or two-winner strategy for conflict management is possible only if feelings of personal victimization are laid to rest and are replaced by a more tempered interpretation of the other's action. Aggressive behavior is suited to the win–lose and the lose–lose models; assertive behavior befits the win–win model. Lange and Jakubowski (1976) regard aggression as being motivated by self-righteousness and as being aimed primarily at hurting the other. In contrast, they view assertion as being motivated by the felt need for change and as being aimed at producing mutually beneficial change. Stuart (1978) has suggested that assertion involves making requests in contrast to the demands made in aggression; it involves taking personal responsibility rather than taking an accusatory approach as in aggression; and it asks for behavior change by the other, not a change in attitudes or feelings. The goal of assertion is equity, while the goal of aggression is a markedly imbalanced outcome.

Clients can be helped to learn how to diagram their conflictual behavior in the same way that their children are taught to diagram their algebra set-theory problems. So-called Venn diagrams and the theory of universal sets and subsets can be used for this purpose. Area I in the diagram below represents gain for the husband; Area II mutual gain; and Area III gain for the wife. In the illustration above, Burt's attempt to berate Margaret and force her to "feel guilty" is an aggressive response that is clearly for his own gain and would belong to Area I. His asking Margaret if they should plan to have dinner a little later is a conciliatory maneuver that is obviously intended to resolve the problem rather than to exact a pound of compensatory flesh, so it would be assigned to Area II. Training clients actually to draw the Venn diagram and locate their goals during conflict can help them to learn how to move from the one-winner to the two-winner model of conflict behavior rather quickly. Each of the remaining guidelines points the way toward additional behavior changes that can make resolution of conflicts a reality.

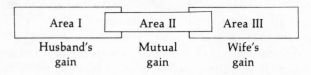

Area I	Area II	Area III
Husband's gain	Mutual gain	Wife's gain

SEEKING SOLUTIONS IN SMALL STEPS

Issues should be addressed one at a time. In international relations, it has long been recognized that smaller substantive conflicts are much easier to resolve than larger conflicts over general principles (R. Fisher, 1964). When spouses conflict, their arguments are much less likely to become overheated if they address issues sequentially rather than all at one time (Rausch et al., 1974). This approach means that couples must avoid counterdemands while each person has an opportunity to express his or her wishes for a change in the other's behavior (Bach & Deutsch, 1970). When counterdemands are expressed, the first speaker is likely to feel as though he or she has been ignored—"disqualified" in the language of Watzlawick et al. (1967)—a feeling that is very likely to force an escalation in demands and thereby intensify the argument. Adding other issues to the conflict also has the effect of increasing the cognitive load, of diverting problem-solving energies, and of forcing the discussion onto side tracks that carry it away from resolution of the dilemma that caused the initial disagreement. It is the frustration that grows from this piling of issue upon issue that leads couples from first- to second-degree fights, from issue-specific arguments to attacks upon each other as people. To help couples learn to maintain focus on a single issue, another pencil-and-paper task can be very helpful. The therapist simply asks each of them to write down at the start of the argument exactly what change each would like the other to make in his or her behavior, to exchange notes, and to limit their discussion only to how the behaviors should be changed, one at a time.

THE NATURAL HISTORY OF MARITAL CONFLICT

The foregoing guidelines are useful during one particular stage of an argument, and it is important to understand the stages of arguments as an aid to timing conflict-containment techniques. Waller (1938), in his classic work, described a four-stage model of conflict: crisis, disorganization, recover, and reorganization. Rausch *et al.* (1974) presented a seven-stage model of conflict resolution beginning with the specification of an issue, followed in turn by exploration of alternative solutions, resolution, practical planning, emotional reconciliation, consolidation of the relationship, and the working out of future coping strategies. A somewhat different description can be derived when the work of Luria (1932) is used as a model. In this approach an initial conflict trigger is believed to generate a reflex of anger. As with every reflex, anger must undergo a period of abatement due to fatigue. The reflex–fatigue stage is then followed by a stage in which one is committed to anger; the physiological emotion is not nearly as strong as the rational decision to remain "angry." This stage is then followed by a time of readiness for reconsolidation and the act of rapprochement itself. The techniques that have already been described can be fit into this model together with adaptation from others:

Trigger—Reflex—Fatigue—Commitment—Reconsolidation—Rapprochement

At the *trigger stage* it is important to recognize the possibility that while some degree of emotional arousal is reflexive, the intensity of the reaction that is expressed is certainly under operant control. Think, for example, about the worker who is offended by something that an employer says or does, but who very prudently holds his reaction in check, while responding with full vigor to the merest provocations of his or her spouse. Clients can be helped to learn to pause before responding and to use this precious time to ask themselves five questions:

1. Exactly what is the issue?
2. Exactly what would satisfy me?
3. Is the goal important?
4. Have I tried to get what I want through problem solving?
5. How much conflict am I willing to risk to get what I desire?

None of these are easy questions to answer. Moreover, many people seem to take pleasure in indulging their anger and in using it to exploit their mates. Therefore, the value of the questions is as much in anticipation of conflict situations as in their execution during crises; they provide each spouse with an opportunity to decide whether to react to a situation with anger and, if so, to rehearse inwardly a measured expression of his or her emotions. Moreover, many of the triggers of conflict occur when spouses are separated: Bill realizes that Mary has not completed some chore and plans to "roast" her when she comes home, or Mary waits impatiently for Bill to pick her up at work and plans to give him "a piece of her mind" as soon as his car pulls up. This time that is normally used to fan the flames of anger could be used much more constructively to plan a more measured response.

During the *reflex stage*, at least a portion of the anger is physiological in origin (Elliot, 1976). Reflexive anger is a sharp physiological reaction, one that "starts rapidly and ends after a relatively short time (less than one second)" (Clynes, 1978, p. 35). While reflexive, this dynamic explosion of anger generally follows learned channels of expression and takes advantage of the resources that each person has for the expression of discontent (Goode, 1969). For example, a spouse who feels thwarted in the use of words may respond reflexively with withdrawal or with violence. The management of reflexive anger therefore depends upon training in two response dimensions: management of the feeling level and management of the words and/or deeds that are chosen for the expression of the emotion.

Training in the management of the feeling level can be accomplished through a combination of skill development in progressive relaxation (e.g., Bernstein & Borkovec, 1973; Sullivan, 1964) and the behavioral rehearsal of assertive rather than aggressive behaviors.

When the feeling tone is under control, control of the words and deeds chosen for the expression of anger can be more readily accomplished. Reflexive anger is commonly expressed as a one-two punch: "you never" or "you always" statements are usually followed with threats. The accusatory statements move the conflict from the first to the second degree; the threats can then carry it to the third degree of intensity.

A threat is "a declaration of the intention to inflict punishment, injury, death, or at least loss upon someone in retaliation for some action or cause" (Milburn, 1974, p. 1). Threats are used at all levels of social interaction, and it is believed that threats are used whenever they are available (Deutsch & Krauss, 1960). The use of threats is not necessarily harmful. Threats may serve as words that inhibit physical aggression (Parke *et al.*, 1972); they may have a signal function that helps each person anticipate the actions that the other might take (Geiwitz, 1967; Kelley, 1962; Shomer *et al.*, 1966); and they can be understood as a definition of the current state of a relationship (Kelley, 1965). Threats have been found to be inhibitors of aggression in some studies (e.g., Baron, 1971; Shortell *et al.*, 1970); they have been found to be ineffective in others (Baron, 1973, 1974; Knott & Drost, 1972). Effective communication between the parties that allows the threats to be understood is one factor that determines their effectiveness (Smith & Anderson, 1975). Their believability is a second factor that affects their effectiveness (Horai & Tedeschi, 1969). Threats that are too large and threats that have not been followed through on in the past are likewise ineffective (Shelling, 1963).

The use of threats is also fraught with danger. Threats are as likely to generate at least covert counteraggression as they are likely to produce compliance. In addition, when threats work, they are likely to induce the successful threatener to rely upon them rather than upon positive inducements as influence strategies in the future. Threats are also likely to involve the core symbols of the relationship and, in so doing, to weaken the forces that bond the spouses together (Coser, 1969).

Just as spouses can be taught to moderate their emotions through tension-control techniques, so, too, can they be taught to temporize their threats. Threats are made by one person, usually "I," against another, usually "you." They are contingent statements that promise to deliver a negative contingency unless some positive act is emitted by the other—hence, they are negatively reinforcing consequences. Choices can thus be made concerning (1) who will do? (2) to whom? (3) what things? (4) unless what things happen? When the threatener qualifies his or her words by stating an emotion—such as accepting ownership of anger as Ellis (1976) suggested—the words that follow are put in a context that qualifies their meaning. If the other person is referred to in derogatory or demeaning terms, the defensiveness that arises is very likely to interfere with reception of the ensuing message. Threats to inflict physical harm or to leave the marriage also seriously impede motivation for problem solving in marital conflicts. And demands for impossible or clearly inequitable changes are more likely to spiral the conflict to greater intensity than to resolve the crisis-causing issue. The checkpoints for threatening messages are therefore well summarized in four questions:

1. Have I qualified my statement by accepting my anger?
2. Have I expressed respect for the other person although communicating my displeasure with his or her actions?
3. Have I made a threat that is modest and therefore credible?
4. Have I asked for a specific and reasonable change?

Unfortunately, when threatening statements are extreme, the attacking individual often feels forced to behave in a more menacing manner than even he or she feels is justified in order to "save face" in the argument (Goffman, 1959, 1967). Therefore, controlling the tension level and utterances during the reflexive stage of arguments can have a very significant impact upon the success of efforts to contain their effects.

Because strong reflexive reactions cannot be maintained very long, the initial surge of anger is almost always followed by a dip in the intensity of the emotion. This is termed *"reflex fatigue,"* and it provides another opportunity to interrupt the conflict cycle.

It is often difficult if not impossible for the listener to interrupt the speaker during reflexive anger. To attempt to do so, in fact, often spurs the speaker to greater wrath. Such an opportunity does occur, however, during the almost inevitable temporary abatement of anger that results from one's inability to keep all bodily systems mobilized at a high state of battle readiness for long (Millenson, 1967). This abatement creates an opportunity not to challenge the reflex but to attempt to redirect it. When partners adopt a win–lose or a lose–lose strategy, they are likely to use this moment to try to steal the offensive. For example, when Burt berates Margaret for arriving home late for dinner, she might seize the floor during Burt's moment of reflex fatigue to accuse him of having consistently shown the same disregard for her, or she might retort that he is not her master and that she is free to come and go as she pleases. Both are maneuvers aimed at sidetracking Burt's anger and at putting him on the defensive. Unless he is a pushover, they will simply intensify his rage. As an alternative, Margaret can make a two-step response that will move the interaction from conflict to problem solving. She can:

1. Express recognition of his anger.
2. Refocus it by asking Burt what he would like her to do in the future.

She will feed his anger if she challenges it head-on, but she can help him to control it if she moves from recognition to redirection in her response to it. She will take these steps, however, only if she adopts a win–win or two–winner orientation, in which her goal would be the best possible outcome for both at the lowest possible cost to each.

The next stage of conflict is the *commitment stage.* It begins when the initial reflexive surge of rage has given way to the fatigue stage; the strong feelings have subsided, but what may be regarded as smoldering feelings of discontent are kept alive not by the original insult but by self-given messages like "I shouldn't stand for that" or "She (he) would never treat me that way if I was truly loved and respected." It is as though one aspect of the person tries to whip the other into prolonged distance from the other person, while that other side might be inclined just to let the issue quietly die. Whereas the reflexive stage of anger is sudden and often unplanned, behavior during the commitment stage is frequently cunning, planned, and highly manipulative.

Men and women have different strategies of action during the commitment stage (Barry, 1970; Cutler & Dyer, 1965), with withdrawal being the most common form of anger commitment among those in troubled marriages (e.g., Locke, 1951; Ort, 1950). The way in which one handles this stage of argument can either greatly shorten the period of estrangement or give rise to unnecessary bitterness as a secondary consequence of the angry encounter.

During the commitment stage, the triggering issue is much less important than the management of the relationship. One partner feels wronged by the other, and it is obvious to everyone that the wrong cannot be set aright. Therefore, the goal at this point in the conflict is to maneuver for relationship gain, generally in the form of greater power in future exchanges. This might be legitimate power gained through the acceptance of one's role needs (e.g., "I can't work if I don't know when you're coming home") or referent power through the expression of righteous indignation ("I never treat you that way"). However, all too often the goal is merely to carve out the right to misbehave in kind in the weeks ahead ("Two can play at that game, you know"). Unfortunately, neither gain can be significant. Concessions gained through coercive anger are quickly repudiated when the rage has subsided, and one's own past mistakes are hardly ever sufficient to buy forgiveness for the errors of others in the future. Therefore, the best thing that can happen to the commitment stage of a conflict is its attenuation; and both spouses can help bring it to a speedy end.

Scoresby's (1977) self-narration strategy is useful during the commitment stage of an argument. It asks the spouse to announce his or her intentions before the fact. He illustrated the suggestion in the following way:

> HUSBAND: I am going to get angry and yell at you because of your mistakes. And, if you try to speak, I'm going to interrupt you because I'm not going to listen to what you say. (p. 154)

This is an effective way to modulate the tension level during the commitment stage. Implicit in this suggestion is the belief that the level of emotion in an argument is directly responsive to—and therefore controlled by—the actions that each person takes. Thus, we can act to nourish our anger, or we can act to weaken it—the choice is always there.

The spouse who is under attack can also take some steps to help bring the commitment stage to an end. Listening quietly without interruption or challenge is important. Respecting the anger of one's spouse is another important step. For example, if Burt withdraws when he is angry and Margaret follows him around the house to get her two cents in, at best Burt will be reinforced by her attention for his sulky withdrawal, while at worst he will be provoked to violence because he has nowhere else to go (Gelles, 1974). Suggesting a change of scene is another useful step. If Burt vents his rage in the living room, Margaret might suggest that they move into the kitchen, or better still, that they go for a walk. If the radio is on when the fight begins, turn it off; if it is off when the first insult is issued, turn it on. Do anything possible to change the stimulus conditions that control the interaction, because any change can break the vice grip of anger.

The commitment stage of an argument can last for minutes or as long as days or weeks. It is never served by the counterwithdrawal of the spouse who is under attack. It is important for both spouses to learn that they gain stature through their mature efforts to keep their composure and to exercise maneuvers aimed at positive control during times of stress. Therefore, neither party should fear a loss of face by admitting to error in anger or by reaching out for reconsolidation.

Arguments end when spouses attempt to *reconsolidate* by shifting into a problem-solving mode. At first, the gestures toward this shift may be tentative, so tentative in fact that they may be overlooked or misperceived. When this happens, the reconsolidating spouse often feels frustrated anew and provoked to a needless new attack. To prevent this sequence from happening, couples should be helped to develop a signal system indicating readiness to renegotiate their differences. The signal should be unambiguous and available at any time and in any place. It should involve the use of both words and gestures. For example, Burt might say he's had enough and wants to find a way to prevent future reruns. To punctuate the words, he might reach for Margaret's hand to overcome the physical distance he seeks at times of anger. Each couple should develop their own style for communicating the end of conflict, for problem solving will begin much more efficiently if both spouses know that they are moving into a problem-solving mode.

Finally, the argument ends with a moment of *rapprochement*. This is not the idle passing of aggression because some other event demands attention. If this happens, the wounds remain only partly bandaged and are apt to fester again. Instead, rapprochement occurs when one spouse summarizes what he or she has learned and the other acknowledges the lesson and agrees to a prophylactic change. For example, Burt might say that he realizes he flew off the handle a bit too much, but that he hopes Margaret will call if she's due to be more than half an hour late. When Margaret acknowledges the change, they will have made a new rule for their relationship and drawn the conflict to its most constructive end.

The steps for conflict that have just been described are based on two major assumptions: conflict is avoidable, and when it occurs, it is containable. Not only can issues that trigger conflict be better handled with problem solving, but the intensity of emotions aroused in conflictual encounters can also be modulated to permit a speedy shifting of gears from attack to issue resolution. Some couples may object that writing down issues and requests or recognizing feelings and relying on redirection are "unnatural." Indeed they are; when conflicts follow their natural course, the joy vanishes from marital relationships, to be replaced by defensive bitterness and rigidity. Conversely, when the natural course of conflict is interrupted, the seeds are sewn for interaction change that can bring new freedom and vitality to any encounter.

C H A P T E R   11

Sex
Therapy

FREIDA M. STUART AND
D. CORYDON HAMMOND

S EVERAL POSSIBILITIES exist in the relationship between sexual and social interactions between couples. Primary sexual problems in either or both partners may give rise to other relationship stresses or they may be accepted without contaminating other spheres of the marriage. On the other hand, sexual problems may result from problems in the social interaction between the spouses. In these situations, couples may either admit to or deny difficulties in their sexual interaction. Whatever the situation, sexual problems are among the more common complaints of couples entering treatment, and it is not uncommon for these problems to be neglected by marriage therapists. This chapter offers an overview of the techniques of sex therapy, beginning with a review of current estimates of the prevalence of problems of sexual adjustment, moving through the description of a multidimensional method of assessing sexual problems, and concluding with a discussion of the therapeutic options available for the treatment of the more common sexual adjustment difficulties. This chapter has been included in the present volume so that readers can make use of it in either of three ways: Some readers who are not trained in sex therapy will find here techniques that can be used to counsel couples with mild sexual disturbances. These readers can also use this material to increase their under-

Freida M. Stuart and D. Corydon Hammond. Codirectors, Sex and Marriage Therapy Clinic, Department of Physical Medicine, School of Medicine, University of Utah. Order of authorship determined by flip of a coin.

standing of the sex therapy process so that they can more effectively refer clients to qualified sex therapists. Other readers, who have completed sex therapy training, will find in this chapter a more detailed presentation of therapeutic technique than is currently available in other publications.

Introduction

Problems in sexual functioning are among the more common marital complaints, but they have frequently been neglected in marriage counseling. In examining 750 couples coming for marital therapy, Greene (1970) found that 80% were sexually dissatisfied, and Sager (1974) has estimated that 75% of couples in marital therapy have a sexual dysfunction.

Although a large percentâge of couples who enter marital treatments may have sexual diffculties, sexual problems *per se* are often not a manifestation of marital discord among the nontherapeutic population. It is not at all uncommon for dysfunctions to be present in otherwise happy marriages. Masters and Johnson (1970) estimated that at some time, one of every two couples struggles with a sexual problem. More recently, Frank *et al.* (1978) studied the sexual adjustment of 100 well-educated, white, middle-class couples. The couples were volunteers who were not involved in therapy, and who, in comparison with the general population, were above average in marital satisfaction—83% of them rating their marriages as "very happy" or "happy." Despite the high degree of marital happiness, 63% of the women and 40% of the men reported a sexual dysfunction, and sexual "difficulties" were described by 77% of the women and 50% of the men. Among the women, 48% had difficulty getting excited, 33% had difficulty maintaining excitement, 46% had difficulty reaching orgasm, and 15% were unable to have an orgasm. Of the men, 7% reported a problem in getting an erection, 9% had a problem in maintaining an erection, 36% ejaculated too quickly, and 4% had a problem in ejaculating. In addition, 47% of the women and 12% of the men were unable to relax during sexual involvement, 35% of the women and 16% of the men expressed lack of interest in sex, and 28% of the women and 10% of the men described themselves as "turned off." This information illustrates that a sexual dysfunction does not always have to cause disruption of the entire relationship nor create marital dissatisfaction. Some couples are successful in tolerating sexual problems, compartmentalizing and insulating them from the rest of the relationship where emotional intimacy and high levels of satisfaction are maintained. Probably the primary factor that determines the degree to which sexual problems negatively influence marital stability is the meaning, value, and importance placed on sex by each of the partners.

In our experience, sexual dysfunction often produces varying degrees of secondary marital discord in otherwise satisfactory marriages because one or both spouses place much significance on their sexual relationship. On the other hand, we also see many cases where preexisting marital conflicts have come to impair sexual function. In these situations, however, the treatment of the marital problems alone is often insufficient to restore sexual function and satisfaction. Once a sexual dysfunction has developed it commonly tends to be perpetuated by the fears of failure that have also evolved, continuing even after the original precipitating stress has been removed. Such cases require sex therapy. But where conflict is severe, resentment impairs a couple's ability to cooperate in therapeutic tasks, and hostility inhibits their erotic desires, marital therapy is the treatment of choice.

It is vital to bear in mind that sexual dysfunctions are invariably caused by multiple determinants and can rarely be traced to a single etiological factor. In our clinical experience, relationship variables and conflicts seem to be associated more often with problems of inhibited sexual desire, secondary orgasmic dysfunction, secondary erectile dysfunction, and possibly delayed ejaculation. In contrast, marital factors appear to be less significant in cases of premature ejaculation, primary orgasmic dysfunction, primary erectile dysfunction, and vaginismus. Negative feelings toward a spouse, demands, quarrels, and pressure are all relationship factors that encourage dysfunction. There are also instances where the sexual problem serves an adaptive function within the relationship. For example, sex may be used as barter in a competitive power struggle or as a weapon to obtain revenge. Dysfunctions may also occur in response to relationship fears, such as the fear of becoming submissive, of being controlled, of being disapproved of, or of being abandoned.

What, then, is the relationship of marital and sex therapy? Certainly, in many cases, a sexual dysfunction cannot be treated in isolation from the general marital system. With most couples, there is a reciprocal influence process between marital and sexual problems. Therefore, the sex therapist should also be a well-trained marital therapist. In cases where marriage conflicts strongly contribute to sexual dysfunction, it is usually necessary to focus initially on enhancing the general marital relationship and to shift the emphasis to sex therapy later. In other cases, where sexual distress predominates, the order of intervention may be to provide sex therapy first and later recommend expanding the focus of treatment to include more general marital conflict resolution, if this is the treatment indicated.

Ideally, all marital therapists would receive advanced training and supervision in sex therapy, facilitating flexible and comprehensive treatment for distressed couples. However, despite the interrelatedness that frequently exists between marital and sexual problems, the vast majority of marital therapists do not have adequate training in the specialty of sex therapy. If they offered sex therapy services, therefore, they would violate professional principles of ethical conduct. Thus, most marital therapists in actuality should sequentially or concurrently refer couples requiring sex therapy services to qualified specialists unless they are in advanced training and receiving regular supervision from a certified sex therapist. Concurrent marital and sex therapy by different practitioners does not have to be disruptive, and, in fact, Sager (1974) stated, "To date, I have seen *no* instances where the process of psychoanalysis, psychotherapy or marital therapy has been interfered with by simultaneous sex therapy conducted by another therapist" (p. 505).

There are, however, some couples with sexual difficulties who do not need intensive sex therapy. Annon (1976) has presented a model for conceptualizing sexual problems and the levels of intervention that are necessary in responding to them. The Plissit model is valuable because it provides a conceptual scheme that acknowledges that therapy must be individualized and that not all sexual difficulties require a highly trained sex therapist. Some couples merely need "permission," the first level of intervention. More specifically, with minimal training, many marital therapists can often provide couples with reassurance that they are normal. This course requires, of course, that the therapist be sexually enlightened and sufficiently free of personal conflict so that he can convey respectful acceptance, affirming the couple's and individual's right to determine the sexual value system that fits for them. With regard to the frequency of sexual activity, sexual thoughts and fantasies, or sexual practices (e.g., oral–genital lovemaking), many couples have fears that they may be abnormal. It is crucial to convey the concept that each person is the world's authority in evaluating what is for him or her "normal," "average," or acceptable. We would also add that sometimes permission giving includes assuring a client that it is acceptable to honor one's feelings about not liking to engage in certain sexual practices.

More sexual education and skill is required at the second level, providing "limited information." If the marital therapist has a broad knowledge of general human sexuality, he or she may be equipped to provide specific factual information that is directly related to client concerns. For instance, limited, relevant information may often ease client anxieties concerning penis or breast size, masturbation, having intercourse during menstruation, birth control, cleanliness of oral–genital contact, or sex and aging. A still higher degree of professional expertise and skill is required at the third level of Annon's system, giving "specific suggestions." At this level, for example, the counselor may discuss with an arthritic couple alternative coital positions that are less painful and may recommend heat treatment, use of physical therapy exercises, and timing of medications prior to sexual involvement. Other suggestions may include recommending concurrent clitoral stimulation with intercourse, openly communicating sexual preferences and desires, and instructing couples in the concept of sex as a natural function. The therapist may decrease performance pressure by dispelling the myth that an erection is necessary for sexual activity, helping the patient to stop catastrophizing his loss of erection, and focus on his attention to other love-play options.

Frequently these three levels of intervention—permission, limited information, and specific suggestion—are also part of the sex therapist's repertoire and are used in conjunction with other treatment strategies for "intensive therapy," Annon's fourth level. The subsequent two sections offer a brief overview of a multidimensional approach to assessment and a detailed view of the treatment of sexual dysfunction, with concentration upon the techniques of intensive therapy. In each instance, the techniques offered are consistent with the marriage therapy techniques presented elsewhere in this volume. For example, the techniques recommended for the assessment of sexual functioning involve analysis of specific sexual interaction behaviors from varied perspectives as well as assessment of individual behavior patterns that might require management prior to undertaking the focal therapy. The intervention procedures are arranged in a hierarchy comparable to that used in the sequence of marriage improvement techniques described herein. For example, the sensate focus technique is designed to allow couples to gain information about their own and each other's desires, to facilitate their making small requests of one another, and to build some commitment to the process of change. These are identical to the goals of the caring-days technique described in Chapter 6. Couples are taught to request, clarify, and acknowledge changes in their sexual interaction precisely as they were taught to communicate more effectively in their efforts to achieve change in the social interaction patterns of their marriage. They are also taught how to negotiate and follow through on agreements to change aspects of their sexual interaction so that each partner can be better able to achieve a more satisfying level of sexual functioning. Therefore, many of the therapeutic techniques useful in managing the social dimension of marital interaction are equally applicable to the management of its sexual dimension.

Assessment

Traditionally, different schools of therapy have tended to emphasize a limited range of determinants of problems. The various orientations, however, have operated on what Goldstein (1969) called the "one-true-light assumption," prematurely presenting themselves as global theories. Other approaches have been viewed as competitive rivals rather than as potential contributors that emphasize different determinants of problematic behavior. Thorne (1967) suggested that preferring a narrow orientation to therapy was analogous to preferring a "one-string violin when actually the whole spectrum of instruments is available" (p. 347). The trend in the field of psychotherapy, and within individual schools, is toward a more broad, multidimensional approach (Hammond & Stanfield, 1977). Nowhere is this more essential than in sex therapy, where Kaplan (1974) asserted her belief that sexual dysfunction has multiple determinants requiring a broad therapeutic approach.

The multidimensional model that we use provides a systematic framework for collecting and organizing assessment data, as well as for comprehensive treatment planning. It is an elaboration of Lazarus's (1973, 1976) multimodal behavior therapy and draws heavily upon Bandura's (1977) notion of reciprocal determinism, among other dimensions of social learning theory. In the remainder of this section, we describe the interrelationship of the six components of this assessment model, as well as giving an overview of the assessment procedures used in our approach. In the following section, we offer an overview of the general considerations in the structure of our treatment approach, and we review the treatment literature on the major categories of sexual dysfunction, concluding each review with an outline of our recommendations for treatment in each area.

MULTIDIMENSIONAL ASSESSMENT APPROACH

The dimensions of the present assessment framework include behavior, affect, sensory–physical responsiveness, imagery, cognition, and the interpersonal and environmental context of the couple's relationship.

On the *behavioral* dimension, the therapist must learn how couples express or inhibit their desires, how they do and do not verify their beliefs about one another's wishes, and how they use touch and other forms of expression in their affectionate and sexual interaction.

On the *affective* dimension, the therapist should be most attuned to levels of depression, which can either prompt and maintain sexual problems or be a consequence of such problems. It is usually recommended that acute depression be treated prior to the undertaking of sex therapy, just as the suggestion is made earlier in this book that the same problem be overcome before the initiation of marriage therapy. In addition to depression, the therapist should be alert to anxiety that may trigger phobic reactions and guilt that may inhibit full sexual expression.

On the *sensory–physical* dimension, the therapist must assess the presence of such problems as misguided stimulation, abrasive touch, sensitivity to odors and moistness, lack of awareness, and an inability to focus on sensations, all of which may contribute to sexual problems. Kaplan (1974) has noted that in males, sexual response is more vulnerable to physiological factors than in females. Also, as suggested by many writers (e.g., Kaplan, 1974; Masters & Johnson, 1970; Reckless & Geiger, 1975), problems with an organic basis generally manifest themselves in a progressive decline and/or are unremitting in nature, while functional disorders occur periodically and situationally.

On the dimension of *imagery*, the therapist must assess the role that fantasy plays in the couple's functioning. Fantasies may increase arousal, or images such as rape and incest may evoke fear. Fantasies are related to the *cognitive* dimension of assessment, which includes awareness of the facts and fallacies that couples bring to therapy. As an added dimension of this component, Masters and Johnson (1970) have referred to "spectorating," in which a person may watch and evaluate his own performance, may become self-absorbed in the process and lose touch with his mate, and often may engender in himself a countersexual reaction. For example, preoccupation with whether or not one's partner is becoming aroused often sabotages one's own arousal. Finally, expectations about the relationship and the meanings of a sensual encounter can bear heavily upon the character of a couple's sex. These expectations should be understood by the therapist, and they lead to the final dimension of assessment, the *interpersonal and environmental context* of the couple's sexual interaction. As recognized in the first chapter of this book, the social interaction between mates sets the stage for their sexual relationship. So, too, does their choice of when, where, and how to be together, their personal mood, their appearance, their level of fatigue, and scores of other details, all of which determine the quality of their sexual relationship.

THE PROCESS OF ASSESSMENT

Assessment consists of collecting, organizing, and interpreting data for the process of treatment planning. Thorough assessment of strengths, deficits, and excesses on each of the multiple dimensions of sexual functioning is a necessary prerequisite for comprehensive treatment.

Sex therapy assessment consists primarily of gathering self-report information about personal, psychological, marital, and physical functioning, sometimes supplemented by a medical evaluation and/or physiological measurements. Our assessment process includes (1) an hour-long conjoint interview focusing on the nature of the couple's relationship, current sexual interaction, and specific sexual complaints, after which the couple complete several tests of inventories and identify in writing their individual goals for therapy; (2) a one-hour individual sex history interview; and (3) a "roundtable" feedback and contracting interview, which includes a review of clinical implications, clarification of goals for therapy, and a structuring of the anticipated course of therapy.

Individuals can be seen without their partners under one of three circumstances: they may not currently have a partner with whom they have a sexual relationship; they may have a current sex partner but be unwilling to ask the other person to participate in treatment for fear that such participation would require escalation of the commitment of both to the relationship; or their partner may be uncooperative. While the partner's participation facilitates therapeutic progress, some clients, such as women learning to experience orgasm through self-stimulation, can be successfully treated in single contacts. In these instances in which only one individual is involved, only two hours of assessment interviewing are required, followed by the roundtable discussion.

Minnesota Multiphasic Personality Inventory (MMPI). The degree of manifest psychopathology influences our decision regarding the appropriateness of sex therapy because the absence of psychological disturbance has been found to be a favorable prognostic indicator (Johnson, 1965; Lansky & Davenport, 1975; Meyer *et al.*, 1975; Lobitz & Baker, 1979; Fabbri, 1976). The MMPI is an excellent screening tool for identifying determinants of sexual dysfunction or factors that could disrupt sex therapy, such as anxiety, depression, thought disorder, distrust, hostility, rebelliousness, impulsivity, low energy level, deficient interpersonal skills, and feelings of inadequacy. In addition, we routinely use the MacAndrew (1965) alcohol and drug abuse scale from the MMPI, which particularly aids in the identification of alcoholism. This is critical because alcohol is a depressant of the central nervous system that impairs arousal, orgasmic capacity, erectile functioning, and sexual attractiveness to partners.

When sexual dysfunction appears to be distinctly secondary to psychological maladjustment, alcoholism, or drug abuse, or where these problems are so serious that they would be disruptive to sex therapy, the patient couple are referred for psychotherapy. They are, however, instructed that our service is available once their more urgent difficulties are resolved. Individuals are frequently accepted for treatment who manifest varying degrees of depression, anxiety, passivity, and impulsiveness that seem unlikely to interfere with therapy. As a general rule, if the patient couple function on an everyday basis and have a relatively stable, even if troublesome, relationship, they will be accepted for therapy.

Dyadic Adjustment Scale (DAS). The nature of the couple's relationship and their motivation for change are the most crucial areas of assessment. Sexual functioning occurs in an interactional context with a significant other. Although there are two individuals with distinct identities, personal philosophies, and values, the couple also forms a system that functions with unique patterns of communication, decision making, values, and interaction, all of which influence sexual functioning. As Masters and Johnson (1970) proclaimed, there is no such thing as an uninvolved partner. Regardless of who exhibits the dysfunction, both partners influence it and will contribute to future change. To maximize the opportunity for successful outcome, the individuals must have a felt commitment to each other and sufficient trust to risk being vulnerable and exposing a sensitive area of their relationship.

The DAS (Spanier, 1976), as described in Chapter 4, is a 32-item inventory addressing couple agreement about varied areas of daily living, varied features of their communication, dimensions of their satisfactions with one another, and their investment in seeing their relationship succeed. At least a moderate level of satisfaction on instruments like the DAS is believed to be a necessary prerequisite for successful sex therapy (e.g., Leiblum *et al.*, 1976), although success may be achieved with couples whose commitment to one another is less than optimal (Leiblum & Kopel, 1977).

We concur with Sager (1974) that serious discord and hostility make sex therapy impossible. Marital therapy is the treatment of choice in such cases, and proceeding with sex therapy may actually result in destructive outcomes rather than in just no change. Thus, it is vital to determine the relationship between marital discord and sexual dysfunction. It is our clinical impression that a couple's capacity for affectionate cooperation is probably the single most valuable predictor of successful outcome. Rather than set couples up for failure, marital rather than sex therapy should be prescribed where serious discord is present. In such cases, couples may be referred for marriage counseling, but increasingly, there seems to be a trend in the field toward combining more marital and sex therapy, although this combination naturally increases the length of treatment. Munjack *et al.* (1976) concluded:

> Since apparently so few sexually dysfunctional couples can be treated solely for their sexual complaints, the present investigators agree . . . that couples must be highly selected for marital harmony (if treatment for a sexual dysfunction is to be attempted directly and immediately) or first be treated for their interpersonal problems. Since marital and sexual problems are most often inextricable, the combined problem should probably be treated by the same therapist or therapy team, as indicated. Time allowance will then have to be made as the goals become expanded. (p. 502)

Sexual Adjustment Inventory (SAI). The SAI (Stuart *et al.*, 1975) provides an evaluation by both partners of sexual satisfaction, sexual communication and decision making, individual responses to different forms of sexual stimulation, and the variety of sexual practices in the couple's repertoire, as well as the degree of pleasure associated with each. The SAI also collects information concerning physical health, use of medications and nonprescription drugs, birth control practices, mood, and marital–personal difficulties. The majority of the SAI questions are asked in the affirmative, channeling the couple's thinking toward positive observation and constructive change, and redirecting their attention from the more common negative characteristics of dysfunctional couples. Use of the SAI decreases the amount of interview time necessary for history taking, thereby minimizing cost for patients. A copy of portions of the SAI may be examined in Figure 1.

Interview Assessment. Our assessment interviews are relatively structured and serve to: (1) delineate the multiple determinants of problems and (2) determine if sex therapy is the treatment of choice. To standardize interview data collection, we delineated specific historical areas of inquiry and questions concerning each major dysfunction. We do allow for flexibility in the interview, however, and during assessment we emphasize to the couple that our treatment is only as good as the information that we receive. Interview data are coded on a three-page form with separate boxes for each interview question and with additional space provided for recording other observations. This procedure was modified from the Crenshaw Clinic's questionnaire (Crenshaw & Crenshaw, 1977), part of which they had in turn adapted from the original Kinsey–Pomeroy interview form. This procedure promotes efficiency in the interview and ensures that essential information will be consistently gathered both for treatment and research.

Although we use a structured interview, it is always necessary to be flexible in exploring leads and asking further questions. It is important for the sex therapist to have internalized a large repertoire of questions that may be called on when the need arises. Abundant and excellent examples are provided in LoPiccolo and Heiman (1978) and Masters and Johnson (1970).

An area of assessment often minimized by nonmedical practitioners is the contribution of physiological factors to sexual dysfunction. In the body's economy, sex is not essential for life or health; thus, under stress, sex is often sacrificed to maintain the efficiency of more vital functions. Hence, a medical history becomes paramount. Also, with any suspicion of organic involvement, the client should be referred to his or her own physician or to a physician who is sensitive to physiological problems in relation to sexual functioning. We often suggest laboratory procedures (urological, neurological, vascular, and/or endocrinological evaluations) that may not be automatically performed, especially when there is absent or diminished nocturnal penile tumescence (NPT). We use NPT monitoring to help differentiate psychogenic from organic erectile failure. Normal male adults have nocturnal erectile episodes every 90–100 minutes during sleep. These episodes last about 20–40 minutes and are closely associated with rapid-eye-movement (REM) sleep (Karacan *et al.*, 1975; Hursch *et al.*, 1972). The NPT monitor is capable of measuring changes in penile circumference by means of two mercury-filled strain gauges. Psychological factors that cause impotence during waking hours may be bypassed during sleep, revealing a normal amount and degree of nocturnal REM erection, and demonstrating the individual's erectile potential.

Prognostic Indicators. Most sex therapists treat a selected population (e.g., Masters & Johnson, 1970; Obler, 1973; Meyer *et al.*, 1975) from which couples with serious marital discord and personal psychopathology are screened out. Sex therapy patients have tended to be very well educated (72% of Masters and Johnson's population were college graduates and 17.5% were physicians) and highly motivated members of higher socioeconomic classes. In two studies among the less-educated and lower-socioeconomic groups (Lansky & Davenport, 1975; Fordney-Settlage, 1975) for which the sample was probably unselected, there were more serious marital difficulties, and the couples were less likely to complete assignments and more likely to drop out.

There is a limited amount of research available about prognosis, but many therapists have shared their clinical impressions. For example, poor prognosis has been suggested for alcoholics and drug abusers, and we accept them into our program only when they have been sober or drug-free for six months. Severe and chronic stress, "excessive vulnerability to stress," and making continuation of the marriage contingent on positive therapy outcome (Kaplan, 1974), as well as hypoactive sexual desire (Kaplan, 1977), are believed to indicate poor prognosis. Caution is recommended in working with patients who are psychotic (Lobitz & Lobitz, 1978).

Favorable prognostic signs may include a high degree of intimacy (Lobitz & Lobitz, 1978), the presenting problems of premature ejaculation or vaginismus (Masters & Johnson, 1970; Kaplan, 1974), and patients suffering with orgasm-phase and excitement-phase disorders, as well as those with performance anxiety (Kaplan, 1974). O'Connor (1976) believed that poor prognosis was associated with excessive sexual guilt, excessive partner anger, traumatic loss of previous partner in males over age 40, sex-specific anxiety or fears, partial impotence, partial anorgasmia, and chronic low libido in men. He did express optimism, however, that penile and vaginal anesthesia may have a good prognosis, particularly if these symptoms are not associated with impotence or orgasmic dysfunction.

Other positive prognostic factors have received tentative research validation. In a sample of 58 women suffering with orgasmic dysfunction and sometimes sexual aversion, dyspareunia, and/or vaginismus, Cooper (1969b) found the following factors associated with positive outcome, some of which have been replicated by others: (1) history of

Figure 1. Portions of the Sexual Adjustment Inventory.

4.(a) Please circle the number which best represents your disatisfaction with each of the following aspects of your sexual relationship.

	Very satisfied	Moderately satisfied			Dissatisfied
1. The way we decide to have sex.	1	2	3	4	5
2. The time of day that we have sex.	1	2	3	4	5
3. The places where we have sex.	1	2	3	4	5
4. The privacy we have.	1	2	3	4	5
5. The length of time spent in foreplay.	1	2	3	4	5
6. The variety of activity during foreplay.	1	2	3	4	5
7. The variety of positions during intercourse.	1	2	3	4	5
8. The man's expression of affection and interest during intercourse.	1	2	3	4	5
9. The woman's expression of affection and interest during intercourse.	1	2	3	4	5
10. The length of time spent in intercourse.	1	2	3	4	5
11. The man's expression of affection and interest after intercourse.	1	2	3	4	5
12. The woman's expression of affection and interest after intercourse.	1	2	3	4	5
13. The way we talk about improving our sexual activities	1	2	3	4	5

(b) Please go over the list once again and place an "X" over the number you think your partner will choose.

5. In the following question, please describe the frequency with which you and your partner do each of the sexual activities listed within your sexual encounters and indicate how much pleasure you derive from these activities by circling the correct number.

How often do you do this?			How often do you get pleasure from doing this activity?		
Often	Sometimes	Never	Often	Sometimes	Never

Check here if you would like this experience more often.

___ 2. Being seen nude by my partner.	1	2	3	4	5		1	2	3	4	5
___ 3. Lip kissing.	1	2	3	4	5		1	2	3	4	5
___ 4. Tongue kissing.	1	2	3	4	5		1	2	3	4	5
___ 5. Touching partner's body except for genitals.	1	2	3	4	5		1	2	3	4	5
___ 6. Having partner touch my body, except for genitals.	1	2	3	4	5		1	2	3	4	5
___ 7. Kissing partner's body.	1	2	3	4	5		1	2	3	4	5
___ 8. Having my body kissed.	1	2	3	4	5		1	2	3	4	5
___ 9. Caressing my own genitals with partner present.	1	2	3	4	5		1	2	3	4	5
___ 10. Caressing partner's genitals.	1	2	3	4	5		1	2	3	4	5
___ 11. Having my genitals caressed.	1	2	3	4	5		1	2	3	4	5
___ 12. Kissing partner's genitals.	1	2	3	4	5		1	2	3	4	5
___ 13. Having my genitals kissed.	1	2	3	4	5		1	2	3	4	5
___ 14. Bring partner to climax with my hand.	1	2	3	4	5		1	2	3	4	5
___ 15. Being brought to climax with my partner's hand.	1	2	3	4	5		1	2	3	4	5
___ 16. Bringing partner to climax with my mouth.	1	2	3	4	5		1	2	3	4	5
___ 17. Being brought to climax by my partner's mouth.	1	2	3	4	5		1	2	3	4	5
___ 18. Just having intercourse with neither climaxing.	1	2	3	4	5		1	2	3	4	5
___ 19. Having intercourse with only man climaxing.	1	2	3	4	5		1	2	3	4	5
___ 20. Having intercourse with only woman climaxing.	1	2	3	4	5		1	2	3	4	5
___ 21. Having intercourse with both climaxing.	1	2	3	4	5		1	2	3	4	5
___ 22. Having anal intercourse.	1	2	3	4	5		1	2	3	4	5
___ 23. Other sexual interests (please specify):											
a. _____	1	2	3	4	5		1	2	3	4	5
b. _____	1	2	3	4	5		1	2	3	4	5
c. _____	1	2	3	4	5		1	2	3	4	5

previously satisfying sexual experiences (Kinsey *et al.*, 1953); (2) short duration of problem (O'Connor & Stern, 1972); (3) positive attitude toward her own and her partner's genitalia; (4) active fantasizing; (5) sexual experimentation; (6) heterosexual orientation (Allen, 1962; Masters & Johnson, 1970); (7) presence of sexual desire (Blair & Pasmore, 1964); (8) self-referral; and (9) feelings of love toward the male partner. Cooper (1969a) also studied prognostic indicators in a sample of 49 males suffering from erectile dysfunction, premature ejaculation, and delayed ejaculation. Positive prognostic indicators (some of which have also been replicated by others) included (1) short duration of the dysfunction (Johnson, 1965; Ansari, 1976; Fabbri, 1976); (2) acute onset of the problem (Johnson, 1965; Ansari, 1976); (3) an affectionate and cooperative partner (Wolpe, 1958; Masters & Johnson, 1970; Fordney-Settlage, 1975; Ansari, 1976); (4) absence of psychopathology (Johnson, 1965; Lansky & Davenport, 1975; Meyer *et al.*, 1975; Lobitz & Baker, 1979); (5) motivation for treatment; and (6) marital happiness. In males with erectile failures, the presence of heterosocial comfort and skill also seems positive (Lobitz & Baker, 1979).

Marital happiness has also been found to be predictive of success with women (McGovern *et al.*, 1975; Leiblum *et al.*, 1976). Also, it appears that, in general, secondary (instead of primary) disorders have a more favorable prognosis.

Abundant evidence now exists for deterioration effects in psychotherapy (Lambert *et al.*, 1977; Yalom & Lieberman, 1971) and marital therapy (Gurman & Kniskern, 1978). In sex therapy, however, studies typically evaluate only change or no-change status. Only a few consider the possibility of negative, destructive outcomes (Kaplan & Kohl, 1972; Cooper, 1969c; Lansky & Davenport, 1975; Powell *et al.*, 1974).

We believe that sex therapists are more likely to create negative effects if they do not adequately assess and screen marital and personal adjustment in addition to sexual adjustment, if they adhere to rigid treatment formats instead of prescribing individualized treatment strategies, if they terminate cases too rapidly, if they do not correct the unrealistic expectations held by some patients concerning sex therapy, and if they mishandle resistance and other reactions to the treatment experience. In future research there is a need for specific rather than global indices of improvement and for multiple outcome measures, including evaluations of marital and personal adjustment accompanying change, lack of change, and deterioration in sexual function.

Diagnosis. Diagnosis has been problematic because there are few discrete categories with standard descriptive behavior. Impotence and frigidity have been catchall terms with varying definitions. Different investigators and clinicians use different language to define subcategories of sexual dysfunction, and there is little uniform agreement.

In our clinic we have adopted the following diagnostic labels: (1) premature ejaculation; (2) ejaculatory inhibition; (3) erectile dysfunction; (4) orgasmic dysfunction; (5) vaginismus; and (6) inhibited sexual desire. When inhibited sexual desire is exhibited in combination with feelings of extreme disgust or revulsion toward sex, we define the problem as (7) sexual aversion, a term we have adopted from Masters and Johnson. All seven disorders may be primary, having existed from the onset of sexual activity, or secondary, occurring after a period of adequate sexual functioning.

After completing assessment and diagnosis, we determine the most appropriate and efficient therapeutic interventions for the particular case. Ideally, we would prescribe completely individualized treatment strategies for each unique couple. However, there are a limited number of techniques available in the repertoire of the sex therapist, and unfortunately, their application is still governed more by clinical intuition and judgment than by research validation.

Next, we will discuss the process of giving feedback to the patient couple and conducting sex education. Afterward, we present an overview of some of the more general and commonly used therapeutic procedures. In the subsequent sections, the treatment of each of the specific dysfunctions is examined separately, and a review of outcome literature and a summary of our therapeutic approach are included.

ROUNDTABLE AND EDUCATION INTERVIEWS

After individual history-taking interviews, the couple are seen conjointly for a roundtable (Masters & Johnson, 1970) feedback session. The purpose of this interview is to provide a brief summary of the assessment information that was gathered and to present a diagnostic and prognostic statement. Identifying the couple's and the individuals' strengths is a particularly vital element of this process. We also reflect to the couple, in a nonjudgmental manner, the determinants of sexual dysfunction and self-defeating patterns that were identified during our evaluation. These may include such elements as problematic communication styles, myths and misinformation, physiological determinants, and individual psychological factors, such as depression. Throughout the process, the couple are invited to participate actively in discussing or elaborating on points, disagreeing, or making corrections, as well as asking questions.

During this interview, we also structure and anticipate for the couple what sex therapy is like and contract with them verbally before proceeding with therapy. Part of the structuring of role expectations includes elaborating on the "change-first principle" (see Chapters 5, 6, and 12) and the concept of self-responsibility. We convey our expectations concerning their active participation and responsibility in therapy. We stress the importance of according their sexual relationship high priority for several months, and state that they will be responsible for reserving three 1½-hour periods each week to complete the assignments that we will prescribe. We accentuate that their faithfulness in following through with assignments will be the most crucial factor in successful outcome, and that the interviews will primarily be spent discussing what transpired during their time together. At the same time, we explain the concept of "neutrality." Essentially, we do not want their past experiences to bias future possibilities. Therefore, we ask them to remain open to the possibility of change and not to predict the future on the basis of past experience (Masters & Johnson, 1970). We also introduce the "world's authority" concept (Crenshaw & Crenshaw, 1978), that is, that each individual is the world's authority on himself or herself. As a result, we request that they try to trust and accept whatever the partner tells them and resist trying to "read in" more than is stated. Finally, the relationship focus of therapy is discussed, including the concept from Masters and Johnson that "there is no such thing as an uninvolved partner."

Basic education about sexuality is also combined with the roundtable discussion and continues into the next interview. An essential component of this process is a presentation about sexual physiology and the sexual response cycle. Couples regularly comment on the value of this material. We use plastic models to illustrate physiology and a series of diagrams in explaining the four stages in the sexual response cycle (Masters & Johnson, 1972). In addition, we discuss some of the common misconceptions and myths. The reader is referred to Zilbergeld (1978), McCary (1978), and Pomeroy (1977) for an extensive elaboration of myths. A fundamental core principle that must be taught to couples is the concept of sex as a natural function. We are indebted to Drs. Roger and Theresa Crenshaw and Masters and Johnson for assisting us in more thoroughly comprehending the paramount importance of this foundation principle for couple education.

Sex is a natural physiological function much like others, such as bowel, bladder, and respiratory functions. The potential to respond to effective sexual stimulation is instinctual, and erection and lubrication are inborn reflexes rather than learned behaviors. These biologically endowed responses occur in male and female infants shortly after birth, and given good health, men will continue to have erections and women will lubricate several times each night throughout the life cycle.

Natural physiological functions are subject to psychosocial learning, however. Thus, children learn bladder and bowel control and table manners, but other natural functions, such as respiration, urination, defecation, sleep, thirst, and hunger, may be subjected to only limited conscious control and delay. In contrast, sex has the capability of being voluntarily delayed indefinitely, and therefore, considerable maladaptive learning often takes place. Men, for example, often assume responsibility for sex and come to believe that it is their duty to be the all-knowing initiator and to arouse women. However, this view takes sex entirely out of the context of a natural function and would be analogous to trying to create hunger, thirst, sleepiness, or perspiration in someone else. When a male believes that it is his job to make his partner orgasmic or the female believes she must create an erection in her mate, they are trying to take over and assume responsibility for someone else's natural function.

A variety of factors will interfere with any natural function, including sexual response: anxiety, stress, poor health, pressure, or fears, such as fear of failure. Sex therapists do not teach patients to respond sexually, they merely assist them to remove those roadblocks that inhibit function.

SUMMARY

Sexual dysfunctions are the result of multiple determinants consisting of behavioral, affective, sensory–physical responsiveness, imagery, cognitive, and environmental–interpersonal factors. Comprehensive assessment must take into account the problems and assets along each of these interacting dimensions, as well as the antecedents and consequences of sexual dysfunction. To facilitate such thorough evaluation, the authors use conjoint and individual assessment interviews; psychological, marital, and sexual adjustment inventories; physiological examination; and laboratory testing when deemed necessary.

Research has indicated that favorable prognostic factors for some of the dysfunctions include marital happiness; short duration or sudden onset of the problem; an affectionate, cooperative partner; the presence of sexual desire; absence of psychopathology; a history of previously satisfying sexual experiences; sexual experimentation; motivation for change; active fantasizing; and a secondary rather than a primary disorder.

Seven diagnostic categories for sexual dysfunction, any of which may be primary or secondary, are identified: (1) premature ejaculation; (2) ejaculatory inhibition; (3) erectile dysfunction; (4) orgasmic dysfunction; (5) vaginismus; (6) inhibited sexual desire; and (7) sexual aversion.

Basic Therapeutic Procedures

The field of sex therapy, much like that of psychotherapy and behavior therapy in general, is still in a prescientific state. We are guided to a large extent by clinical wisdom and the art of clinical practice, not unlike medical practitioners in the 19th century (Thorne, 1968). The efficacy of many individual treatment techniques has not been evaluated. Moreover, most technique combinations and many of the nonspecific therapeutic factors are yet to be studied. In the absence of data that fully substantiate the effectiveness of any procedure singly or in combination with others, treatment planning remains something of an art. While space limitations preclude our summarizing all of the research on each recommended procedure, in this section, we present an overview of the kinds of data that support the use of each technique with each designated disorder.

SEXUAL TASKS

The most distinctive feature of sex therapy is the assignment of graduated sexual tasks for couples to perform in the privacy of their home. To the outsider, these may appear but a grab bag of calculated erotic tricks. However, they are systematically structured experiences, carefully interwoven into the fabric of an established relationship. The emotional feelings of both partners that are stimulated by the experiential assignments are vital to the progress of therapy and must be openly explored, shared, modified, and cultivated. The activity prescribed and the defined hierarchy of erotic experiences, though essential, are of no greater importance than the couple's feelings about the experiences. Except for sensate focus, a description of which follows, the other sexual tasks that may be recommended are reported in the next section, which describes the treatment strategies for each dysfunction. Although some tasks may sound mechanical, sexually dysfunctional couples who have been in therapy can attest to the highly emotional, intimate opportunities they discovered as they involved themselves in the directed erotic exercises.

SENSATE FOCUS

Masters and Johnson's (1970) introduction of sensate focus is undoubtedly the single most significant therapeutic technique that has been developed in sex therapy. Regardless of the presenting problems of our couples, we find that there is great value in instructing them in sensate focus, the goal of which is sensual pleasure, not sexual arousal. Often couples in sexual distress have reduced physical contact to a minimum, and sex has become merely rapid coitus, unless the male has erectile problems, in which case there is often barely a caress between the pair. Sensate focus provides the opportunity to restore natural sexual responsivity through the enhancement of sensory awareness. Without pressure to perform, with the only directive being to tune into the senses, sensate focus experiences break down ingrained patterns and perceptual stereotypes regarding what sexual interaction "should be," freeing the individual simply to experience what occurs. Couples may become aware that they "try to push the river" and force responsivity, instead of accepting and enjoying sensual input and allowing it to "flow by itself."

There are several guidelines that we suggest before explaining the procedure to the couple. Depending on the couple's comfort with their existing pattern of initiating, we determine whether they should alternate the responsibility for inviting their partner for the sensual date or if one of them should be placed in charge temporarily. We strongly urge the couple to plan the time for the date at least 12–24 hours in advance. Most clients have busy social and work obligations, and therefore, we even suggest that they schedule their three experiences for the subsequent week en route home from the therapy session. Also, we expect them to set 1½ hours aside three times each week for the task assignments. Although we do not want them to continue sensate focus until they get tired or bored, we do want them to have sufficient time to feel unhurried and unpressured. We suggest that they begin their sessions when they feel as relaxed as possible, offering ideas as to how to create a pleasant mood for the experience. The activities may entail showering together, listening to music, cuddling in front of the TV, quietly talking, playing a game together, having a snack, etc. We forewarn them that their early sessions may seem awkward and artificial, but we explain that any awkwardness is due to unfamiliarity and will soon pass.

The temporary prohibition against intercourse that may have been discussed at the roundtable is reiterated again. The instructions for sensate focus may then be given as follows:

In a private, softly lit, comfortable place, usually the bedroom, undress and *take turns* touching each other's bodies, excluding breasts and genitals. You may touch, hold, kiss, lick, suck, or otherwise caress your spouse's body in a way that is pleasant and interesting for you. Your responsibility to each other is from time to time to communicate how you feel: "Your rubbing makes me feel warm and secure"; "I like what you are doing now"; "Your kisses makes me tingle." If your partner caresses you in a manner that does not please you, you must take the responsibility for indicating this. However, instead of making a complaint, you might say, "It feels better when you press my lips more gently," or "I would enjoy a soft touch more." You may even communicate nonverbally by guiding your partner's hand over any part of your body or in any manner that suits you. You may want to try using lotion, oil, or even caressing with feathers or material. Feel free to experiment if you choose. While you are receiving, selfishly soak up every sensation. Enjoy your here-and-now experience, focusing on sensory awareness. Try not to let your mind wander beyond what you are feeling. If it does, bring yourself back to the experience. Remember, though, that whatever or however you feel is ok. The only requirement is to be aware of your feelings and sensations. Either of you may start. We will let you decide who goes first. But remember to *take turns*. The sensual time is to be for yourself. By taking turns, you are able to concentrate on your own feelings, whether giving or receiving. When simultaneously touching each other, too often you get lost in pleasing the other. Although pleasing your mate is an important part of a sensual encounter, pleasing yourself is equally important. Often, taking responsibility for yourself is neglected, so we prefer that you concentrate on that for the time being. Remember to plan ahead, to allow yourself at least 1½ hours for each session, and to get together three times this week. Bob, will you take responsibility for initiating the first session this week? Are there any questions?

When working with an individual who is unusually inhibited and/or more able to become aroused while fully or partially clothed, the assignment is modified. The clothing may remain during sensate focus, or it may be necessary to begin with only kissing, nuzzling, and holding, with body exploration reserved for a subsequent week.

Couples' reactions to sensate focus tend to be very positive: "At first I felt silly, but what fun after we became involved"; "What a relief, I felt relaxed. I didn't have to perform"; "We were giggly, like adolescents again." Although the exercise may not arouse erotic sensations, it generally evokes an emotionally pleasant response. The experience often proceeds without the tension typical of the couple's usual sexual transactions and generates a closeness that creates optimism for change in their sexual relationship.

Occasionally, however, the reaction may be negative: "We started, but it seemed so silly and artificial that we quit after a few minutes"; "It was kind of boring so we only did it once"; "I fell asleep." In some instances, a couple never even begin. We listen carefully to their account of their reactions and inquire about what would help them to complete the assignment three times the next week. Fear of rejection and fear of failure based on the history of their sexual transactions tend to be the major obstacles usually encountered. Reassurance, support, encouragement, and giving the assignment again, perhaps with increased structure, usually assure that the prescription will be followed. While they are in the interview, we may set the day, time, and place that they will meet for the assignment, as well as determining the order for giving and receiving. In some cases, we may also set a brief time limit (e.g., 15-minute turns) for the first session.

Whether positive or negative, it is important to discuss in detail and depth what occurred, how each felt about the experience, and how they interacted. Open discussion of the procedure and their feelings during the interview models the kind of communication that couples must learn in order to facilitate free sexual expression. Other procedures for the resolution of resistance are presented later.

RECORD OF ASSIGNMENTS

We request that all couples in sex therapy write a commentary on each of their therapeutically prescribed sexual experiences. As soon as possible after the encounter (immediately or the following morning), we instruct each of them to record separately her or his remembrance of the activities that occurred. They are to be specific and to indicate how they felt about the various events that occurred and about the experience as a whole. We request that they bring these notes to therapy, and we review them prior to inviting the couple into the office for the interview. This procedure alerts us to progress and to the obstacles that may occur, pinpoints topics for discussion during interviews, and assists us in planning subsequent assignments. For the couple, keeping a record crystallizes their experience and helps them identify more specifically how they feel, which is an important dimension of any sensual encounter.

MANAGEMENT OF RESISTANCE

The techniques of sex therapy are always applied within a therapeutic relationship. Refined skills in establishing a warm relationship and finesse in working through patient resistance are very crucial to success. The skillful management of resistance is what distinguishes the sophisticated and highly effective therapist from the novice with modest outcomes (Hammond et al., 1977, pp. 241–248). Kaplan (1974) recognized the importance of the therapist's skills in neutralizing resistance, as well as the complexity of the process:

> He must know when to refrain from interpreting an obviously neurotic conflict because the patient's sexual functioning can be improved without such intervention, and when vigorous and persistent interpretation is necessary because the patient will not be able to function sexually until the conflict is resolved. . . . He must know when to "leave well enough alone," and when to attempt to modify their mode of communication. He must be able to support one spouse without mobilizing fear and defensiveness in the other, to work with both together, and to work with each spouse separately. (p. 222)

Common manifestations of resistance in sex therapy include complaints of feeling "nothing," being "too busy" to complete prescribed assignments, anger and fights with the spouse, persistent tardiness to appointments, repeated requests for changes in appointment times, fatigue, having intercourse despite prohibitions, and experiencing ticklishness, mind wandering or sleepiness during sexual assignments. Munjack and Oziel (1978), in an excellent article, concluded that resistance most often stems from misunderstandings, deficits in skills, lack of motivation, discouragement and anticipation of failure, anxiety, guilt, or secondary gains from the dysfunction. Spouse resistance is most commonly encountered when improvement becomes evident, whereas resistance appears more often in the symptomatic patient just prior to remission of the problem (Kaplan, 1974).

The following guidelines may suggest some alternatives for working through resistance. Mild resistance may often be ignored or bypassed or overcome by reassignment of the therapeutic task. When anxiety related to interview topics or task assignments evokes resistance, temporarily diverting the subject or proceeding at a slower pace may reduce the intensity and thereby resolve resistance. For example, for some unusually inhibited couples, sensate focus exercises may be too threatening, and their behavior must be shaped through more gradual approximations, such as having them begin by holding and cuddling while fully clothed. In many other cases of mild resistance, roadblocks may be removed simply through empathically recognizing and acknowledging the presence of the resistance and accepting it. This may especially be true with patient feelings of pessimism, fearfulness, or embarrassment. Normalizing such emotions may likewise be beneficial, for instance, by explaining that "many people in this kind of situation experience similar feelings." In still other cases, a clarification of misconceptions may be all that is necessary. When resistance is pointed out, but denied, the therapist may often obtain success by temporarily bypassing the issue with the injunction that perhaps she or he was in error in interpreting the behavior as an avoidance or manifestation of fear, but that if it occurs again, he will begin to question if it is not more than coincidence.

If none of these procedures successfully resolves the resistance, the therapist encourages the patient to interpret the possible purposes served by the resistance. When the patient is unable or unwilling to analyze the possible reasons for resisting, the therapist may have to offer tentative interpretations. Inquiring about the consequences of improvement will also aid in determining if the sexual problem also serves an adaptive function. Consequences that are sometimes identified include fears of failure, of being controlled, of being hurt, of being exposed as inadequate and deficient, of being taken advantage of, of becoming emotionally close, and of abandonment. Also common are fears of disapproval, ridicule, pain, pregnancy, divine disapproval, and loss of control (either in the sense of fear of becoming promiscuous from enjoying sexuality, or of loss of bladder or bowel control with orgasm). Resistance often defends against some feared catastrophe. Resistance may also function to maintain a type of self-image or self-definition, to save face, to declare inadequacy, to demonstrate moral superiority, to distract attention, or to excuse retreat or failure. In other cases, resistance or sexual problems may elicit attention or sympathy, may serve as a means of power and control, or may function to express vindictiveness and to obtain revenge. A more thorough elaboration of these offensive and defensive functions of behavior is found in Hammond and Stanfield (1977).

It is also often possible to create incentives and motivation for the client to proceed, regardless of the resistance. The therapist may provide encouragement and inspire the client's hope for improvement, citing the positive gains that may accrue. Defensiveness may also be pierced through the therapist's expression of caring, reassurance, and affirming his or her belief in the patient's ability to cope with the situation and to succeed. Another method of encouraging movement through resistant impasses is to aid the client to save face. One way of doing this is through attributing positive intentions to the individual despite undesirable actions with the spouse. There are several ways of crediting clients with positive goals. For example, in some cases, it may be possible to reinterpret "demandingness" as an insensitive but well-intentioned desire to be closer and an eagerness to provide pleasure. Positive relabeling is discussed below. It is probably one of the most powerful therapeutic tools for resolving resistance.

When other methods fail, the therapist may often enhance motivation by confronting the patient with the undesirable consequences of his or her actions and the discrepancies between his or her original goals and the current self-defeating behavior. If this method is unsuccessful, the therapist may want to reexamine objectives with the couple. In some cases, resistance stems from a discrepancy in therapist–couple goals, often because of the therapist's imposition of values on patients. Another alternative, if a single therapist has been seeing the couple, is to invite an opposite-sexed cotherapist to join the case. There may also be situations where paradoxical intention may be a useful technique. When all these methods fail, termination or referral may be necessary.

POSITIVE RELABELING

This procedure is a valuable treatment technique for all therapists, regardless of orientation. The words we use reflect how we perceive the world around us, and, in turn, interpretation influences how we feel. Couples experiencing sexual distress are attuned to deficiencies in their lives, and thus, they frequently express disappointment in the way in which they handle their sexual time together. In order to encourage them to see themselves as successful, with a firm conviction that feeling successful increases the opportunities for being successful, we always ask, "Which encounter this week was best for you?" "What did you like about it?" "How did it make you feel?" "Can you see ways to sustain the benefits?" Inevitably, couples also identify what went wrong. We indicate that they are in therapy to learn, and that one of the best ways of learning is from mistakes: "What has this experience taught you?" "It sounds like a good lesson, so the experience was worthwhile after all!" "Let's examine ways to prevent the difficulty from recurring in the future." "But if this does happen again, how would you handle the situation differently?" Through our questions and positive relabeling we are able to reframe positively what the couple originally perceived as a negative encounter. Whenever possible, we reinterpret failure as success or a positive opportunity to learn, demand as request, feelings of being controlled as expressions of caring, anger as disappointment, and insult as hurt. Surface statements of feeling often hide a deeper, more meaningful expression or desire.

BIBLIOTHERAPY

Many of our clients have not had the opportunity to review straightforward, authentic material about sexual expression. They may be versed in anatomy, reproduction, or even typical newstand erotica, but until the last 15 years or so, written sex information seemed mostly to be pornographic or to deal with the process of reproduction. There was no middle ground. Now there are a number of readings that offer a realistic view about sex that we believe may be helpful to couples in distress. Also, since for many people the printed word carries an aura of expertise and authority, prescribed readings may be a therapeutic adjunct to the treatment process. Some volumes not only normalize experiences but also give permission and reinforce therapeutic directives. A few examples include Nancy Friday's *My Secret Garden* (1973), Albert Ellis's *The Sensuous Person* (1974), D. W. Hastings's *A Doctor Speaks on Sexual Expression in Marriage* (1972), and Heiman *et al.*'s *Becoming Orgasmic: A Sexual Growth Program for Women* (1976).

COMMUNICATION TRAINING

Depending upon the couples' level of communicational effectiveness, they may or may not be referred for marriage counseling to build their skills in this area. Techniques such as those outlined in Chapter 7 may also be incorporated into our work with the couple, including training in making self-statements and in listening skills, and training in giving and receiving feedback and clarification. Often, too, we include coaching in the use of a feeling vocabulary (Hammond *et al.*, 1977) and in the daily dialogue as it is used in the marriage encounter movement (Calvo, 1975; Demarest *et al.*, 1977; Smith & Hammond, 1980).

Communication training in the sexual area requires a willingness to take the responsibility for one's own sexual pleasure. We facilitate this willingness by discussing its importance and structuring opportunities to practice. We will ask one or both partners to express their sexual or sensual preferences, desires, and pleasures, either in words or through nonverbal guidance, such as body positioning or directing their spouse's touch with their own hand. We follow up with an inquiry as to what was requested, how it felt to ask, and how the request was received. We role-play initiation and refusal in order to develop client skills in how to ask and also in how to feel the freedom to say no in the manner least likely to make the partner feel rejected.

MAINTENANCE AND FOLLOW-UP PLANS

After about two-thirds of the treatment has elapsed, we enlist the couple's assistance in determining the prescribed tasks for the following week. By doing this, they become involved in learning to shape their experience and to think through what makes sexual sense to them at a given time. Thus, they cultivate a skill that they may need in the future when a problem occurs. In the next to last interview we request that couples evolve their own maintenance plans for discussion and refinement in the final interview. These plans should include an identification of what they were doing that contributed to their problems, ways to correct these problems, danger signs that may signal impending relapse, and the actions they may take to prevent relapse. As standard policy, we also schedule a follow-up interview six to eight weeks after termination, and we make routine telephone contacts six months after termination.

In the interview preceding our final visit, we also give the couple the DAS (Spanier, 1976) Test, Sections C through H of the SAI (Stuart et al., 1975), a general evaluation sheet, and a copy of the goals they originally set for themselves. We also request that they answer the following questions: (1) To what extent do you feel that you have changed in the ways that you wished? (2) To what extent has your mate changed in the ways that you wished? (3) Did any changes (sexual or nonsexual) take place in yourself that were not part of your original hopes? (4) Did any changes (sexual or nonsexual) take place in your mate that were not part of your original expectations? (5) In what ways would you still like to change? We repeat the DAS (Spanier, 1976) and SAI (Stuart et al., 1975) at six-month follow-up. These materials are gathered so that we may have data about the immediate effect of the therapy and the sustaining effect of the therapy.

During the process of sex therapy, we have observed an interesting phenomenon exhibited by a majority of our clientele. When a couple come for the initial interview, they often express awkwardness about discussing sex, tend to be embarrassed and closed, and answer questions with the least amount of elaboration possible. As assessment and therapy proceed, even the most inhibited and shy persons often become open and straightforward, giving details about whatever sexual matter needs to be discussed. Then, again, toward the end of treatment, after the couple's sexual interactions have been modified, sex again becomes a personal affair. The notes that are part of their required assignment become shorter or neglected. Oral descriptions of their sexual encounters become general and loose. They are hesitant to reveal private and intimate details. They seem to be separating themselves from the therapist, bonding more closely together, and assuming shared secrets about their sex. But this time, the secrets are pleasures, rather than problems.

SUMMARY

There are a variety of therapeutic strategies that the authors frequently use in the treatment of all diagnostic categories of sexual dysfunction. These procedures include graduated sexual tasks, of which sensate focus is most common; making a record of assignments; positive relabeling; bibliotherapy; communication training in both marital and sexual areas; and enlisting the couple's assistance in evolving their own maintenance plans. Periodic resistance must also be skillfully managed. In addition, when assessment indicates that a couple's general communication skills need improvement, several strategies may be employed to enhance their interaction.

Treatment Methods

OVERVIEW AND CRITIQUE OF SEX THERAPY RESEARCH

A comparative evaluation of the effectiveness of different modes of treatment is difficult because of methodological deficiencies and differences between studies. Because of space limitations, we have not offered a critique of the methodology of each individual study. However, there are common deficiencies that plague the literature. The field of sex therapy has lacked a standard nomenclature, and different definitions of sexual dysfunctions predominate in the literature. There has also been wide variability in criteria for patient selection and for the evaluation of improvement. Studies have not controlled for the chronicity of dysfunctions, the severity of marital adjustment, or the experience level of therapists. Enough research data have been compiled so that it seems safe to state that sex therapy, conducted by trained professionals, is often an effective method of treatment, but we are still unable to evaluate the therapeutic elements that are most effective with different disorders and those that are dispensable and irrelevant embellishments.

Although a few attempts have been made to compare more than one treatment modality (O'Connor & Stern, 1972; Lazarus, 1961; Obler, 1973; Kockott *et al.*, 1975; Reisinger, 1978; McMullen, 1976), common methodological errors include assigning severe subjects to a specific treatment and lumping erection and ejaculation problems together as one entity, and small sample sizes mitigate against drawing reliable conclusions about differential effectiveness. For example, Masters and Johnson (1970), despite their large numbers of clients and exceptionally long follow-ups, did not include control groups or assess personal or marital adjustment. Their follow-up data are also incomplete. They did not include initial therapy failures in the follow-up, and 12% of the remaining sample could not be located for follow-up. In sum, 28% of the original treatment population did not receive follow-up.

Another serious problem is that most studies have not adequately described treatment techniques, with a resultant deficiency in the standardization of therapeutic procedures. For example, there is considerable variation in the instructions given for the sensate focus procedure, and a similar diversification exists in the application of the "squeeze technique." However, there is no research evidence comparing the variations in these methods. In addition, on close scrutiny it may be observed that many investigations that were purportedly studying the efficacy of a specific technique included a variety of other therapeutic procedures in the treatment, such as education and enhancing social skills, without ever considering their influence or outcome. For these and other reasons, the recommendations made below must be taken to be reasonable hypotheses but by no means techniques whose effectiveness has been fully established.

TREATMENT OF PREMATURE EJACULATION

Because the time necessary for orgasmic response is highly variable in women and approximately 10% never or rarely experience coital orgasm (Gebhard, 1966), we do not concur with Masters and Johnson's (1970) transactional definition of a premature ejaculator as one who reaches orgasm before his partner does more than 50% of the time. According to Kaplan (1974), the crucial aspect of premature ejaculation seems to be the absence of voluntary control, regardless of whether the woman reaches orgasm or how many thrusts occur. Therefore, the goal of treatment is to foster an increase in ejaculatory control through assisting the male to concentrate more fully on his preorgastic sensations.

Stop–Start Technique. The stop–start procedure for the treatment of premature ejaculation was originated by Semans (1956). Patients were instructed by him to have the female partner stimulate the penis until the male experienced sensations premonitory to ejaculation, at which point stimulation ceased until the sensations disappeared. After some degree of control was attained, the penis was lubricated prior to stimulation. This method was successful at follow-up in each of the eight case reports that Semans presented. Cooper (1968) and Kaplan *et al.* (1974) also used the stop–start method in combination with other therapeutic techniques and reported improvement ranging from 10% to 100%.

Therapy Programs Using the Squeeze Technique. Masters and Johnson (1970) originated the use of the squeeze technique in the treatment of rapid ejaculation. Their intensive two-week dual sex-therapy team program includes reassurance and instillation of hope, individualized education, sensate focus exercises (with and without genital play), instruction in communication principles, and instruction in the use of the squeeze by the female partner. At five-year follow-up on 186 patients, they reported success in 97.3%, and more recently (Masters *et al.*, 1978), after a two-year follow-up of 179 patients, they found a success rate of 93.3%.

Other researchers (Lobitz & LoPiccolo, 1972; Yulis, 1976) have also incorporated the squeeze while modifying or changing other aspects of Masters and Johnson's therapy for premature ejaculation. In these studies, the range of success varied from 85% to 100%.

Group Treatment Programs. Group formats have also been used to treat premature ejaculation (Zilbergeld, 1975; Leiblum *et al.*, 1976; Zeiss *et al.*, 1978). Some of the groups have been male only; others have included partners. The squeeze and stop–start techniques were combined with other therapeutic strategies, for example, masturbation, relaxation and/ or assertiveness training, education, and encouraging communication between partners. Effectiveness rates were around 66%.

Bibliotherapy. Zeiss (1977) recently reported substantial improvement both at termination and eight-month follow-up in the uncontrolled treatment of two high-school-educated, working-class couples who used a self-directed therapy program. A written manual (Zeiss & Zeiss, 1978) was used that included troubleshooting guides concerning commonly encountered programs (as in Zilbergeld, 1978) that accompanied each week's assignment. The program lasted 12 weeks and included three nonsexual communication exercises and instructions in the use of sensate focus, the squeeze technique, and the stop–start procedure. Brief (three- to five-minute) weekly telephone contacts by the therapist and a refundable penalty deposit encouraged follow-through.

An earlier control-group study (Lowe & Milulas, 1975) has also supported the value of a self-directed therapy program with a similar written treatment guide for premature ejaculators and their spouses. Impressive changes in ejaculatory control occurred with all 10 subjects; these changes showed significant differences from waiting-list controls. Similar to the troubleshooting procedure of Zeiss (1977), quizzes in each section determined comprehension of the instructions before the patients proceeded, and "depending on the subject's experiences with any section, he was either instructed to continue on to the next section or was sent back through the same section with additional instructions" (p. 297).

Systematic Desensitization. Friedman (1968) used desensitization with Brevital-induced relaxation to treat six cases of premature ejaculation, with an 83.3% "cure" rate at termination. However, only 50% maintained their improvements at 6-month to 12-month follow-ups. Kraft and Al-Issa (1968) successfully treated two cases of rapid ejaculation with Brevital-induced relaxation and desensitization. In addition, however, the patients were also instructed in sexual technique.

Hypnosis. Three men with rapid ejaculation were successfully treated by Shazer (1978) in three to five sessions. He used a specialized hypnotherapy procedure based on Milton Erickson's "reorientation to the future" technique. Ten clients fantasized themselves successfully functioning in a future sexual interaction and receiving positive feedback from their pleased partner. The future fantasy was then forgotten, except for the memory of telling the therapist about a successful encounter. The criteria for improvement were not reported.

Implications and Treatment Strategies. A stop–start technique seems to have some therapeutic usefulness but has received only modest research support thus far. It may be helpful to assign stop–start masturbation to the male, which he could practice concurrently with sensate-focus couple assignments. This procedure may provide a means for the male to gain confidence and focus totally on developing control prior to the more anxiety-laden situation with a partner, where he must communicate to receive a squeeze. Abundant evidence now exists to support the value of treatment programs that include the squeeze technique, and especially the Masters and Johnson (1970) format, which seems to be the treatment of choice. We believe that the utilization of a modified Masters and Johnson program in a couples' group format may also be used effectively with premature ejaculation, and the results thus far seem encouraging.

Outcomes with male-only groups are definitely positive enough to recommend them where cooperative partners are unavailable; but with our limited research evidence, these groups appear less effective than conjoint therapy if cooperative mates are available.

Further research is needed to determine the types of persons for whom self-directed bibliotherapy is indicated. At present, self-directed therapy with a carefully prepared written manual seems to be a promising treatment format, but we feel that the technique is indicated primarily with individuals who have a high school education and positive marital adjustment, a cooperative partner, and an absence of concurrent sexual dysfunctions in the relationship. Also, a refundable penalty deposit, brief weekly telephone contacts with a therapist, and the encouragement of patient telephone calls if problems are encountered are all recommended to encourage follow-through as well as to alert the therapist to difficulties. Further, it is recommended that such a manual contain a "troubleshooting" procedure similar to that of Zeiss (1977; Zeiss & Zeiss, 1978). Finally, posttherapy follow-up should be conducted, and brief sex therapy services should be available if needed either in case of failure with the written program or to consolidate therapeutic gains.

In our clinic, men usually learn ejaculatory control in a rather straightforward, uncomplicated manner. Like Kaplan (1974), we find that this condition is generally independent of marital factors and may be treated with minimal attention to relationship improvement. We begin by advising the couple that the prognosis is excellent, but that the success of the treatment rests on their willingness to follow faithfully the prescribed assignments. The initial focus of therapy, it is explained, will be on the male. If the female partner is nonorgasmic, she is told that after ejaculatory control is gained by her spouse, then additional procedures will be introduced to assist her. Initially, however, we request that she give her partner "permission" to ignore her needs temporarily in order to overcome his problem.

The initial therapeutic task, following the roundtable and sex-educational interviews, is sensate focus without genital or breast stimulation. Intercourse is prohibited at this time. Following several experiences with this exercise, the couple is instructed to include genital play. However, the female partner is to provide only the minimal amount of sex play necessary to establish an erection in her husband. He is requested to lie back while she manually stimulates his penis. His sole responsibility is to concentrate on the erotic sensations. He need not concern himself with her reactions or allow irrelevant thoughts to distract him. He is asked to think of a 0–10 arousal scale where 0 is no arousal and 10 represents ejaculation. We explain that we want him to tune into his erotic sensations and continuously judge where his arousal level is on this scale.

At the same time that the above instructions are given, the couple are taught the squeeze technique and are provided a handout illustrating the method. In addition, we use a lifelike dildo to model the correct positioning of the fingers, afterwards asking the woman to squeeze the dildo to check comprehension. The therapist then asks the woman to squeeze his or her hand to be sure that she is squeezing firmly enough. She must squeeze very firmly for four seconds and should be reassured that her husband will not be injured and will give her feedback if he experiences discomfort. We request that the male signal his spouse to apply the squeeze when he rates himself between levels 6 and 8 on the arousal scale. It is explained that following the application of the squeeze, part of the erection is sometimes lost and that it will return with stimulation. After a pause of usually about 30 seconds, when the male feels that arousal has decreased, he signals his partner to again begin stimulation of his penis. When arousal increases to the same range, he again signals her to squeeze. At no point should he ever try to exert conscious control to impede ejaculation, such as through tensing muscles. He should only request a squeeze. He is further instructed not to practice "brinksmanship" by trying to attain levels 9 or 9½ of arousal before requesting a squeeze. If he finds that he must ask for another squeeze almost immediately after stimulation is resumed, he is probably not waiting long enough after a squeeze to let his sensations subside. After three squeezes have been provided, his partner may stimulate him to ejaculation. He is also advised to attend to his sensations and arousal level while being stimulated to orgasm. In order to give attention to the female's sexual expression, after he ejaculates or on another occasion during the week, he may provide her with sexual pleasure short of intercourse.

During the second week of these exercises, we typically suggest that the couple experiment with having the male guide his partner's hand to vary the speed, pressure, and location of stimulation (Kaplan, 1974). The squeeze continues to be employed on his request, but we urge that his level of arousal be between 8 and 9 before he requests a squeeze. At this time, if control was maintained during the prior week's experiences, we further suggest the use of a lubricant (K-Y Jelly) during penile stimulation. However, we caution the male that this procedure will more closely approximate the vagina and produce greater excitement. Therefore, he must pay close attention to his physical sensations and the gradually mounting arousal. When successful control has been reported during the use of the squeeze technique with a lubricant, we request that couples transfer from the use of the squeeze technique to the stop–start technique (Semans, 1956). In the initial one or two sessions together, the couple is asked to perform stop–start with a dry penis. If ejaculatory control is maintained, they are then instructed to use stop–start with a lubricant and to have the woman also rub the penis against the vulva.

Increased confidence in the ability to maintain ejaculatory control is gained through these successive experiences by both the man and the woman. The next step is to allow intromission from a female superior position. Entry should occur when male arousal is low, and the woman is instructed to give the penis a squeeze before making entry. She should also be the one to guide penile entry. We instruct the *female* (not the male) to engage in slow, nondemand thrusting. The male may place his hands on her hips and stop her as arousal becomes high, remaining motionless until arousal subsides. After stopping three times, they are allowed to proceed to ejaculation, but the thrusting should still remain slow while the male focuses on his sensations. An alternative procedure, proposed by Masters and Johnson (1970), allows more gradual progress for couples who have had difficulty maintaining control earlier in the treatment process. In these cases, instead of proceeding to female superior stop–start intercourse, the couple initially only make intromission, remaining motionless afterwards. If the man fears loss of control, he should signal his partner to withdraw and give him a squeeze. The next intermediate step is for the female to thrust until the male instructs her to withdraw, and she then applies the squeeze. This procedure is used three times prior to thrusting to ejaculation.

After the couple have successfully used stop–start intercourse in a female superior position, they are allowed to repeat this procedure in a side-to-side position. At this time, we also suggest that they experiment with varying the pattern of thrusting. For example, we suggest occasionally shifting from thrusting to having the woman rotate her pelvis in a circular motion, and we allow the man to begin participating in slow thrusting. If at any time during this process the man experiences unusually high excitement prior to desired ejaculation, he is instructed to ask for a squeeze. It also continues to be a positive procedure to have the woman always apply a squeeze just prior to entry.

Masters and Johnson suggested using the squeeze once a week prior to entry, recommending regular sexual contact and advising a monthly manual stimulation session of 15–20 minutes' duration with several applications of the squeeze as a maintenance plan. Kaplan (1974) advocated that couples have one stop–start session weekly. We frequently recommend some combination of these procedures, see the couple for a six-week follow-up interview to check maintenance, and again have a routine follow-up contact in six months.

There are cases where relationship conflict creates resistance. Most often this may be bypassed, but occasionally the treatment process also includes short-term communication training and relationship enhancement procedures. These may be prescribed prior to or concurrently with the graduated sexual tasks.

TREATMENT OF EJACULATORY INHIBITION

Ejaculatory inhibition may be defined as "a specific inhibition of the ejaculatory reflex" (Kaplan, 1974, p. 316). Like the other dysfunctions, inhibited ejaculatory response may range from mild to severe. Some males reach orgasm through masturbation but rarely if ever ejaculate intravaginally. Intravaginal ejaculation may not even occur after 45 minutes to an hour of continuous thrusting. Many times the man is also unable to masturbate to ejaculation if he is in the presence of a woman.

Some men retain their sexual interest and responsiveness, experiencing pleasurable sexual sensations despite the absence of ejaculation. Other men may refrain from sexual involvement to avoid the psychological pain and embarrassment of not ejaculating.

It appears that delayed ejaculation is rarely due to organic causes. However, it has been hypothesized that pharmacological agents producing alpha-adrenergenic blockage may temporarily interfere with contraction of the seminal vesicle, ampulla, and ductus deferens (Kedia & Markland, 1975). Even if substantiation is found for drug impairment of ejaculation, this factor would account for only a limited number of the cases of delayed ejaculation. Psychological causality also remains speculative. Based on clinical inference, Masters and Johnson (1970) discussed a multiplicity of factors that may inhibit ejaculatory response: religious orthodoxy, male fear of pregnancy, lack of desire for the female partner, or homosexual orientation. Kaplan (1974) has received psychoanalytical, systems-theory, and learning-theory formulations of causality. We are, however, reticent to draw any conclusions concerning etiology from the limited population we have treated. Regardless of etiology and despite the lack of firm support for our approach, we find that multidimensional treatment is relatively effective in reversing the problem.

Eclectic Treatment Programs. Masters and Johnson (1970) treated 17 cases of "ejaculatory incompetence" with a dual sex-therapy team in an intensive two-week format. Therapy included individualized education, sensate focus, and lubricated manual penile stimulation by the female partner, followed later in therapy by intromission in a female superior position just prior to ejaculation, and then demanding thrusting. After several occurrences of intravaginal ejaculation with this procedure, intromission gradually occurred at lower levels of arousal. Masters and Johnson reported a success rate of 82.4% at five-year follow-up. Between 1972 and 1975, they treated 36 cases of delayed ejaculation and on two-year follow-up were successful with 61.1% (Masters *et al.*, 1978).

Tuthill (1955) reported treating six men who had never ejaculated during either masturbation or intercourse, though they had experienced nocturnal emissions. He provided brief advice on technique, encouraged the use of fantasies, provided a vasodilator for application to the penis, and gave them a drug containing a combination of amphetamine sulphate, strychnine, arsenic, and yohimbine. In a postal follow-up, all six men were "satisfied with improvement."

Cooper (1968) treated 13 delayed ejaculators with a combination of relaxation training, sex education, superficial psychotherapy, and provision of novel and optimal stimulation by the female partner. Improvement or cure was reported in 46% (6 of 13).

Systematic Desensitization. Systematic desensitization using Brevital-induced relaxation was used by Friedman (1968) to treat three cases of delayed ejaculation, but despite prolonged treatment ($\bar{x} = 29.3$ sessions), only slight improvement was reported. However, Razani (1972) successfully treated a case of delayed ejaculation and coital anxiety in only five sessions. He used a combination of deep-muscle relaxation, education, brief systematic desensitization to the image of intravaginal ejaculation, and stop–start penile stimulation. No recurrence of ejaculatory overcontrol had occurred by six-month follow-up. Jones and Park (1973) also used desensitization with Brevital-induced relaxation and "discussion" to treat a case of delayed ejaculation successfully.

Vibrator. Erotic photographs and a phallus-shaped vibrator with a stiff extension sheath that fit around the glans of the penis were used by Newell (1976) in treating a case of primary "ejaculatory incompetence." The subject experienced ejaculation within three weeks; this generalized to coitus and improvements were maintained at one-year follow-up.

Implications and Treatment Strategies. It is already evident from this brief review that very little research evidence exists on methods of treatment for ejaculatory overcontrol. Without question, the only treatment strategy with significant research support is that of Masters and Johnson (1970), and their latest statistics are rather poor. This is an area where some of our most important contributions in innovative approaches to treatment and research are yet to be made.

Following the roundtable and educational discussions, we prescribe task assignments, usually commencing with sensate focus. For couples who have remained sexually active, sensate focus provides nondemand pleasurable and arousing experiences in which both partners have an opportunity to increase their sexual communication skills. For couples who have avoided sexual contact for some time, sensate focus presents an opportunity to begin knowing each other again physically, without the demand for performance.

Concurrently with other prescribed tasks for the couple, the male is trained in fantasy enhancement. We have adapted ideas from Flowers and Booraem (1975) for imagery training, including practice increasing the vividness and detail of mental imagery, using erotic literature, and building fantasies from *in vivo* situations. The use of fantasy and absorbing oneself in perceiving erotic sensations mentally preoccupies the patient and keeps him from engaging in anxiety-provoking spectatoring while simultaneously increasing arousal.

We follow Kaplan's (1974) pattern of gradually shaping ejaculatory behavior. The male is instructed to ejaculate initially under circumstances where he has previously been able to ejaculate (e.g., through masturbation while alone). Ejaculatory behavior is gradually shaped until he can masturbate in his partner's presence. Intermediate steps may include sensate-focus caressing followed by male masturbation alone;

subsequently masturbating with his partner in the next room but with the door open; masturbating to ejaculation with his partner across the room, but not visible to him; and finally, masturbating on the bed while his partner is simultaneously masturbating. Masturbating in each other's presence decreases the performance pressure that is placed on the male if only he is requested to masturbate in front of his partner.

The next process goal of therapy is for ejaculation to occur through partner stimulation. The first step toward this goal is usually to combine partner and self-stimulation, having the man finish stimulating himself to ejaculation. The couple are requested to use a lubricant on the penis, and he is instructed to show her how he masturbates and effectively stimulates himself. He may both model this and guide her by placing his hand over hers, guiding and giving her feedback on the pace and pressure of stimulation. Fellatio is also an option, although we find that many clients prefer manual manipulation. We often have the man masturbate himself almost to ejaculation and then signal his partner to take over stimulation to ejaculation. Gradually, she can provide more and more of the stimulation to orgasm. When he is being stimulated, we instruct the man to focus on his physical sensations and, if he becomes anxious or notices his arousal decreasing, to absorb himself in fantasy. LoPiccolo (1977) has also suggested that during a state of high arousal, ejaculation may be facilitated by having the male cup the scrotum and testicles and press them against the perineum. Similarly, increasing muscle tension (e.g., tensing the abdomen, tensing the legs and pointing the toes, holding one's breath, and pelvic thrusting) may help "trigger" orgasm in some cases. Use of an electric vibrator may also be suggested when other procedures have been unsuccessful.

After the male has been brought to ejaculation by the female, solitary ejaculation is no longer permitted. His partner must then participate in all further stimulation to ejaculation. Ejaculation is now shaped gradually closer to the vaginal entrance. Initially, this may involve penile–vulva stimulation. The next step may involve a combination of manual stimulation and coital stimulation, but withdrawing and ejaculating through partner stimulation. Finally, the male may be brought close to ejaculation through manual stimulation, and then make entry and rapidly thrust to ejaculation. Again, cupping the scrotum and testicles, increasing muscle tension, and fantasy are all procedures that may facilitate ejaculatory response.

Kaplan (1974, p. 324) also suggested female manual stimulation during coitus, having the man signal at the point of impending orgasm so that her hand may be withdrawn and ejaculation brought on by thrusting. In the event that ejaculation does not occur almost immediately, the female may withdraw and repeat the process of manual stimulation almost to ejaculation followed by entry. Patients who continue to ruminate and spectate when they are highly aroused could be advised that when this occurs, they should withdraw, cease further stimulation, and not ejaculate on that occasion.

As in the treatment of other male dysfunctions, the woman's sexual needs may be temporarily neglected while she focuses on her mate. We have discovered, however, that taking her needs into account not only avoids frustration on her part but also facilitates improvement in her partner. Men often feel uncomfortable when placed in the position of receiving without giving in return. It is our clinical impression that the man feels more secure in the sexual relationship when he is able to give some, if not equal, attention to his partner. Therefore, although we give his needs first priority, we structure sexual tasks to provide for her pleasure also, thereby preventing the feeling that she is merely "servicing" her mate. Time for her may be allotted either through a weekly "lady's day" or through reserving time for her after her partner is stimulated.

Treatment for delayed ejaculation may involve resistance, particularly with severe dysfunction and where it is accompanied by avoidance of sexual contact. In such cases, it may be necessary to examine the adaptive function of the sexual symptoms (Hammond & Stanfield, 1977). Facilitation of insight will not resolve the problem, but it may neutralize resistance to sex therapy assignments. Supportive therapy and marital enhancement techniques are often necessary also, along with gentle but firm confrontation about avoidance maneuvers.

TREATMENT OF ERECTILE DYSFUNCTION

Erectile dysfunction, also referred to as impotence, is the inability of the male to obtain or maintain an erection sufficient for the completion of coitus. Erection may or may not occur at any time throughout sexual stimulation and may or may not be available for penetration and minimal thrusting. Some men are functional with one partner, but not with another, and are able to attain erection with masturbation, but not with a partner. In some cases, the male gets partial erections but never achieves a firm erection. In other cases, he does not attain an erection under any circumstances. Erectile dysfunction may be primary or secondary. In the former category, the male has never had successful intercourse with a woman; in the latter, he was functioning adequately for some time but is presently having difficulty. According to Kaplan (1974), the prognosis for primary erectile failure is poor because it is likely to be associated with a psychiatric disorder or an endocrine disorder, but the prognosis for secondary erectile failure is usually excellent, especially for the man who has a cooperative partner.

Systematic Desensitization. In the literature, there are a number of successful single-case studies for the treatment of erectile dysfunction through systematic desensitization. Studies with a larger number of subjects had success rates varying from 25% to 85.7%, but often there seemed to be other techniques incorporated along with the systematic desensitization, including reeducation, support, fantasy, and chemically induced relaxation (Friedman, 1968; Jones & Park, 1972; Lazarus, 1961; Kockott et al., 1975).

Eclectic Treatment Programs. In studies for eclectic models, therapy consisted of several of the following techniques in combination: education, instruction in improving communication, muscle relaxation, specific suggestions for sexual tasks, use of a tranquilizer, support, encouragement, fantasy, and attempts to decrease performance anxiety and enhance sexual experimentation (Masters & Johnson, 1970; Cooper, 1969c; Ansari, 1976; Lobitz & LoPiccolo, 1972). Ansari (1976) found no significant difference between patients he treated and control patients. The other studies did not have a control group, and the reported success rates varied between 37% and 85.9%, depending upon onset of the problem and whether the erectile failure was primary or secondary. Masters and Johnson (1970) reported the largest treatment numbers. They successfully treated 59.4% of primarily impotent patients ($n = 32$) and 72.7% of secondarily impotent patients ($n = 213$), although 11.1% of the latter had relapsed at five-year follow-up. More recently (Masters et al., 1978), they reported 76.9% and 85.9% success rates with primary and secondary impotence cases, respectively, at the end of two-year follow-ups.

Testosterone Therapy. Testosterone therapy is a controversial area. Uncontrolled studies (e.g., Margolis et al., 1967) have reported a significant improvement in impotent patients administered testosterone. Although flawed by methodological deficiencies, double-blind studies (e.g., Sobotka, 1969; Jakobovits, 1970) consistently show that testosterone seems to provide a definite psychophysical uplift over and above placebo effects. However, significant psychological factors are also involved in treatment response, and patients also significantly improve under placebo conditions. It also seems possible that the increased number of erections that occur with testosterone therapy may reflect an increased sex drive and interest level, which result in a greater number of attempts to have intercourse.

Testosterone is often administered to patients with normal serum testosterone levels, despite the fact that hormonal causes of erectile dysfunction are extremely uncommon. When testosterone is administered to patients without hormone deficiency, especially when organically caused by vascular insufficiency or neurological damage, the patient may frustratingly experience increased sex drive without a concurrent increase in erectile capacity. Even when testosterone levels are low, this may not be a significant etiological factor. Erection occurs in infant monkeys and humans despite very low androgen levels (Beach,

1967; Karacan, 1968), and erection normally occurs even in some surgically castrated patients (Roen, 1965). Clearly, further research is needed to delineate the types of patients for whom testosterone therapy may be effective.

Hypnosis. A few successful single-case studies exist on the use of hypnosis in treating impotence, and Crasilneck and Hall (1975) claimed improvement in 80% of more than 400 patients in uncontrolled treatment using "psychotherapy and hypnosis," while Alexander (1974) similarly achieved full recovery in 6 of 10 patients. Mirowitz (1966) claimed a 52% success rate in treating "psychic impotence."

Group Treatment. Lobitz and Baker (1979) used multitreatment strategies, including stop–start masturbation, progressive relaxation, graduated assignments, a female cotherapist as a facilitator, role playing to increase communication skills, sex education, and fantasy training, with a group of six men with secondary erectile dysfunction and three with primary erectile dysfunction. At four- to nine-month follow-up, 83% of the former and 33% of the latter indicated successful sexual functioning.

Implications and Treatment Strategies. After reviewing the research evidence, Masters and Johnson's most recent outcome statistics are clearly the most impressive in the field. Despite the lack of a control group and the methodological flaws noted earlier, their work is outstanding in terms of low failure rates, lengthy follow-ups, and the large number of patients treated. Even taking into account a well-educated and highly motivated population, their statistics are still exceptional. Lobitz and Baker's study (1979) offers tentative encouragement that all-male group treatment may also be beneficial with secondary erectile dysfunction when cooperative female partners are available. However, temporary inclusion of a female cotherapist to role play, give feedback, and dispel myths may be an important element in the success of such groups. Future research may also be improved if patients could be screened with the monitoring of nocturnal penile tumescence (NPT) and lab testing to determine that the dysfunction is psychogenic, as some failure rates may reflect the inclusion of patients with organic etiology in psychological treatment (Cooper, 1968).

Systematic desensitization appears to have some effectiveness, most likely where there is high sexual anxiety. From the information available, however, we believe that many of the studies using desensitization have also used a variety of other methods that have been deemphasized or not even acknowledged in the published reports. Contaminating procedures have been found to include sexual reeducation, instruction in communication principles and assertiveness, ventilation, guided fantasy, and thought stopping and substitution. Nevertheless, desensitization does appear to have value and may prove particularly useful as part of a treatment package for difficult cases of men without partners.

Insufficient research evidence allows only tentative conclusions, but it is our current impression that hypnosis may be beneficial if integrated into a broader treatment program. We are favorably impressed by the model of Alexander (1974), who used hypnosis to decrease a performance orientation while facilitating sensory awareness and giving permission. When used in this manner, perhaps also to enhance sexual fantasies and in combination with other methods, hypnosis may increase confidence and remove roadblocks to natural function. In the vast majority of cases, however, we are skeptical of the value of hypnosis when used to explore and uncover historical conflicts.

With the limited current knowledge, our conclusion is that testosterone *may* be beneficial and indicated under certain conditions: (1) when laboratory evaluation determines a low testosterone level or high luteinizing hormone levels, and where other organic conditions have been ruled out through NPT monitoring (Karacan *et al.*, 1975), sex history, urological and neurological examination, and vascular examination with the Doppler method (Abelson, 1975); (2) with patients under 60 years of age (Margolis & Leslie, 1966); and (3) with patients who have a low sex drive and/or are not responsive to or only partially improve with sex therapy, and who meet criteria 1 and 2. Even in these conditions, however, therapists and patients should be aware of possible adverse effects (e.g., risk of prostatic cancer, coronary thrombosis, atherosclerosis, sodium retention, hepatic dysfunction, gynecomastia, and prostatic hypertrophy). In cases not meeting the above conditions, the physician may consider giving a placebo to obtain psychological placebo effects.

The essential therapeutic goals with erectile dysfunction are to diminish a performance orientation and anticipated failure, to restore confidence, and to enhance stimulation. It is vital during the education and roundtable discussions to teach the concept of sex as a natural function, emphasizing that erectile response cannot be taught or "willed." Rather, like breathing, bowel, or bladder functions, erection is a reflex reaction and will automatically occur in response to sexual desire and effective stimulation.

After assessment and education, we instruct the couple to maintain ejaculatory abstinence and engage in sensate-focus pleasuring, without breast or genital play. The emphasis is on mutual enhancement of pleasure and having an opportunity to think and feel sexually, rather than on sexual performance. Rejection of the myth that sex is synonymous with intercourse must often be reemphasized. During sensate focus, the couple are instructed not to anticipate an erection or be concerned if erection occurs but is lost. They cannot force responsivity, and lubrication or erection is not the goal. This is merely an opportunity to learn and communicate what is pleasurable. When spontaneous erections are reported, they can be interpreted as demonstrating that there are no physiological problems, and that under conditions of relaxation and enjoyment, erections will occur (Kaplan, 1974). If erections come and go, this reaction can be noted as evidence that loss of an erection is not crucial, and that erection will be regained if the focus is on enjoyment, not genital performance.

Concurrent with nondemand sexual pleasuring with his partner, the male may be instructed to use stop–start masturbation while alone to enhance erectile confidence and build fantasy. In an excellent and detailed discussion, Zilbergeld (1978) identified four exercise variations. The first step consists of practice in losing and regaining erections. The man is instructed to masturbate with a lubricant and to stop once the penis is firm and allow it to become flaccid. The second step consists of masturbating while fantasizing an entire sexual encounter with his partner, and then masturbating while imagining the point in the love-making process when he tends to lose erections. The final steps consist of masturbating to erection, stopping and fantasizing losing or gaining an erection, and picturing oneself coping in fantasy with this situation and making the necessary adjustments. With each exercise, Zilbergeld anticipated possible obstacles and presented suggestions for the problems that arise.

After a positive response is obtained with sensate focus (one to two weeks), instructions for sensate pleasuring are expanded to include breast and genital play, *after* more generalized body touch has occurred. We caution couples against reverting to the genital focus of "rushing for the crotch," instead of enjoying nongenital erotic pleasure. They are instructed to use a teasing type of genital touch, rather than the more familiar rhythmic, pushing-for-orgasm type of stimulation. Again, it is emphasized that erection, lubrication, and orgasm are not the goals of the assignment. The goals are awareness of physical sensations, pleasure, and sharing this information with each other. The female partner is instructed to fondle the male's "flaccid penis," and if he should get an erection, to allow it to subside. If couples need to remain in this step for another week, they may be instructed to use K-Y Jelly to lubricate the penis and to demonstrate how they masturbate to their partner.

Particularly when the man becomes involved in spectatoring, we provide instructions in fantasy building. He is told to explore a variety of erotic literature to ascertain what is especially exciting to him. The imagery does not have to be an elaborate story but may simply consist of a scene or brief mental pictures that are arousing. In some cases, these mental pictures may be more romantic and sensual in nature than explicitly sexual. More vivid imagery may be facilitated by having the man look at the details of an erotic picture that he enjoys and then close his eyes and try to visualize as many details as possible. This process may be repeated several times with a single picture, while the man tries each time to imagine more vivid details. After the man has gained proficiency in developing sexual fantasies and imagery, he may call on them whenever he is aware of becoming anxious or spectatoring during love play. Absorption in fantasy is a competing response with spectatoring, and one that may simultaneously enhance arousal.

During this time, we also use cognitive restructuring to emphasize that if the man loses an erection, it is not catastrophic. Much of the fun of sex is exploration and pleasure, which do not depend on erection. The male has "10 erect fingers" and a mouth over which he has voluntary control and that may be used to bring pleasure to his mate. Also, erection often occurs when he is absorbed in stimulating his partner. While some men are preoccupied with how loss of erection affects them, others continually worry about how lack of erection affects their mate. If the male expresses overconcern for his partner, we indicate that he must learn temporarily to be "selfish," that is, to disregard her sexual gratification and to enjoy his own pleasure for the time being. Although this is never an end goal, it frequently is a necessary intermediate step. Also, it permits another opportunity to stress that sex is more than performance of intercourse. After several weeks of noncoital interactions and structured masturbatory experiences, the man frequently has both improved confidence and erectile response.

Preparatory to resuming coitus, we suggest that the woman assume a female superior sitting position and caress her genitals with his penis. Whether or not erection occurs, insertion is prohibited. The next step is intromission and vaginal containment without orgasm. It is again stressed that erection is not necessary for this assignment and that the female may "stuff" a flaccid penis into the vagina. Immediately after intromission is often a time characterized by catastrophic fears about loss of erection, and he is instructed not to ejaculate intravaginally. The couple are also instructed that from this time forward, the woman should always be the one to insert the penis. This procedure prevents the anxiety that may occur if the man fumbles to locate the vaginal opening. After one or two experiences with vaginal containment, slow thrusting is permitted, but ejaculation, if desired, should take place extravaginally. The sequence of entry, vaginal containment, slow thrusting, withdrawal, and extravaginal stimulation may be repeated several times before ejaculation.

After successful completion of this phase, coitus is permitted from a female superior position to readily facilitate mounting and avoid distraction. The woman is instructed to lean forward at a 45-degree angle and lower herself onto the penis. She should thrust in a slow, nondemanding manner, since forceful thrusting may be threatening. The man is told that he may ejaculate intravaginally if he desires, but that if he experiences any anxiety or doubts about his ability to perform, he should withdraw and ejaculate only extravaginally. To decrease performance demands, the couple is told that as more restrictions are removed, he may have some fears of performance. Following the model of William Masters, we explain that from time to time such fears will reappear and that they are probably too deeply ingrained ever to be totally eliminated. Therefore, we ask the couple to develop a word or a phrase that they can use as a cue between themselves. Immediately upon experiencing performance fears, he uses this signal. If the couple accept this feeling and share such anxiety openly, rather than fighting against it, pressure will decrease. At that point, they reinvolve themselves in a different activity, and the female partner is instructed to use his body for her pleasure and enjoyment, rather than withdrawing. Later, the man is also encouraged to begin slow thrusting, emphasizing a focus on pleasuring and being pleasured, not on his performance.

Other optional strategies include using the male's morning erection for intercourse to establish confidence, or having the female partner stimulate the penis extravaginally until he is close to the point of ejaculatory inevitability and then to make entry and allow him to ejaculate before catastrophic fears can disrupt performance.

Many couples also need assistance in developing initiating and refusal skills. For this purpose, we have modified the reverse role-play exercise of Heiman *et al.* (1976). Couples are requested to set a scene, taking turns play acting how they prefer sex to be intiated. Emphasis is placed on being positive and specific. The mate is asked to practice making good initiations several times, with assistance and reinforcement from the spouse and the therapist. The same procedure is used to develop refusal skills. Discussion and role playing focus on how to say no in a sensitive manner. Frequently, sexual refusal is perceived as a personal affront. Practice in making a nonhurtful refusal and accepting such a refusal minimizes the feelings of being personally rejected.

There may be occasional male patients who experience a revulsion to female genitals. For these persons, systematic desensitization may prove useful, or they may respond favorably to *in vivo* procedures. For instance, the man may be instructed to thumb through erotic magazines until he finds pictures that he enjoys that include exposure of the genitals. He is taught relaxation training and/or the use of masturbation as the medium for counterconditioning. He may be instructed to relax and look at other parts of the woman's body and then to look at the genitals for as long as he can comfortably do so, trying each time to look at the genitals somewhat longer. Later, the *in vivo* desensitization should include examination of his partner's genitals and genital touch.

Unlike premature ejaculation, which is often amenable to change even when the mental interaction is problematic, in men with erectile failure the tenor of the relationship is more crucial. While emphasis may still be placed on intervention through structured sexual tasks, inevitably therapeutic strategies must be implemented that deal with the relationship. The techniques we most commonly introduce are caring days (Stuart, 1976) and exercises to increase communication skills and to build trust. As the relationship is enhanced, the man's emotional vulnerability diminishes, thereby freeing reactions that in the past would have impaired sexual response.

TREATMENT OF INHIBITED SEXUAL DESIRE (ISD)
AND SEXUAL AVERSION

Sexual desire may be conceptualized as a continuum, and in some extreme cases, there is an absence of desire, rather than an inhibition, accompanied by strong aversion and general phobic reactions to anything sexual. At a less extreme point on the gradient, there may be an acceptable attitude toward sex, especially after actual arousal, but the individual is seldom desirous of sexual contact. As with other sexual dysfunctions, ISD and sexual aversion may be primary or secondary, situational or generalized. These conditions are usually present within the context of a marriage, for while occurring in nonmarital relationships, such liaisons usually dissolve before reaching therapy (Crenshaw & Crenshaw, 1977). When desire is inhibited with a spouse but is present with another partner, the problem is interactional and more appropriate for marital than for sex therapy. However, ISD may coexist in an otherwise caring, affectionate relationship as well as in a conflict-ridden marriage.

In sexual aversion, sex is avoided not merely from a lack of interest but because it is keenly experienced as distasteful and revolting. Frequently, any physical touch that could progress to sexual contact is totally avoided. Crenshaw and Crenshaw (1977) descriptively identified the characteristics of sexual aversion. Primary sexual aversion is characterized by a negative response to all sexual interaction from earliest remembrance to the present and usually coexists with other dysfunctions (e.g., vaginismus, primary orgasmic dysfunction, erectile dysfunction). In secondary aversion, there is also continuous avoidance of sexual activity, but sexual involvement was pleasurable at some time in the past.

Sexual desire is complex and is influenced by multiple determinants. Kaplan (1977, 1979) noted that the physiology of sexual desire is not yet clearly defined. Clinical evidence suggests that desire may in some cases be physically impaired through hormone imbalance or deficiency or by central nervous system depression from medications, illness, or surgery. Psychological factors such as stress, conflict, depression, fear, and anxiety, as well as traumatic sexual experiences such as rape and incest, may also inhibit libido. Sexual ignorance, religious prohibitions, low self-esteem, disturbed couple communication, hostility and destructive interactional patterns, and excessive demands and fatigue are other factors that have been implicated in low sex drive.

Hypnosis. Several uncontrolled case studies have been reported in the treatment of sexually unresponsive female patients, but they also included varied therapy procedures in addition to hypnotic suggestions encouraging sexual interaction. Araoz (1980) successfully used hypnosis to treat ISD in 10 patients, and an increased frequency of enjoyable sexual activity was found at four- to eight-month follow-up in 9 of the patients. However, sampling procedures were not described, and there was no control condition. Thus, it is totally impossible to determine the role of hypnosis in effecting the successful results. It is our clinical impression, however, that hypnosis may have definite potential as one component of a broad treatment program for ISD and sexual aversion. Research is needed to confirm this speculation and to define the specific patients with whom it may be most beneficial.

Systematic Desensitization. A variety of desensitization methods have been studied. For example, Winzce and Caird (1973, 1976) learned that video desensitization was superior to standard systematic desensitization, and Husted (1975) found imaginal desensitization more efficient than *in vivo* desensitization. Numerous case reports are also present in the literature. The research literature is suggestive and encouraging, but it rests primarily on uncontrolled studies. Only Husted's (1975) study, in which the number of subjects was not stated, indicated that desensitization for women with ISD or sexual aversion may result in positive outcome. Furthermore, only Lazarus (1963), Cooper (1969b), and Husted (1975) unequivocally recognized the category of sexual aversion by their descriptive definitions. Lazarus (1978), however, personally identified a variety of other contaminating interventions that may have contributed to his earlier success rate of 56%, thereby confounding the role of systematic desensitization.

Eclectic Treatment Programs. Eclectic approaches include those of Kaplan (1979) and Cooper (1969c). Cooper's (1969c) treatment package included relaxation training, optimal sexual stimulation provided by the partner, sex education, and superficial psychotherapy. His success rate was very low—only 25% cured or improved.

Kaplan (1977, 1979), reviewing clinical evidence, hypothesized that among clients with sexual problems, those who present with inhibited sexual desire have the least favorable prognosis and are likely to need psychotherapeutic help that extends beyond the area of sexuality. Therapy tends to be lengthier (20–30 sessions) and requires more flexibility. Kaplan often deals with such etiological causes as fear of pleasure and romantic success, and fear of intimacy. Contrary to popular stereotypes, ISD also commonly afflicts men, and in our clinic, the ratio of males to females with this problem is 4:5.

Because of the multiplicity of influences that are often involved in these cases, careful and broad multidimensional assessment is especially required. As may be seen from the research review, however, the varied treatment strategies that we are employing are primarily a result of clinical judgment rather than documented evidence. Once organic factors have been ruled out, we find that marital factors often appear to be involved, especially in secondary ISD. Therefore, relationship-enhancement treatment methods are used. Sometimes couples lack prerequisite communication and affectional skills for establishing intimacy and closeness. If these deficiencies appear to lend themselves to brief therapy, we offer the necessary training. One valuable procedure for creating an atmosphere conducive to intimacy is Stuart's (1976) caring-days assignment, described in Chapter 6. We particularly emphasize identifying and increasing affectional behaviors. In addition to the caring-days assignment, dating sessions (Annon, 1976) may be implemented as a means of rekindling feelings of anticipation, pleasure, and interest. We structure these dates with the couple so as to take into account personal preferences and finances.

Enhancement of couple communication involves many of the techniques outlined in Chapter 7. In some cases where the relationship is not seriously conflicted, we have referred couples to a marriage encounter weekend or to a marriage enrichment (Acme) program, and the intensity of these experiences tends to be beneficial. Some couples also need assistance with conflict containment, using techniques like those presented in the preceding chapter of this volume.

When lowered self-esteem, most often occurring in the female, appears to be related to ISD, the therapeutic management of these feelings must precede sexual task assignments. Assertiveness training may be prescribed. We may give the woman permission to be somewhat "selfish" each day, for example, by visiting a friend, taking a half hour of free time from children and spouse to have an uninterrupted bubble bath, delegating household chores to other family members, or becoming involved in interests outside the home. She may also become more active outside the home in civic activities, school, and making plans to return to work.

Relatedly, environmental factors may influence sexual desire. We have encouraged couples to rearrange furniture in the bedroom, agree to a purchase that would pertain to their sexual interaction (e.g., a lamp for special lighting, candles, a vibrator, a subscription to erotic literature), or purchase a lock for the bedroom door to maintain privacy from children. Altering stimulus conditions may also include modifying the time and place, as well as the atmosphere, surrounding sexual involvement.

When the ISD or aversive client has high sexual anxiety or sexual phobias, desensitization seems particularly recommended. This may include imaginal desensitization followed soon afterwards by *in vivo* assignments. As with all of the other dysfunctions, the therapist must create a nondemanding, relaxed, and sensual atmosphere where sexual response may unfold naturally in the course of physical contact. We repeatedly refer to the concept of sex as a natural function, encourage tender and affectionate gestures that do not "lead to sex," and carefully graduate sexual assignments. At the beginning, imaginal desensitization rather than sensate focus, may be prescribed in cases of strong aversion, or less threatening *in vivo* assignments may precede sensate touching.

During *in vivo* assignments, it is particularly important to encourage the patients to focus on their feelings and physical sensations. We do not pressure them for sexual arousal, but merely to be aware of current experiencing. We encourage couples to create a relaxed atmosphere, which may mean bathing or showering together, reading poetry, listening to music, taking a walk, or simply finding uninterrupted quiet time to talk. Initially, it is important for their time simply to be pleasurable, even if it is not perceived as sexual. For some individuals with ISD, the thought of becoming aroused can create anxiety, but they can tolerate the intermediate step of enjoyment and relaxation. To take turns pleasuring may also be valuable, because with clients who avoid sexual contact, giving is often much less anxiety-producing than receiving. Thus, even if the client's own sexual feeling is not significant, he or she can appreciate the chance to give pleasure to the partner and perhaps share pleasure in being together, without sexual excitement for himself or herself. Tolerance and appreciation of giving may be a reasonable and satisfactory goal.

In the treatment of ISD and sexual aversion, resistance is almost inevitable. One of the major problems is that task assignments are simply not done. The inhibited partner often refuses to invite the spouse for sessions, and the less inhibited partner, after years of rejection, feels that if the mate will not initiate activities, it means that he or she is still not desired. It is necessary to help the less inhibited partner to refrain from personalizing the ISD and to agree to assume temporary responsibility for beginning the sessions. The therapist must bear in mind that the pace of assigning tasks will be much more gradual with ISD and aversion.

Cognitive restructuring, education, and bibliotherapy may all be important with some clients. Readings such as *The Hite Report* (Hite, 1976), *McCary's Human Sexuality* (McCary, 1978), *A Doctor Speaks on Sexual Expression in Marriage* (Hastings, 1972), and *My Secret Garden* (Friday, 1973) may be prescribed. Bibliotherapy is merely one more tool for producing attitudinal changes. With some patients, we further suggest the use of newsstand erotic literature, especially as an aid in fantasy training (Flowers & Booraem, 1975).

It is our clinical impression that one of the favorable prognostic indicators with ISD–sexual aversion in the female is her willingness to participate in the gradual nine-step masturbation program (LoPiccolo & Lobitz, 1973). Initial resistance sometimes yields with explanation of a rationale with gentle support. Reinterpretation may also be valuable.

Among primarily aversive women, however, self-stimulation may arouse even more anxiety in some cases than genital touch by the partner. In such situations, we do not pressure. We will, though, encourage nudity on nonsexual occasions such as dressing and undressing, allowing the partner in the bathroom while bathing, and even remaining naked in bed together just to talk. It is imperative, however, that the sexually interested partner not violate established limits by attempting sexual involvements that would destroy the trust and the degree of comfort that is slowly acquired. Males with ISD are usually more acceptant of a masturbation and fantasy training program (Zilbergeld, 1978). They also do not hide behind the concept of modesty as much and tend to be more open to nudity. Related to fantasy training, masturbation and fantasy may be used in a program for conditioning or reconditioning erotic desire (Marquis, 1970; Davison, 1968).

In sexual aversion, the inhibition seems so pervasive and deep at times that we have learned to respect less than optimal goals. For example, with one couple, intercourse was rarely permitted by the wife. She refused all but the slightest amount of hugging and kissing, submitted to intercourse only with considerable pressure and resistance, and then avoided all touch for long periods. With treatment, she learned to accept body massage, cuddling, and kissing. In time, she would also tolerate having her spouse masturbate in her presence or rub his penis against her body until he ejaculated. Finally, she was even willing to stimulate him manually to ejaculation. Although this couple may not have reached an ideal goal of mutual pleasure in intercourse, they both viewed their situation as acceptable. The therapist must be cautious to respect patient values and rights to self-determination. In some cases, the goal may be tolerance rather than enjoyment, and an accommodation between the partners that lessens distance and creates the possibility of minimal to moderate levels of sexual contact.

TREATMENT OF VAGINISMUS

Vaginismus is the result of an involuntary spasm of the muscles surrounding the vaginal introitus. Upon attempted penetration, the vaginal entrance tightly closes, and intercourse is impossible in many cases. Frequently, women who suffer from this condition have never had a pelvic examination or even inserted a finger or a tampon into the vagina. Women with vaginismus may phobically avoid sexual contact of any kind, or they may be sexually responsive and indulge in all varieties of sex play short of penetration.

Hypnosis. Using a combination of sex education and posthypnotic suggestion, Leckie (1964) successfully treated 13 of 15 patients (87%) with vaginismus. Fuchs *et al.* (1973) treated 9 patients with hypnotic desensitization, education, and graduated home-task assignments that consisted of successfully completed anxiety hierarchy scenes. Of the 9 patients, 6 (67%) achieved penetration. However, 34 other women were taught autohypnosis and instructed to use dilators with self-hypnosis. They also received a partial gynecological examination, which included digital dilation while under self-hypnosis. This program resulted in a 91.2% success rate, and the 3 patients who were unsuccessful were all individuals who prematurely terminated after the first few interviews.

Muscle Exercises. S. P. Hall (1952) described an inability of women with vaginismus to contract their vaginal muscles voluntarily. He assigned "Kegel" muscle contraction exercises to 24 women, requesting that they perform them twice daily. Success was obtained with 67% of the women, and another 17% showed improvement after a period of time. However, the patients were told to do contraction exercises against a finger or a large test tube, thus confounding whether the mechanim of change was the contraction exercise or the dilation procedure.

Dilation Exercises. Elgosin (1951) described the successful treatment of one case by therapist digital dilation and another where digital self-dilation was used. In a study of unconsummated marriages, Dawkins and Taylor (1961) treated 43 women with moderate to severe vaginismus primarily by instructing them in digital self-dilation, occasionally combined with dilators. The husbands were not involved in the therapy. Of these patients, 77% successfully consummated their marriages, and there was improvement in all 4 women treated exclusively with dilators. Despite successful penetration, however, in many cases a satisfactory sex life did not ensue, perhaps because the husbands were not included in the therapy, and because many misconceptions, fears, and inhibitions were not treated.

Friedman (1962) treated 100 women with a combination of dilation and supportive psychotherapy and reported a 71% success rate. Ellison (1968) reported an 87% success rate in 100 cases using dilators and insight therapy. Most case studies using dilation exercises also report successful outcomes.

Masters and Johnson (1970) used sensate focus exercises and insertion of graduated dilators in the treatment of vaginismus. They encouraged the husband's involvement in inserting the dilators under the wife's manual control. Educational information was also routinely provided. After treatment and five-year follow-up of their first 29 patients, they reported a 100% success rate (Masters & Johnson, 1970). Between 1972 and 1975, they treated another 36 women, and at two-year follow-up, they found a failure rate of only 2.8% (1 case). Dubble (1977) used vaginal dilation along with sensate focus exercises to treat 32 women with vaginismus and unconsummated marriages: 72% consummated their marriages, 21% could not be located after treatment, and there was 1 treatment failure where the husband also had primary erectile dysfunction.

Implications and Treatment Strategies. Clearly, the treatment of choice with vaginismus is a therapy program that includes vaginal dilation exercises. Although the combination of self-hypnosis and dilation seems successful, dilation without the time-consuming instruction in autohypnosis seems comparably effective. Autohypnosis and hypnotic systematic desensitization could, however, conceivably be beneficial prior to vaginal dilation exercises in the infrequent case where phobic avoidance is so high that dilation exercises are firmly resisted, despite interpretations fostering examination of the adaptive function of such avoidance.

Lamont (1977) discovered physical factors that may have been related to the onset of vaginismus and that required correction prior to dilation therapy in 29% of his patients. Some form of vaginitis (caused by atrophy, *Monilia*, or *Trichomonas*) was present in 11% of cases, 8% had problems with an episiotomy, and other factors noted in 3% of cases included constipation, retroversion, previous surgery (vaginal hysterectomy), and pelvic congestion. It is essential that a physician screen for organic factors during the pelvic examination, which is done to document the presence of the involuntary spasm. Prior to proceeding with sex therapy, the patient should receive medical treatment for any physical factors that are discovered.

Several less specific factors are rarely discussed but are undoubtedly influential in the treatment of such a strong avoidance reaction. Fuchs *et al.* (1973) have stressed the importance of establishing a good relationship between the therapist and the couple and of providing an understanding, warm, and noncritical atmosphere. Kaplan (1974) likewise described the importance of using reassurance and support but, when necessary, confronting the women with the consequence that if they do not "stay with" their uncomfortable feelings and insert something into the vagina, they will not overcome their problem.

Several authors have stressed the etiological role of ignorance and misinformation (Blazer, 1964; Ellison, 1972), finding it present in over 90% of vaginismus patients. Therefore, we believe that routine education about anatomy, physiology, the sexual response cycle, and common myths is indicated with this dysfunction. As part of the education process, we prescribe self-examination of the genitals as a home exercise, along with assigned reading about this exercise (Heiman et al., 1976, pp. 32–39). In explaining the conditioned vaginal response, we often use the analogy of someone salivating when a person describes tantalizing foods. Both are conditioned involuntary reflexes. A useful analogy to facilitate understanding in husbands is to liken vaginismus to the difference between voluntarily flexing one's calf muscle versus having an involuntary spasm (cramp).

In our clinic, we use Young's rectal dilators and show them to the patient one at a time. We explain that she will not feel pain but may experience some anxiety or tightness. She should tolerate and "stay with" these feelings, and they will diminish. If the woman is exceptionally anxious, she is provided with tape-recorded instructions for tensing and relaxing muscle exercises (Goldfried & Davison, 1976), which may be used prior to dilation. She is instructed to lubricate the dilator with K-Y Jelly and slowly insert it toward the coccyx. She should insert the dilator for 15 minutes three times a day, doing Kegel muscle contraction exercises immediately before insertion and around the dilator after insertion. It may also be suggested that she gently move the dilator back and forth in the vagina prior to concluding the exercise. The last exercise should be done at bedtime, and she is requested, if it is not too uncomfortable, to try to sleep with the dilator inside the vagina. After she is comfortable inserting one size of dilator, she is given the next larger size. If problems are encountered, the therapist should double-check the method of insertion and whether contraction exercises are being done immediately before insertion is attempted.

Prior to or concurrently with dilation exercises, the couple is assigned sensate-focus pleasuring exercises. Later, genital play may be included, at at that time the male is requested to examine his partner's genitals in full light, using a drawing to identify each part. He is then included in observing the dilation procedure and begins inserting the dilator, with his spouse holding and guiding his hand. The next step calls for the husband to insert the dilator unassisted and then to move it in and out slowly and gently under his partner's guidance. Throughout this time there should be absolutely no attempt at penile penetration.

After all five dilators can be used with comfort, a "quiet vagina" exercise is prescribed. The couple may engage in sensate love play initially, and then they are instructed to dilate the vagina with the largest dilator. Next, the penis is lubricated, and the woman assumes the female superior position and guides entry of the penis in the same manner she used for inserting the dilators. We instruct couples that henceforth the woman is always to guide entry. After insertion, they should merely rest quietly and then withdraw. The next progressive step includes slow thrusting and then more rapid thrusting, with instructions to stop if she experiences pain. The woman, however, is instructed to distinguish between mild "discomfort" or "pressure" and acutal pain. Prior to this time, birth control measures should be discussed.

TREATMENT OF ORGASMIC DYSFUNCTION

Orgasmic dysfunction is an inhibition of the orgasmic phase of the sexual response cycle. The condition is primary in the female who has never experienced orgasm through any manner of sexual stimulation. The condition is secondary if the woman has reached orgasm in the past but is currently nonorgasmic. Situational orgasmic response may refer to a woman who can reach climax through some methods of stimulation (e.g., manual stimulation, masturbation, or oral–genital sex) but not through others (e.g., partner stimulation or coitus). It is important to note that coital orgasm is in large measure produced by indirect stimulation of the clitoris or with direct stimulation of the clitoris while thrusting and is not defined as equivalent to "vaginal orgasm."

Women who have difficulty with orgasm may also experience inhibited sexual desire or vaginismus and avoid physical contact, or they may have a strong sex drive and enjoy all aspects of their sexual relationship.

Hypnosis. Short-term hypnotherapy was employed by Richardson (1963) to treat 76 cases of "frigidity." In 61 cases, direct suggestion was used while the patient was under hypnosis, and hypnoanalysis was used with 15 patients. Dramatic improvement (experiencing coital orgasm in over 35% of opportunities) was reported in 94.7% of the cases (72/76), and 61 of these women were reporting attainment of orgasm more than 80% of the time.

Alexander (1974) used a combination of hypnotherapy and psychotherapy in the treatment of seven women with orgasmic dysfunction. Five of the seven women reported complete or partial success with orgasmic return. The central focus of his therapeutic techniques was to decrease overconcern with pleasing the male partner and to decrease other types of thought processes that inhibit natural, involuntary sexual responses. Hypnotherapy was also used by Shazer (1978) to treat successfully five of seven women (71%) who did not have a partner available for therapy.

Eclectic Treatment Programs. Masters and Johnson (1970) used a two-week dual-team therapy approach with education and sensate focus exercises to treat orgasmic dysfunction in highly motivated, well-educated, middle- and upper-class couples. They reported an 83.4% success rate, with 2.6% relapse at five-year follow-up, in treating primary orgasmic dysfunction ($n = 193$). However, after a two-year follow-up of patients seen between 1972 and 1975 ($n = 45$), they found a success rate of only 66.7% (Masters et al., 1978). With situational orgasmic dysfunction ($n = 149$) they originally reported a 72.2% success rate at five-year follow-up, and their more recent statistics ($n = 176$) are a 64.2% success rate at two-year follow-up. In treatment of random orgasmic dysfunction, Masters and Johnson (1970) were originally successful with 62.5% of their patients ($n = 32$), but their most recent cases have shown a 77.5% success rate ($n = 71$).

Munjack et al. (1976) described the treatment of 12 primary and 10 secondarily anorgasmic women with relatively harmonious marriages. The treatment package was individualized for each couple but usually included systematic desensitization, assertion training, modeling and behavioral rehearsal, education and correction of misconceptions and unreasonable expectations, graduated assignments to overcome performance anxiety, and communication training. Masturbation training and vibrators were occasionally used. At termination, 22% of the primary and 40% of the secondary orgasmic dysfunction patients were orgasmic in 50% or more of coital opportunities. But at nine-month follow-up, none of the primarily anorgasmic women was still orgasmic 50% or more of the time, although the secondarily anorgasmic women continued to improve, and 60% of them met this criteria.

Blakeney et al. (1976) treated 10 couples with primary and 28 couples with secondary orgasmic dysfunction. They used an intensive 2½-day workshop format, and on lengthy follow-up, total symptom reversal was found in 70% of the primary women and 57.1% of the secondarily anorgasmic women. The treatment incorporated methods of Masters and Johnson and Hartman and Fithian.

Masturbation Training. Several investigators have either primarily used masturbation as a treatment procedure for orgasmic dysfunction or have included it as a significant component in a broader treatment package. Lobitz and LoPiccolo (1972) developed the most thorough masturbation program using a dual team for 15 treatment sessions. It consisted of sensate focus exercises and a graduated nine-step masturbation program for the woman, beginning with visual self-examination of the genitals and culminating in the partner's manipulation of the female genitals (manually or with a vibrator) only and during intercourse. The treatment package also included training in sexual communication skills through role playing and modeling, the use of fantasy and pornography, the role playing of exaggerated orgasms to encourage disinhibition, therapist self-disclosure, a refundable penalty deposit to enhance motivation, and client participation during final sessions in planning task assignments and a maintenance program. The success criterion was attaining orgasm in 50% or more of coital opportunities, and 100% of the 13 primary patients were successful at termination and six-month follow-up. With secondarily anorgasmic women, however, the program resulted in only a 33% effectiveness rate ($n = 9$).

McGovern et al. (1975) used Lobitz and LoPiccolo's (1972) treatment format with six primary and six secondarily anorgasmic women. Following therapy, all of the primarily dysfunctioning women had experienced orgasm, although only 50% were orgasmic in 50% or more of coital experiences. In contrast, however, the secondary women demonstrated almost no increase in frequency of orgasmic response to partner manipulation or coitus. The investigators found significantly more marital dissatisfaction among the secondary couples, which required therapy time for conflict resolution and communication training, leaving less time to concentrate on formal sex therapy. They also discovered that most of their secondary-dysfunction women had long histories of masturbating in very restrictive ways, bringing orgasm under tight stimulus control. Although the patient sample was small, they suggested that secondary anorgasmia may respond better to a combination of marital and sex therapy, a prohibition on masturbating by previous methods while encouraging new methods, and by gradually shaping the focus of self-stimulation to approximate coital behaviors.

Self-directed treatment with primary orgasmic dysfunction was attempted by McMullen (1976). She used an automated masturbation program in which 60 subjects either read six booklets, viewed six videotapes, or were assigned to a 10-week wait-list control group. An unexpected finding, with potential implications for the use of media in sex therapy, was that there were no differences in outcome between video and booklet subjects on any dependent measure. Of treatment subjects, 60% became orgasmic with vibrator masturbation, while no controls experienced orgasm. The effects of erotic media, masturbation training with fantasy, and a combination of the two procedures was tested by Reisinger (1978) with situational orgasmic dysfunction. The data seemingly indicated that erotic media alone are insufficient to resolve this problem. Masturbation training was more effective, but the combination of erotic stimulation and masturbation training appeared more effective than either procedure alone. However, only six subjects were used, and the population consisted of young, well-educated women, with little or no religious practice, who indicated that some types of pornography were sexually stimulating to them. Thus, religious women with negative reactions to pornography may be more responsive to masturbation training alone, which seems to be the more powerful of the two procedures.

Group Treatment Format. There have been a number of studies using group formats (Barbach, 1974; McGovern et al., 1976; Leiblum et al., 1976, 1977; Schneidman & McGuire, 1976), some with women only, others with both partners. A combination of treatment techniques was used. Examples include masturbation training, home tasks, Kegel exercises, education, and relaxation training. Rates of success ranged from 33% to 92% and varied depending on whether the orgasmic experience occurred during masturbation, clitoral manipulation, or coitus.

Kegel Exercises. Incidental to treating women for urinary stress incontinence, Kegel (1952) found:

> Whenever the perivaginal musculature is well developed, with a contractile strength of 20 mm Hg or more, as measured with the perineometer, sexual complaints are few or transient. On the other hand, in women with a thin, weak pubococcygeus muscle, with a contractile ability measuring zero to 3 mm Hg, expressions of indifference or dissatisfaction regarding sexual activity were frequently encountered. (p. 522)

He concluded that sexual feeling in the vagina is closely related to muscle tone, and "muscle education and resistive exercise" enhanced sexual feelings and resulted in some women's experiencing orgasm for the first time, but no specific statistics are provided.

Numerous studies and treatment programs routinely include Kegel exercises, but only one other study provides suggestive evidence to support the value of muscle exercises. Kline-Graber and Graber (1978) reported a retrospective review of 281 women seen in a sexual dysfunction clinic. For statistical analysis, the subjects were divided into three groups: primarily anorgasmic, noncoitally orgasmic, and orgasmic during both coitus and noncoitally. They found significant differences between these groups on measures of sustained strength and atrophy of the pubococcygeal muscle, providing correlational support for Kegel's (1952) report on the role of this muscle group in enhancing female sexual arousal and facilitating orgasmic release. However, no controlled studies are available on the efficacy of this technique, and opinions also differ on whether a perineometer is necessary in doing the exercises and on the length of time required in practice sessions (e.g., Kline-Graber & Graber, 1978).

An unspecified number of dysfunctional women were treated by Husted (1975) with either imagery desensitization or *in vivo* desensitization. Half of the women in both conditions had their partners included in treatment, and both groups used identical anxiety hierarchies. Outcomes for the two groups were not significantly different, but there was a difference in efficiency with the imaginal desensitization requiring an average of 7.8 sessions, while the *in vivo* method lasted an average of 13.3 sessions. Partner participation did not influence outcome or the number of sessions required. Husted found an 80% decrease in anxiety scores at termination and six-week follow-up, as well as an increase in the frequency of intercourse. Secondarily dysfunctional subjects, who had experienced orgasm at some time in the past, reported an increase in orgasmic frequency after treatment, but neither program was effective in increasing the orgasmic frequency of women with primary dysfunction.

Education and Media. Although the imparting of sexual information is a routine component in the majority of therapy programs, this aspect is often neglected or minimized as a mechanism of change. Jankovich and Miller (1978) found, however, that an audiovisual sex-education program presenting anatomy and physiology, the sexual response cycle evoked by manual stimulation, and a film on intercourse seemed to be influential in facilitating female sexual response. With no other interventions, 7 of 17 (41.2%) primarily anorgasmic women became orgasmic within a week of viewing the materials. Four were orgasmic with masturbation, two with partner stimulation, and one with coitus and simultaneous manual stimulation.

Robinson (1974) examined the effects of vicarious and observational learning through videotape programs on orgasmically dysfunctional women in contrast with untreated controls. The tapes showed a male therapist presenting either a wide variety of sexual information to a role-playing couple or providing information about masturbation along with specific suggestions for the model female patient. Results indicated that sexual behaviors may be acquired or may increase in frequency as a result of media modeling. Outcomes suggested that the videotapes were very effective in promoting positive attitudes toward masturbation, though not necessarily orgasmic return in primary dysfunctional subjects. Appropriate media materials may shorten the time required in therapy.

Implications and Treatment Strategies. There is suggestive evidence available that both Kegel muscle contraction exercises and hypnosis may hold promise as valuable techniques to be integrated into treatment packages, at least with certain clients. Controlled research is still necessary, however, to evaluate their therapeutic potential. Education and media have also tentatively been shown to be valuable components of a treatment program, although they seem insufficient by themselves for the resolution of orgasmic dysfunctions (Jankovich & Miller, 1978; Robinson, 1974). But with the abundance of new media resources available to sex therapists, a temptation may exist for unsophisticated therapists to use media indiscriminately, and ill-trained therapists may use media as a flashy gimmick to conceal their deficit in skills. We believe that education should be a standard component in the treatment of orgasmic dysfunction, but that media must be used discriminatingly, with the value systems of the clients being taken into account. Furthermore, McMullen's (1976) finding of no differences between videotape and booklet presentation of information on masturbation suggests that expensive (and with some clients, potentially offensive) video and film materials may respond more to therapist than to client needs. Further research is clearly needed in this area, particularly to determine if videotapes and films add anything over and above what therapist and/or bibliographical explanation provides, and to specify for which clients such materials may be therapeutic rather than offensive or even psychonoxious.

Imaginal systematic desensitization has been found to reduce sexual anxiety and to disinhibit sexual communication and response, especially in secondarily anorgasmic women (Husted, 1975; Jones & Park, 1972). On the other hand, programs using masturbation training (McGovern et al., 1975, 1976; Schneidman & McGuire, 1976; Lobitz & LoPiccolo, 1972) have produced very significant positive changes in women with primary orgasmic dysfunction but have proved relatively ineffective with secondary anorgasmia. Systematic desensitization seems most indicated where sexual anxiety is a determinant in secondary orgasmic dysfunction, whereas programs that include masturbation training are the treatment of choice with primary orgasmic dysfunction. There are also suggestive indications that marital factors may be significantly involved in many cases of secondary dysfunction. Therefore, an emphasis on relationship enhancement and sexual communication training may often be vital to success with secondary dysfunction (McGovern et al., 1975).

For women without partners, women's groups seem to be a viable treatment option. When women have available and cooperative partners, however, couples group therapy as used by McGovern et al. (1976) is still a cost-effective procedure, and one that is also anticipated to reduce the threat frequently observed in men with female partners who are involved in women's groups (Schneidman & McGuire, 1976). Concurrent with reducing threat, couples therapy groups may increase mate cooperation, support, and understanding; provide more enhancement of the general relationship between partners; and increase the chances of facilitating coital orgasm. Coital orgasm may not be a realistic goal for all women (Kaplan, 1974) and may be justifiable as an alternative but not the only way to sexual expression. Although female-only groups have problems in maintenance of change and lack of generalization to partner stimulation and intercourse, in general the results of group treatment studies provide encouragement but appear on follow-up to be less effective than conjoint therapy in the treatment of primary orgasmic dysfunction.

The therapeutic management of women with orgasmic dysfunction varies according to whether their condition is primary or secondary. A description of our treatment strategies with females who have never experienced orgasm under any conditions is presented first, followed by a discussion of the way our treatment proceeds with the secondarily dysfunctional woman.

Primary Orgasmic Dysfunction. In primary orgasmic dysfunction, the objective is to achieve orgasm under any circumstance possible. We begin sexual tasks with a dual approach that runs parallel through the course of treatment. There are assignments for the couple that must be practiced twice weekly and assignments for the female alone that must also be practiced twice a week. For the couple, we begin with sensate focus, and concurrently we start the woman alone on a masturbation program (Lobitz & LoPiccolo, 1972) to minimize the inhibitions that often occur in the presence of a partner.

Recognizing that women who have never masturbated are likely to feel uncomfortable and anxious about attempting such an experience, we often must deal with guilt, misinformation, and negative attitudes about masturbation. We educate and offer permission, support, and encouragement. If the anxiety level remains high, we provide relaxation training. In a few cases, the woman's inhibitions are too great, her guilt too pervasive, and her sexual value system too rigidly opposed to tolerate masturbation. We must respect her decision not to proceed, and help her in the framework of the heterosexual interaction. Our clinical impression is that the woman who refuses masturbation training is not necessarily a poor prognostic risk.

When suggesting that the female begin a masturbation training program, it is important to stress that self-stimulation is a vehicle for growth and also a means of sexual learning that may be shared later with her partner. Also, we insist that the self-stimulation be attempted only when the woman is alone and free from interruption. The first instructions are for the woman to look at herself in the mirror after a bath or a shower, which tends to be a relaxed time. She is to think about what she sees, what she likes and dislikes about her body, and how she feels about herself sexually. Since most women feel dissatisfied with some parts of their body, we anticipate critical self-statements and gently remind our clients that "no body is perfect." Often, women also surprise themselves by discovering parts of themselves that are "not so bad" and even find other body parts quite attractive. After this assignment, tasks are graduated from looking at her genitals and comparing them to a drawing of the anatomic parts of female genitals, to exploring them by touch without expectation of arousal, to touch for pleasure and arousal. Early in the sequence, we introduce Kegel exercises and provide the woman with written instructions on how to perform them correctly.

Often the woman becomes increasingly in tune with her body and reaches higher and higher levels of arousal, yet is unable to release orgasm. At this point, we discuss "orgasm triggers" (Heiman et al., 1976), such as voluntarily increasing muscle tension, breathing heavily, or exaggerating pelvic thrusting. This is also a time when a vibrator may be introduced, since it can offer more concentrated, intense stimulation. We recommend a type such as Prelude 3.

Throughout this process, another essential ingredient is the use of erotic fantasy. For women who already fantasize, encouragement of this activity validates a rarely discussed sexual expression. For women who have not allowed themselves the privilege of sexual fantasizing, we recommend imagery building. The use of erotic material, such as Friday's *My Secret Garden* (1973), assists in accomplishing this directive. Fantasy is a particular aid for nonorgasmic women because it is a stimulant that enhances sexual arousal, as well as a distractor that competes with inhibitory throughts.

Another means of maximizing stimulation and avoiding performance orientation is focusing on the sensual and sexual feelings that the body is experiencing. By remaining present-centered and concentrating on bodily sensations, a woman may learn the types of sexual stimulation that are effective in her arousal.

Not only do some women have difficulty accepting masturbation training, but some husbands also have problems with the notion of their wives' masturbating, feeling threatened that they may learn to bring themselves sexual enjoyment that the husbands have been unable to provide. In these situations, we interpret masturbation as a learning experience that will benefit both husband and wife. We discuss it as a means to a very positive end, as a way that the wife can learn to appreciate her body responses and then teach him to provide the stimulation she needs.

Some men are also threatened by the use of a vibrator, perceiving it as a mechanical device that may bring pleasure they do not, reflecting their inadequacy as lovers. We assist the couple to perceive the vibrator as another way of sharing, of exploring and enriching sexual expression, and of using a convenience that can help in reaching their objective. The vibrator need not only be used for female genital stimulation. It may be used on the rest of the body for relaxation and enjoyment and also to stimulate the male. Kissing, hugging, caressing, and close body contact provide extra warmth and emotion to make the vibrator more effective. Once recognizing that he will eventually be part of the experience helps the concerned spouse to be more accepting.

As the female is exploring on her own, she is also involved in sensual time with her partner. As mentioned, we start with sensate focus, exploring the body first while prohibiting genital and breast contact, and then later including these parts of the body. The purpose of the shared experience is to enrich sexual expression, to encourage the communication of sexual preferences, and to encourage the freedom to enjoy each other sensually, without the pressure to perform. Unless suffering from inhibited sexual desire, almost every woman feels relief and renewed enjoyment in experiencing sex play without coitus. Women inevitably comment on feeling that "the pressure was off" or "I didn't have to worry about disappointing him because I couldn't climax." They also, however, are concerned about providing satisfaction for the mate.

With some reassurance from him, and by providing him with orgasmic release through manual or oral stimulation, the women tend to accept the shared time as an opportunity to learn to be together in a different way. Also, many couples comment on the fun of similar premarital sexual activity that they enjoyed but have neglected since.

After the woman has learned more about her sexual response through masturbation, she is encouraged to share the information with her partner. She may do this by telling him what pleases her or by guiding his hand with hers, indicating place, pace, and pressure, or she may model for him how to stimulate her. It is our experience that asking for pleasure is, on the whole, more difficult for women than for men. Even if the woman is reticent to express requests openly when alone with her partner, she will frequently discuss her preferences with the support of the therapist. We use part of the therapeutic session to be certain that the male knows what is likely to please his spouse. However, sexual arousal is not always contingent on a preference announced in advance. Nevertheless, the wife usually appreciates her husband's attention to her earlier requests and is more likely to acknowledge spontaneously what is pleasing once she has openly discussed her desires with him.

Once they are able to masturbate to orgasm reliably, some women make a rather quick transition to orgasmic response through partner stimulation. Like Kaplan (1974), we minimize the pressure to perform by suggesting that after making love in their usual way, and when the husband has ejaculated, he may concentrate on stimulating her.

For other women, the presence of the partner still provokes anxieties and fears of performance. In such situations, because she better understands her own erotic needs, we suggest self-stimulation in his presence. Clinical experience has taught us that acceptance of this recommendation is facilitated by discussion and by the man's willingness to masturbate in her presence. In discussion during the interview, we explore the cultural meanings of masturbation, personal values and feelings, and how it may be used by the married individual. Husbands often offer their spontaneous support of this concept, while recognizing that the experience may not be an easy one. In cases where the couple are strongly opposed, we revert to having the woman teach her partner about her needs through verbalization and guided stimulation, while she employs fantasy for distraction.

Early in treatment with primarily anorgasmic women, we explore the woman's conceptions of female orgasm, as well as potential fears (e.g., of loss of control, injury, going crazy, becoming promiscuous, passing gas, and appearing ridiculous or ugly). We explain that orgasm is merely an involuntary reflexive reaction and describe what it feels like, ranging from mild to intense sensations, from a gentle warmth to a loud pulsing, from local genital sensations to a total body sensation. We talk about muscle tension, rhythmic contractions, and relaxation. We indicate that the woman may desire to read about other women's experiences with orgasm (Hite, 1976, pp. 81–84), stating that these represent to the intense end of the scale but are nevertheless valuable. Hite also has two pages (pp. 78–80) where women express their shy feelings about having orgasm with their partner. Our patients can readily identify with these feelings and have some sense of shared experience that normalizes some of their thoughts and concerns. Kaplan (1974) emphasized that orgasm is only a reflex and instructed the woman that her life would not be dramatically different simply because she has had an orgasm. This reassurance helps to dispel the symbolic qualities often attributed to climax by anorgasmic women. Also, role-playing orgasm may be used with those women who become apprehensive of approaching orgasm, who can masturbate to orgasm but are coitally anorgasmic, and who seem inhibited and afraid of embarrassing themselves by uttering involuntary noises and displaying muscle contractions (Lobtiz & LoPiccolo, 1972). In this procedure, the woman, with the involvement of her husband, playacts a grossly exaggerated orgasm, complete with screaming, moaning, and violent convulsions. They should have fun with the experience, making it into a game. Initial anxiety and embarrassment soon turn to amusement and are finally desensitized.

Another common fear of primarily anorgasmic women is that they will take "too long" to become sexually aroused. They become preoccupied with thoughts such as "He must be getting bored," "His hand will get tired," "I'm taking too much time," and "I'm getting nowhere and he's already aroused." When questioned about what is a proper amount of time for becoming sexually aroused, it is rare for the anorgastic woman to suggest more than 15 minutes as an appropriate amount of attention for her. Even when alone in masturbation, 10–15 minutes' time often seems enough. We have to encourage women to indulge themselves, to be "selfish" about their pleasure, and to allow a minimum of one-half hour and, if necessary, even an hour to focus on themselves. Sexual feelings rise and fall, spectatoring interferes, and they need sufficient time to practice staying with their sensations, identifying pleasures, and viewing erotic material to precipitate arousal. We assure them that once orgasm is attained, it tends to become progressively easier to experience.

In heterosexual situations, nonorgasmic women often feel even greater pressure concerning time because they measure themselves against their husband's erection. In fact, many women, even those who are orgasmic, feel pressured by their partner's erection and proceed to intercourse when they would prefer to continue other forms of sex play. In general, sex is frequently governed by what the female *thinks* the man needs, rather than by an acutal expression of his or her desires. We propose that erections are always to be admired but are not always to be used for intercourse. When these issues are openly discussed, we find that many men are amenable to taking more time in sex play before proceeding to coitus.

Our experience is that primarily dysfunctional women and their partners feel a sense of accomplishment and satisfaction once her orgasm is part of their shared experience. It does not seem to matter to most couples whether the orgasm occurs with manual stimulation, with oral–genital sex, or with intercourse. We recommend to those, however, who do want to have orgasm during coitus that they allow themselves six months to consolidate their gains and establish a pattern of reliable female orgasmic expression by whatever means available to them, suggesting that in time coital orgasm may occur. We explain to them several techniques that they may try, such as stimulation to the point of orgasm and then making immediate entry; clitoral stimulation by the partner or by the woman herself concurrent with intercourse; and vibrator stimulation concurrent with intercourse. However, whatever stimulation parallels coitus, a moment before orgasm, the simultaneous stimulation should cease to allow thrusting to trigger orgasm. At the six-month follow-up, we may evaluate the sexual relationship again, and if the couple desire further help, we arrange another few sessions to work with them toward their goal of orgasm with intercourse.

Secondary Orgasmic Dysfunction. Secondarily anorgasmic women fall into three distinct categories: those who can masturbate to orgasm but cannot at present climax in any manner with their partner, those who attain orgasm with their partner but not during intercourse, and those who at an earlier time experienced orgasm with the mate but no longer do so. Our clinical experience indicates that marital dissatisfaction is often greater in this third category than in the other two. Often, a large portion of our treatment time for these couples is used for conflict resolution, decision making, and communication training.

Generally, the women in the first category, like primarily anorgasmic women, want to experience climax with the mate in whatever manner is possible. We use the same treatment strategy with them that was used in treating primary dysfunction, except that there is no need for the masturbation training program. The therapy commences with the couple's beginning sensate focus.

For women in the second category, we find it important to explore the stated desire for coital orgasm. Is it indicative of a relationship problem? Does the male feel that he fails as a lover when the woman does not climax with intercourse? Is her lack of orgasmic response because of his poor technique or because of his rapid ejaculation? Does she feel less feminine or inadequate, or does one or both of them merely assume that intercourse is how orgasms are "supposed to be" experienced? Are the couple simply seeking to enrich their sexual experience?

Whatever the need, we inform all such couples that the woman's present orgasmic response is considered normal and that millions of women do not experience coital orgasm. We explain that only mild sexual stimulation is provided for the woman through intercourse, and that physiologically, she may personally need the more intense clitoral stimulation for orgasmic release. We reassure both that the wife's response is not "second best" unless they choose to regard it that way and that some women actually prefer to achieve orgasm by manual or oral stimulation.

A general discussion regarding sexual physiology, reassurances of normality, and brief descriptions of techniques that may help are sufficient for some couples to feel satisfied with their current adjustment. They may try the suggestions on their own, and if these are not effective, perhaps they will return later. We inform those couples who choose therapy that they may attain their goals, but that it is also possible that coital orgasm will not occur. Nevertheless, they will probably learn greater sexual appreciation of one another and increase the openness and communication between them.

Although these women already reach orgasm with the partner, we usually find that therapy is facilitated by beginning with sensate focus. For couples who feel some concerns about their sexual relationship, these pleasuring exercises create a low-keyed sensual experience in which they are free to explore at their leisure without pressure to reach a goal. Further, when genital touch is prohibited, communication regarding likes, dislikes, and requests is less threatening. Also, when breast and genital touch is included for the purpose of communicating and learning about sensual pleasures, the couple has the opportunity to explore lovemaking techniques that heighten sexual arousal. This may mean introducing oral–genital sex, discovering new rhythms and pressures, using teasing touches, etc. Frequently, caressing the erect penis against the vulva and barely inserting it into the introitus, making rotating motions and again rubbing it against the vulva, is highly arousing.

Concurrent with the sensate focus experiences, we request that the woman involve herself in three exercises to enhance vaginal sensation. In addition to the Kegel exercises already discussed, we suggest that while sitting, she tense and release her buttocks, noting the vaginal sensations. Also, when lying down, she is instructed to tense her legs and arch her pelvis upward, again noting the sensations in her vagina. These exercises may be done two or three times daily for a few minutes at a time. They may create additional vaginal awareness, and they should also be used during intercourse to grasp the penis and increase pleasurable feelings.

Following sensate focus, coitus is prescribed. Kaplan (1974) described two ways in which it may be performed. One is in a stop–start, teasing manner following sex play to high arousal. The penis is inserted, and the male thrusts for a brief period in a slow, teasing manner, withdraws for a brief period, and then reenters and slowly thrusts. If orgasm does not occur with this teasing technique, clitoral stimulation may be prescribed during the interruptions of intercourse. We suggest that the husband lie on top of the wife, and she may then tense or rub her pelvis against his pubic area or, as in sensate focus, rub his erection against her vulva. The couple is encouraged to have as many stop–start periods as needed or desired. If orgasm does not happen, they may try "brinksmanship," whereby during interruption, he stimulates her to the edge of orgasm and then quickly penetrates.

The bridge maneuver suggested by Kaplan (1974) is a combination of fantasy and clitoral stimulation with penile thrusting. The clitoral stimulation may be provided by either partner or with a vibrator. When the woman is near orgasm, clitoral stimulation stops and hard thrusting is done. The process may have to be tried repeatedly to be effective. When it does trigger orgasm, some of the women may become progressively more easily orgasmic with intercourse alone. Others will continue to require some direct clitoral stimulation in combination with coitus.

One of the changes that occurs when an anorgasmic women experiences orgasm with her partner, or a secondarily dysfunctional women achieves coital orgasm, is the recognition that she is a sexual being with needs, desires, and a sexual rhythm that may differ from her mate's. For sex to remain a mutually pleasurable and deeply meaningful experience, she will have to take active responsibility for her own gratification, openly communicating her interests and responsivity. By establishing for herself a more egalitarian role, she may stir new emotions in her mate that will need special attention in the therapeutic process. If, however, the marital relationship is viable, the new sexually assertive role she has adopted will not only be accepted but will be preferred by her partner. Ultimately, sex is more satisfying when both partners are free to explore, initiate, request, give, and receive pleasure.

Summary

In this chapter we have defined each of the major sexual dysfunctions and have briefly summarized a sampling of the outcome research currently available. Despite the limited experimental evidence, research has specified several therapeutic procedures that appear to be effective with certain dysfunctions, and there is at least suggestive evidence for others. Table 1 summarizes the techniques used in varied combinations to treat the seven varieties of sexual disturbances covered in this chapter.

Table 1. Summary of treatment techniques

Nonspecific therapist factors	Cognitive interventions	Anxiety-reduction techniques

Empathic understanding
Respect
Warmth and caring
Encouragement and support
Instillation of hope
Resolution of resistance
Permission giving
Therapist self-disclosure
	1. Reinterpretation
	  a. Normalizing and universality
	  b. Postitive relabeling
	  c. Feedback
	  d. "World's authority" concept
	2. Concept of self-interest and self-responsibility ("selfish")
	3. Avoid spectatoring —thought-stop and use of competing cognitive activities
	4. Cognitive restructuring
	  a. Facilitating resolution of historical factors
	  b. Sex more than intercourse (other myths, unrealistic expectations, sex as a natural function, neutrality)
	  c. Hypnosis
	5. Education about anatomy, physiology, male and female response cycles
	6. Bibliotherapy, education, and modeling through audiovisual aids
	7. Roundtable: cognitive conceptualization of problems
	8. Stay with the feelings of discomfort
	9. Involvement of clients in planning assignments
		1. Graduated presentation of assignments (*in vivo* desensitization to decrease performance anxiety)
		2. Deep-muscle relaxation
		3. Systematic desensitization
		4. Relaxation via medications
		5. Hypnotic relaxation
		6. Cognitive restructuring (meditation, autogenic training)

Relationship enhancement and communication training	Techniques for enhancing imagery and sensory awareness	Task assignments and instructions
1. Couple communication training a. Perception-of-feeling training b. Constructive expression of emotions (e.g., "I language") (1) Anger-management procedures c. Empathic communication training (1) Ticket-to-talk exercise d. Daily dialogue e. Cotherapist modeling of interaction 2. Caring days: increase of affectional interaction 3. Sexual communication training a. Assertion training (1) Expression of preferences, desires, and pleasure (2) Initiation and refusal skills (3) Nonverbal guidance b. Sensate focus assignments	1. Directed attention: focus on erotic sensations 2. Imagery and fantasy building 3. Erotic literature, pictures, and media	Squeeze Stop–start Graduated masturbation Masturbation during vaginal containment Body or genital self-examination Mutual manual stimulation Dilators and digital dilation Come and go Kegel exercises *In vivo* assignments, for example, sensate focus, sensate focus with genital stimulation, varied positions, controlled intercourse Prohibition of intercourse Use of lubricants Exaggerated (role-play) orgasm Vibrator Vaginal containment ("quiet vagina") Experimentation Increased frequency of sexual contact Altering stimulus conditions (atmosphere, mood enhancers) Diary Female guidance of entry Scheduling intimate contacts Writing summary of learnings and maintenance plans Self-stimulation during partner love-play and intercourse

Although we are acutely aware of the limited state of our knowledge, we have presented many of the details of our clinical practice in the hope that these may be useful to the therapist who must provide service while awaiting definitive guidelines from the researchers. The strategies described are applicable in principle to many couples, but all therapists must guard against the simplistic notion that any technique or approach is necessarily the treatment of choice for a particular dysfunction. Although there are only a circumscribed number of techniques currently available in the field, their use in combination and according to empirical indications allows the clinician to prescribe an individualized course of therapy geared to the needs of each couple within the confines of their sexual value system. Mechanistic application of sex therapy techniques in a rigid and unvarying format and without regard for the individual couple may hold the potential for destructive outcomes. Finally, we would remind the reader of our belief that technical knowledge is insufficient unless it is combined with expertise in establishing a therapeutic relationship, working through resistance, and working with the social interaction of the couple. No program of sex therapy can hope to be successful unless it includes a thoughtful and individualized plan of intervention that addresses these focal concerns in service delivery.

Maintaining Results

THE GENERAL PROBLEM of the maintenance of therapeutic outcome is reviewed here, with recommendations offered for building into active treatment steps that will work toward perpetuation of treatment-mediated changes. Inherent in the service-delivery strategy of this approach, with its emphasis upon educating clients as to the rationale and techniques being utilized, is an important component of the initiation of sustainable change. To this can be added specific techniques that prompt self-corrective actions by the spouses when therapeutic guidance is no longer available. This chapter offers a review of these techniques.

As will be recalled from Chapter 4 (see Table 1 in that chapter), follow-up evaluations are the critically important but all-too-often neglected stepchildren of marriage and family researchers. This neglect is a reflection of several factors. For example, the collection of follow-up data is costly, and their collection often requires compromising the rigor used in collecting the initial experimental data. Moreover, as follow-up intervals are often several times greater than the number of weeks used to produce initial changes, the collection of these data requires considerable delay in the publication of the original results. Finally, many researchers may fail to collect follow-up data because these researchers do little in promoting initial changes that will make these changes maintainable over time. This is a serious flaw because building skills in maintaining positive therapeutic outcomes is fully as important as promoting change in the first place.

While Stuart (1973b) has noted elsewhere that effective treatment requires three technologies—service delivery, focal treatment, and maintenance—that are separate and distinct sets of skills, maintenance programs are almost never discussed in the clinical literature, and they tend to be ignored in clinical training programs. Therefore, therapists are almost never equipped to deal with the challenge of helping their clients maintain therapeutic gains. In addition, clients and therapists alike almost always have a short-term orientation in approaching treatment. Clients seek immediate relief from their distress, and therapists recognize that in order to have any long-term success to measure, they must first produce short-term change. Moreover, when successful treatment is concluded, clients refocus their attention to other pressing challenges in their lives, and therapists invest their energies in efforts to assist other clients; the hard-won gains, therefore, tend to recede into the background and are all but forgotten. Finally, when clients do begin to slip back into their old ways, they often have a tendency to consider this slip their failure and wish to hide it from their therapist, or they consider the treatment a failure and seek help elsewhere—in either case, masking relapse as far as the therapist is concerned.

Therapists and clients alike hope for the "final solution"—the intervention method that will cause the problems to vanish, with no further effort required. The reality is, however, that marital strife, like so many other behavioral disorders (Stuart, 1980d, in press), is an expression of a lifestyle disorder. The correction of flawed interaction patterns, therefore, depends upon the comprehensive change reviewed in Chapter 3: modification of labels, of expectations, and of molecular and molar reciprocal interaction patterns. The efforts of the therapist provide at least some of the energy and much of the skill to effect these changes, with the clients' commitment to relationship improvement and their skill development providing the rest. When treatment ends, it is the hope that the partners will self-apply both the motivation-building and the problem-solving skills learned during treatment. In many instances they do, but obviously in others they do not. The challenge faced by the therapist is thus to potentiate clients' self-application of the therapeutic methods, which she or he can do by:

1. Helping the clients to learn the rationale for each therapeutic instigation.
2. Selecting instigations that are suitable for self-application.
3. Including in the treatment training in interaction analysis and relationship change so that the clients can be effective intervenors in their own behalf.
4. Providing clients with a foreknowledge of the times at which stress can be expected to occur.

5. Building any necessary external supports for the maintenance of change.
6. Helping clients to develop skills specific to resisting relapse and maintaining change.

The first three of these points pertain to the way in which short-term change is planned, while the latter three are designs for posttherapeutic actions. All, however, comprise the technology for maintenance, and all should be considered integral parts of every service undertaking. As suggested in Chapter 5, the best-conceived focal treatments can fail through inattention to efforts to induce clients to change their behavior in prescribed ways. So, too, can these exceptional programs fail if they do not build into focal intervention a technology for maintaining change.

Training Clients to Maintain Change

TEACHING THE LOGIC OF ALL CHANGE-INDUCING TECHNIQUES

Teaching clients the rationale for each step in treatment helps them to understand its logic and builds their ability to generalize the application of the method across the challenges that arise in their relationship. Carpenters learn that the strength of joints between pieces of lumber is directly proportional to the amount of contact of glued surfaces and to the resistance of the joint to stress. Knowing this principle, a carpenter can choose wisely when to use overlaps, full or half laps, plain or stopped dadoes, mortice and tenon, dovetails, or other forms of joints. As apprentices, they may practice only three or four of these, but as journeyman carpenters, they will apply this principle to the completion of a wide range of construction projects. Couples undergoing therapy for marital distress likewise have an opportunity to learn principles of relationship management in the context of the specific issues raised in their therapy, with the expectation that they will generalize this learning to situations that arise *de novo* in the therapist's absence.

Each of the stages of the present treatment is based upon a pool of identifiable, teachable, and learnable principles—principles that can be stated at varied levels of abstraction commensurate with the level of the client's ability and interest. A summary of some representative principles is found in Table 1, which constitutes one way of summarizing the major theoretical underpinnings of the action side of this approach. As a way of introducing clients to each instigation, the therapist is well advised to state the principle in the mnemonic terms used in the table, and then to ask the clients to restate the principle before she or he finally offers a recommendation for change. To build into treatment an orientation to generalization, it is also helpful to ask clients to project other situations in

Table 1. Principles of relationship change

1. IN UNDERSTANDING RELATIONSHIPS:

A. *The open-system principle:* All relationships change constantly as a result of reactions to external demands and shifting desires on the part of all people in the relationship. Therefore, change is the norm of all relationships.

B. *The best-bargain principle:* The behaviors that all parties in relationships display at any given moment represent the best means that each person believes he or she has available for obtaining desired satisfactions.

C. *The instability principle:* All relationships are intrinsically unstable in that any party may decide that the reward–cost balance of opting out of the relationship may be greater than the reward–cost balance of remaining within it.

2. IN CHANGING RELATIONSHIPS:

A. *The change-first principle:* To overcome polarities in relationship struggles, all parties must assume the responsibility for changing their own behavior first in order to prompt behavior changes in others.

B. *The positive-change principle:* Relationships can be changed best through a search for positive behaviors that can take the place of (i.e., provide the satisfactions earned by) negative exchanges.

C. *The small-steps principle:* Complex relationships can be changed only through small, planned, sequential steps.

D. *The as-if principle:* To prompt the initiation of small, assertive, positive changes, it is important for each person to act as if the others have a definite interest in promoting relationship change.

E. *The fear-of-change principle:* In virtually all areas of human behavior, it is wise to expect that people will be fearful of change even if by any objective standard that change is toward the relief of pain and the provision of pleasure. Therefore, some resistance to all change efforts is to be expected and cannot be taken as a negative sign.

F. *The testing principle:* All parties can be expected to test especially the most positive of changes in order to make certain that they can be trusted over time. Testing takes the form of a time-limited return to earlier behaviors that can be overcome by reaffirmation of the desire for change.

G. *The predictability principle:* Relationships produce more comfort and more freedom for all principals when their norms are expressed as rules.

H. *The principle of irreversibility:* No act of any kind can ever be completely withdrawn, nor will it ever be completely forgotten. Therefore, tact and timing should be the benchmarks of all behavior.

I. *The all-win or no-win principle:* In every bargaining situation in all relationships, no person can make more than a temporary gain unless all parties win.

J. *The principle of shared responsibility:* All parties to the relationship are jointly responsible for everything that happens between them, good or bad; and therefore, all parties must participate in any successful effort to promote relationship change.

K. *The principle of behavioral essence:* We are all what we do in the eyes of others. Therefore, we are "loving" only if we act in lovable ways; we are "trustworthy" only if our behavior supports this label, etc.

L. *The principle of the urgent present:* It is necessary to concentrate attention on the present, forsaking the opportunities to exact penalties for the past in all efforts to promote or maintain relationship improvement.

3. IN UNDERSTANDING AND CHANGING COMMUNICATION:

A. *The principle of constant communication:* One cannot not communicate, as every behavior, verbal or nonverbal, expresses both a specific content and a comment about the relationship between the parties.

B. *The principle of level consistency:* Because all communications have at least two levels, and because communicators often attend more closely to one level as opposed to the other(s), there are frequent inconsistencies between the varied levels of each comunication.

C. *The principle of the whispering words and shouting gestures:* When there are inconsistencies between the levels of the messages expressed, the nonverbal message almost always has a greater impact than the spoken message.

D. *The princess-and-the-pea principle:* Any negative dimension of any communication is likely to have a greater impact than the sum total of all of the positive dimensions of the communication.

E. *The ownership principle:* It is important to take active ownership of every message sent whether in the form of a statement or in the form of a question, for that is the only way to enter into responsible communication.

F. *The principle of incomplete communication:* Because one can never be sure that the message sent is the message that will be received, no communication cycle is complete until the message is sent and acknowledged.

---

which the technique might be helpful at the time that it is introduced into their therapy.

BUILDING WITH SELF-APPLICABLE TECHNIQUES

Consistent with the second requisite of maintainable intervention, every step that the clients are asked to take during treatment is one that they can take independently after their treatment ends. Absolutely none of the procedures depends upon therapeutic artistry; each is a skill. Making requests and acknowledging small and positive changes, as was done during caring days, and making and clarifying self-statements, as was undertaken as part of communication change, are illustrations of such specific techniques.

The analysis of intention, action, interpretation, and reaction offered in the chapter dealing with communication change (Chapter 7) is a model of the kind of interaction analysis that clients can be profitably taught and can learn with interest and great benefit. Teaching the couple to use certain key terms such as "one-winner" versus "two-winner" orientation during their negotiation or "first," "second," or "third degree" in commenting on each other's fight tactics can be most effective in helping each person both to identify and to change the strategy each is using.

The chapters dealing with focal behavior and communication change (Chapters 6, 7, and 8) alluded to what might be termed "the natural history of interaction change." The phases of this adjustment process can be identified as follows:

1. Initially, each person labels the other and expects him or her to change.
2. The problem is relabeled as one that has been reciprocally caused, and both parties accept the responsibility for change.
3. Each begins to make a somewhat tentative and self-conscious change effort.
4. Positive results tend to reinforce commitment to the changes that are being accomplished.
5. Doubt about the ability of such simple behavioral change to promote such complex affective and cognitive change then weakens confidence in the procedure.
6. This phase is followed by a period of testing in which either or both parties stop delivering on their part(s) of the bargain, as if to test the other's motivation.
7. When the other continues to deliver, the faith is partially restored.
8. A "second-honeymoon" period is then rudely interrupted by a second and more mild testing period.
9. The couple who survive this second test then enter a prolonged period during which the new method is consolidated into their repertoire.

A review of these steps indicates the fragile chain of events that must precede the consolidation of successful relationship-change efforts. A failure in any of these nine steps can doom to failure the best of intentions. The therapist is instrumental in moving the clients away from their use of terminal language and toward process descriptions of their interaction so that each can correctly identify his or her role in the change process (see Chapters 4 and 8). The therapist initially models the formulation of change requests, a skill that successful clients assume during the course of therapy.

HELPING CLIENTS TO ANTICIPATE RELAPSE CHALLENGES

The therapist then has the responsibility of helping the clients learn to interpret the meaning of data descriptive of their more constructive behavior. Where maintenance is relevant, the therapist is responsible for helping the spouses to anticipate that they will test the stability of the changes they have been working so hard to produce, not one time but twice. The spouses should be helped to see that this testing is predictable and normal—that it is, in fact, an almost inevitable dimension of the way in which humans respond to stages of the evolution of their relationships. To make this point, it is often helpful for the therapist to share with clients the graph found in Figure 1, for it is an approximate representation of what they can expect in association with many of their change efforts.

In explaining this graph to clients, it is important for the therapist to stress that the line at every point is wavy, implying that the rates of all good things fluctuate constantly. It is also important to point out that the first testing phase may bring the rate of positive change all the way back to baseline, but that persistence by one spouse can bring it back to the therapeutic level. The couple should note, too, that the second testing phase tends to bring a more shallow dip in the rate, a dip that is overcome in less time than was true during the first period of testing. Finally, when the challenge of the second test has been overcome, the changed behavior can be consolidated into the couple's normal routine—it is no longer a "new action and reaction pattern."

IDENTIFYING EXTERNAL SUPPORTS FOR NEW BEHAVIOR

A certain humility about the change potential of the currently available intervention technologies is essential in meeting the fifth prerequisite of maintainable change: the provision of external supports for the main-

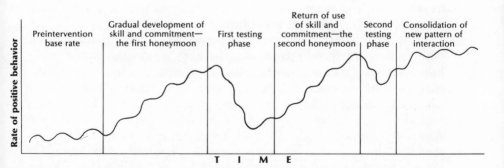

Figure 1. An approximation of the natural history of efforts to produce positive interaction changes.

tenance of change. Stuart and Guire (1979) have pointed out that it is naive to approach weight control as though it were a long-term problem amenable to a short-term solution. Efforts to do so continually result in relapse. Instead, when weight control is viewed as a challenge to develop a dramatically new lifestyle in which important situational and personal changes are undertaken in order to reduce the urge to overeat and to minimize overeating when it does occur, the futility of expecting long-lasting results from minimal intervention clearly comes to light. In the same vein, it is perhaps more in keeping with the facts to conceptualize marital therapy as beginning with an intensive change effort followed by planned booster contacts, much as is being done in services to the overweight.

Two forms of booster sessions have proved helpful in efforts to maintain changes made through this approach. First, clients have been asked to plan to devote one hour each month to an assessment of their efforts to sustain their gains and to plan any new changes that either desires. They are asked to plan these discussions well in advance, writing them in their appointment books or on their calendars, much as they would have done in an effort to remember appointments with the therapist. They are asked to have these discussions after their children are in bed or in a place where they can relax in privacy, even if this means sitting in their car while it is parked at a scenic overlook. They are asked to structure this time with each other by filling in every cell of the chart provided in Figure 2. Clearly, this chart prompts them to provide each other with systematic positive feedback about one another's functioning in each of the areas addressed during active treatment. They are then asked to list any positive and specific goals for change in each area, entering only those upon which both agree. In achieving these goals, each person is asked to indicate the changes that he or she will make. In every instance, both spouses must commit themselves to make some change in an effort to attain the listed goal. They may or may not wish to record such changes in the manner described in Chapter 6, which introduced the caring-days procedure.

It is often helpful to supplement these client-implemented sessions with semiannual "good relationship checkups" analogous to the "well-baby" clinics offered in many hospitals. It is important to stress that the purpose of these sessions is to review accomplishments and plan any additional changes that either partner desires. It should be stressed, also, that the purpose is not to find fault with anything that has been done by either spouse, but to find, reinforce, and build on their constructive changes. It is often sufficient to allow only 30 minutes for these contacts, and just as each regularly scheduled session should begin with a review of the prior weeks's data (see Chapter 5), it is helpful for the therapist to review the self-assessment and planning forms that the

Date: _____

Area of interaction	Steps we have taken to maintain positive exchanges in this area		Additional positive changes we would like to make in this area	Steps toward this goal that will be taken by:	
	Husband	Wife		Husband	Wife
Maintaining each other's commitment to our marriage through small, positive behaviors					
Efforts to try to make certain that we send and receive important messages accurately					
Efforts to meet our designated role responsibilities well					
Efforts to respect each other's areas of decision-making authority					
Efforts to contain conflicts when they do arise					

Figure 2. Self-assessment planning form.

couples have completed during the intervening months. Also, just as telephone prompts prove useful in initiating compliance with the caring-days procedure, so, too, do such calls often pay rich dividends during the posttherapeutic period. Calls three months after each booster session (which the therapist must schedule just as appointments are scheduled so that they will not be forgotten) can prove to be very helpful indeed in reminding the clients of the therapist's interest and in prompting reapplication of any aspects of the technology that may have fallen into disuse.

ANTICIPATING STABILIZING MANEUVERS

The final plank in the maintenance technology advocated here is the help offered to clients in developing skills specific to this critically important time in their lives. In understanding testing, they have already acquired a realistic prediction of things to come. Now they must be helped to develop the coping skills needed to keep their relationship on a steady, positive, and improving course.

Two techniques have been found to be useful in this effort. At the conclusion of their treatment, each couple is given a written summary of the intervention as it is viewed by the therapist. A sample of this summary is presented as Figure 3. Note that it summarizes in the therapist's words the nature of the presenting request, a reformulation of this request as a set of positive change goals, and a summary of the instigations that were offered during each of the phases of intervention. The couple are asked to review this document each time they find their uneasiness about their marriage rising and each time they undertake a monthly review of their success in maintaining the changes achieved through therapy. Parenthetically, this document also serves as a record of the treatment for use by the therapist as a closing summary and as a quick review prior to making contact with the clients for maintenance therapy.

As a second maintenance skill-building intervention, couples can be asked to complete a "what-if" exercise such as that found in Figure 4. Note that the situations portrayed in this form are commonly experienced by couples during testing, when crises arise that may not have been discussed in treatment, or when either partner contemplates a major change in his or her personal life. It is useful to present several of these probes to clients during each of the final two or three sessions, asking them to assume complete responsibility for either role-playing or discussing possible solutions as if they were actually confronted with each dilemma. It is best for the therapist to help to structure the early discussions, perhaps modeling the role that either partner might play. An audio tape has been prepared expressly for that purpose (Stuart,

Figure 3. Summary of therapeutic progress.

Bruce and Carolyn O'Dwyre, December 19, 1979

A. WHY DID THE COUPLE BEGIN THERAPY?

Both felt burned out. Both had been having casual relationships with other partners. Carolyn began to have a serious interest in Hank and felt that she should evaluate her marriage before moving into a deeper outside relationship. Bruce sensed Carolyn's withdrawal and interpreted it as depression and grew progressively more angry because he felt that she was withholding her love for selfish reasons. He hoped that therapy would help Carolyn realize she had been remiss in their relationship.

B. HOW DID THEIR CONCERNS TRANSLATE INTO PROBLEMS TO BE SOLVED?

It was agreed that treatment would offer an opportunity to test the positive potential of their relationship. It was further agreed that should the initial three-week experiment yield positive results, they would terminate or at least interrupt the outside relationships in their "open marriage" and would concentrate upon building some long-term shared goals that might fire them up and then improve the quality of their interaction to help them move toward these new objectives.

C. WHICH OF THE FOLLOWING STEPS WERE THEY ASKED TO TAKE AND WHICH DID THEY TAKE SUCCESSFULLY?

	Success	
Step	Bruce	Carolyn
1. Caring days	x	x
2. Communication change, including:		
a. Listening skills	x	x
b. Self-statements		x
c. Feedback		x
d. Clarification	x	
3. Behavior exchange, including:		
a. Two-winner bargaining	x	x
b. Holistic contract	x	x
4. Problem solving, including:		
a. Powergram	x	x
b. Problem-solving methods	x	
5. Conflict containment		x

D. WHAT ARE THE MAJOR CHANGES EACH PERSON MADE DURING TREATMENT?

Bruce

1. Learned to maintain present focus in all disputes and problem solving.

2. Learned to encourage Carolyn's dancing.

3. Learned to take some of the responsibility when things went poorly in place of old pattern of sulking and laying blame on Carolyn.

4. Learned that he alone is responsible for changes that help to overcome his "blues."

5. Learned to seek means of intimate expression other than genital intercourse.

6. Learned to adapt personal pastimes to include activities that he and Carolyn could enjoy together.

7. Agreed to make promises sparingly and only when he is sure he can follow through, relying on expressions of desire at other times.

Carolyn

1. Learned to use process instead of terminal labels.

2. Learned to interpret Bruce's questions about her activities as interest and not efforts to establish control.

3. Learned to take responsibility for planning at least those cultural activities she enjoys.

4. Learned to express respect for Bruce's efforts to earn a good living and to develop new skills.

5. Learned to move into a problem-solving mode ("What would I like us to do differently?") during conflict instead of relying on negative labels.

Figure 4. "What if . . . ?"—Preparing to maintain change.

You will find described below a series of situations fairly common in the experience of couples who complete marriage therapy. Read each description aloud along with the alternative responses that are coupled with each. Discuss the way in which you would like to see one another handle the situation, were it to arise in your relationship. Finally, agree to prompt each other in making the agreed-upon response if and when the challenge arises.

1. June had been complaining for years that Alan consistently came home late for dinner without calling. During their treatment, this was one of the items that June asked to have built into their behavior-change contract, and Alan was careful to grant this request consistently. Almost since the last week they saw their therapist, however, Alan has reverted to his old ways and has come home late several times each week. Finally, when June was due at an important business meeting after dinner, Alan was late again, and she was beside herself with anger.
   a. What should June do?
      (1) Just leave the house as she had planned and let Alan fend for himself?
      (2) Call him at the store and tell him how angry she feels?
      (3) Accuse him of having essentially lied to her during treatment, as proven by his immediate return to his poor behavior?
      (4) Tell him she feels upset about his behavior and ask that he go back to complying with their agreement?
   b. What principle(s) guide(s) this action?

2. When Alan heard June's concern, he decided she was being overbearing and coercive. He had been working late because his store was caught in a squeeze: the prices he pays for the goods he sells have been rising, but two competing stores have opened in his area, so he has actually had to cut his prices. Therefore, he felt that while he was struggling to make a go of it, June paid little heed to his efforts.
   a. What should Alan do?
      (1) Tell June he thinks that the contract is no good and say that he wants to start a new one?
      (2) Accuse June of being utterly self-centered?
      (3) Ask June in what other ways he can express his concern for her because he does need extra time in the store now?
      (4) Discuss the "deeper meaning" of his failure to follow through on this item of their agreement?
   b. What principle(s) guide(s) this action?

3. Several months after she and Rob finished their marriage therapy, one of Maxine's old boyfriends turned up in town sporting a recent divorce. He invited Maxine to have dinner with him to "talk over old times." It was her discovery of Rob's relationship with another woman that prompted Maxine to suggest that they both get outside help.
   a. What should Maxine do now?
      (1) Meet her old beau for lunch and possibly have an affair with him just to balance the books with Rob?
      (2) Tell Rob about the call and ask if he would mind her meeting her friend just to hash over old times, calling him back to make certain he knows her feelings?
      (3) Just tell Rob about the call without asking approval, also calling to clarify her intentions with her friend?
      (4) Have just a friendly lunch without mentioning it to Rob?
   b. What principle(s) guide(s) this action?

4. Paulo and Rosa were on the brink of divorce when they entered therapy. With the help of their counselor, they greatly improved their interaction. Within two months of their last session, however, each believed that the other had begun to let things slide, and they

began to drift further and further apart. One Sunday Paulo felt alone and angry—the fearful combination of feelings that had originally led him to think about divorce.

a. What should Paulo do now?

(1) Decide that his original feelings were correct and that his marriage to Rosa really is burned out, leaving divorce as the only option?

(2) Decide that this is the best he can hope for in this or any other relationship, so the best he can do is hold his peace and suffer through?

(3) Tell Rosa that he feels she has let him down and ask her to resume doing the things he appreciated her doing while they were in therapy?

(4) Tell Rosa how he feels and that he would like to begin their therapy over, this time without outside help, by resuming the steps that helped them earlier, beginning with caring days?

b. What principle(s) guide(s) this action?

5. When Sammy and Ellen were in therapy, they agreed that one of the strong points of their relationship was the fact that they were both very responsible parents who had few disagreements about how to manage their children. Since the end of their therapy, the once-fought-about issues have been fine, but they have had a number of conflicts about how to respond to their children.

a. What should they do now?

(1) Decide that this is a major problem and call upon their therapist for additional help?

(2) Decide that with the loss of this major source of unity, their marriage is weaker than either one believed?

(3) Dust off the problem-solving skills they learned in therapy in order to treat this as just another challenge in a challenge-filled life?

(4) Accuse one another of dirty fighting because each appears to be trying to undermine the other's relationship with the children?

b. What principle(s) guide(s) this action?

6. Kurt and Marta have a long history of outrageous fighting, with their conflicts often including violence. Therapy put a stop to their arguing, but now, some months after its end, they have not only begun fighting again, but Marta almost took out one of Kurt's eyes when she threw a plate at him during their last fight.

a. What should Kurt do?

(1) Express his concern and remind Marta that he loves her and hopes that they can contain their conflicts as they had learned to do in therapy?

(2) Express his concern and tell Marta that he thinks she should remember the things they learned about conflict containment in therapy?

(3) Express his concern and tell Marta that he thinks they could not love each other if they fight this way?

(4) Express his concern and hope for the best?

b. What principle(s) guide(s) this action?

7. Mary Ellen has become very depressed, a problem that began to get serious about 10 months after she and John completed marriage counseling. Several things have come together: she discovered a suspicious lump in her left breast; she was laid off from her job because the firm decided its legal staff was too large; and her closest friend moved to Boston because she, too, had been laid off.

a. What should John do?

(1) Allow Mary Ellen to fend for herself as a growth experience?

(2) Complain that she has been neglecting him?

(3) Offer to solve all of her problems?

(4) Express his support, ask how he can help, and tell Mary Ellen that he is counting on her to remain active in their marriage?

b. What principle(s) guide(s) this action?

1980c). For later enactments, however, it is best for the therapist to remain silent during the problem-solving interaction, offering comments and suggestions only when the couple have carried it as far as they can. During these sessions, the therapist can play and discuss with clients portions of the maintenance-technique-modeling tape designed for this purpose. Clients can also be given a copy of the tape and can be invited to play it at home, stopping the tape after each situation is described before listening to the way in which the illustrative couple attempt to rise to the challenge.

Conclusion

Readers of this book have been offered a "soup-to-nuts" view of one approach to marriage therapy. Great care has gone into providing a rationale for each stage of the treatment and into a presentation of implementation details that can guide therapists in the successful delivery of services consistent with this approach. Convincing cases can be made for the adoption of other approaches, but an attempt has been made here to adopt from these alternative strategies their more well-tested techniques and to provide original stratagems where critical issues have generally been ignored in the published literature. All of the techniques recommended here have in common that they are aimed at the achievement of positive and specific changes through reciprocal actions by the spouses in a stage-specific sequence. Each technique can be viewed as the independent variable in an experiment in which the short-term dependent variables are the prescribed changes in the clients' behaviors and the long-term dependent variables are changes in the clients' thoughts and feelings. Because absolutely every aspect of this approach is clinically data-based, and because its major tactics are amenable to experimental testing, it is certain that some aspects of this approach will be firmly supported while others will fall victim to adverse findings, being replaced by alternative procedures that hopefully will withstand the test of validational testing. Therefore, this approach, like every other responsible intervention program, must be classified along with the other "unfinished business" in human services. It is a program that is undergoing revision, that will change in important ways because it must always remain responsive to the experiences of the therapists and the clients who are its constituents, and that hopefully will be one of the instruments that proves valuable in our heroic efforts to help the protagonists in modern marriages to find what they struggle so hard to experience in their relationships.

R E F E R E N C E S

Abdallah, W. P. A comparison of spouses' perceptions of their mates, opposite sex, acquaintances, close friends, and parents. *Dissertation Abstracts International*, 1974, *34*, 6187.

Abelson, D. Diagnostic value of the penile pulse and blood pressure: A Doppler study of impotence in diabetics. *Journal of Urology*, 1975, *113*, 636–639.

Abramowitz, C. V. Blaming the mother: An experimental investigation of sex-role bias in countertransference. *Psychology of Women Quarterly*, 1977, *2*, 24–34.

Adams, J. S. Inequity in social exchange. In L. Berkowitz (Ed.), *Advances in Experimental Social Psychology* (Vol. 2). New York: Academic Press, 1965.

Adams, J. S., & Romney, A. K. A functional analysis of authority. *Psychological Review*, 1959, *66*, 234–251.

Adams, M. *Single Blessedness: Observations on the Single Status in Married Society*. New York: Basic Books, 1976.

Adams, S. Some findings from correctional caseload research. *Federal Probation*, 1967, *31*, 48–57.

Addeo, E. G., & Burger, R. E. *Egospeak*. New York: Chicago Books, 1973.

Adelson, J. P., & Talmadge, W. C. Tips for clients: How to screw up your marriage counseling. *Family Therapy*, 1976, *3*, 93–95.

Adler, A. *Superiority and social interest* (H. L. Ansbacher & R. Ansbacher, Eds.). Evanston, IL: Northwestern University Press, 1964.

Aldous, J. A framework for the analysis of family problem solving. In J. Aldous, T. Condon, R. Hill, M. Straus, & I. Tallman (Eds.), *Family Problem Solving*. Hinsdale, IL: Dryden Press, 1971.

Alexander, L. Treatment of impotency and anorgasmia by psychotherapy aided by hypnosis. *The American Journal of Clinical Hypnosis*, 1974, *17*, 33–43.

Alexander, J. F., Barton, C., Schiaro, R. S., & Parsons, B. V. Systems-behavioral intervention with families of delinquents: Therapist characteristics, family behavior, and outcome. *Journal of Consulting and Clinical Psychology*, 1976, *44*, 656–664.

Alkire, A. A. Social power and communication within families of disturbed and nondisturbed preadolescents. *Journal of Personality and Social Psychology*, 1969, *13*, 335–349.

Allen, C. *Textbook of Psychosexual Disorders*. London: Oxford University Press, 1962.

Allen, G. J. *Understanding Psychotherapy*. Champaign, IL: Research Press, 1977.

Allen, V. L. Situational factors in conformity. In L. Berkowitz (Ed.), *Advances in Experimental Social Psychology* (Vol. 2). New York: Academic Press, 1965.

Allport, G. W. *Personality: A Psychological Interpretation*. New York: Holt, Rinehart and Winston, 1937.

Allred, G. H., & Kersey, F. L. The AIAC, a design for systematically analyzing marriage and family counseling: A progress report. *Journal of Marriage and Family Counseling*, 1977, *3*, 17–25.

Andes, D. A. An evaluation of a couple's relationship-building workshop: The use of video and small group feedback in teaching communication skills. *Dissertation Abstracts International*, 1975, *35*, 4637–4638.

Annett, J. *Feedback and Human Behavior*. Baltimore, MD: Penguin Books, 1969.

Annon, J. S. *Behavioral Treatment of Sexual Problems*. New York: Harper and Row, 1976.

Ansari, J. M. A. Impotence: Prognosis. *British Journal of Psychiatry*, 1976, *128*, 194–198.

Ansbacher, H. L. Adlerian psychology: The tradition of brief psychotherapy. *Journal of Individual Psychology*, 1972, *28*, 137–151.

Araoz, D. L. Clinical hypnosis in treating sexual abulia. *American Journal of Family Therapy*, 1980, *8*(1), 48–57.

Ardrey, R. *The Territorial Imperative*. New York: Dell Publishing Company, 1966.

Arensburg, C. M. The American family in the perspective of other cultures. In E. Ginzberg (Ed.), *The Nation's Children: The Family and Social Change* (Vol. 1). New York: Columbia University Press, 1960.

Arkowitz, S. A study of unrealistic and realistic expectations of marriage. *Dissertation Abstracts International*, 1973, *34*, 2918.

Aronson, E. Some antecedents of interpersonal attraction. In W. J. Arnold & D. Levine (Eds.), *Nebraska Symposium on Motivation, 17*. Lincoln, NB: University of Nebraska Press, 1969.

Aronson, E., & Linder, D. Gain and loss of esteem as determinants of interpersonal attractiveness. *Journal of Experimental Social Psychology*, 1965, *1*, 156–172.

Ashby, W. R. *An Introduction to Cybernetics*. New York: John Wiley and Sons, 1963.

Association for the Advancement of Behavior Therapy. Ethical issues for human services. *Behavior Therapy*, 1977, *8*, 763–764.

Attneave, F. *Applications of Information Theory to Psychology*. New York: Holt, Rinehart and Winston, 1959.

Ausubel, D. P. *The Psychology of Meaningful Verbal Learning*. New York: Grune and Stratton, 1963.

Ausubel, D. P. The use of advance organizers in the learning and retention of meaningful verbal material. *Journal of Educational Psychology*, 1960, *51*, 267–272.

Averill, J. R. Personal control over aversive stimuli and its relationship to stress. *Psychological Bulletin*, 1973, *80*, 286–303.

Ayllon, T., & Azrin, N. *The Token Economy: A Motivational System for Therapy and Rehabilitation*. New York: Appleton-Century-Crofts, 1968.

Azrin, N. H., Naster, B. M., & Jones, R. Reciprocity counseling: A rapid learning-based procedure for marital counseling. *Behaviour Research and Therapy*, 1973, *11*, 365–382.

Bach, G. R., & Deutsch, R. M. *Pairing*. New York: Avon Books, 1970.

Bach, G. R., & Wyden, P. *The Intimate Enemy*. New York: William Morrow, 1969.

Bachrach, L. L. *Marital Status and Mental Disorder: An Analytical Review*. Rockville, MD: U.S. Dept. of Health, Education and Welfare, 1975.

Baekel, N. G., & Mehrabian, A. Inconsistent communications and psychopathology. *Journal of Abnormal Psychology*, 1969, *74*, 126–130.

Bakan, D. *Pain, Sacrifice, and Disease*. Chicago: University of Chicago Press, 1968.

Baker, E. Brief psychotherapy. *Journal of the Medical Society of New Jersey*, 1947, *44*, 260–261.

Baldwin, D. A. The costs of power. *Journal of Conflict Resolution*, 1971, *15*, 145–155.

Bales, R. F., & Strodtbeck, F. L. Phases in group problem solving. *Journal of Abnormal and Social Psychology*, 1951, *46*, 485–495.

Ball, R. A. Sociology and general systems theory. *The American Sociologist*, 1978, *13*, 65–72.

Balogun, B. Marriage as an oppresive institution: Collectives as solutions. In L. B. Tanner (Ed.), *Voices from Women's Liberation.* New York: New American Library, 1971.

Baltes, P. B. Longitudinal and cross-sectional sequences in the study of age and generation effects. *Human Development,* 1968, *11,* 145–171.

Bandura, A. *Principles of Behavior Modification.* New York: Holt, Rinehart and Winston, 1969.

Bandura, A. *Social Learning Theory.* Englewood Cliffs, NJ: Prentice-Hall, 1977.

Bandura, A. The self system in reciprocal determinism. *American Psychologist,* 1978, *33,* 344–358.

Bandura, A., & Walters, R. H. *Social Learning and Personality Development.* New York: Holt, Rinehart and Winston, 1963.

Bane, M. J. Marital disruption and the lives of children. *Journal of Social Issues,* 1976, *32,* 103–117.

Bannester, E. M. Sociodynamics: An integrative theorem of power, authority, interfluence and love. *American Sociological Review,* 1969, *34,* 374–393.

Barbach, L. G. Group treatment of preorgasmic women. *Journal of Sex and Marital Therapy,* 1974, *1,* 139–145.

Barnlund, D. C. *Interpersonal Communication.* Boston: Houghton, Mifflin, 1968.

Baron, R. A. Exposure to an aggressive model and apparent probability of retalization from the victim as determinants of adult aggressive behavior. *Journal of Experimental Social Psychology,* 1971, *7,* 343–355.

Baron, R. A. Threatened retalization from the victim as an inhibitor of physical aggression. *Journal of Research in Personality,* 1973, *7,* 103–115.

Baron, R. A. Threatened retalization as an inhibitor of human aggression: Mediating effects of the instrumental value of aggression. *Bulletin of the Psychonomic Society,* 1974, *3,* 217–219.

Barry, W. A. *Conflict in Marriage: A Study of the Interactions of Newlywed Couples* (Doctoral dissertation, University of Michigan). (University Microfilms, 1968, 68–13, 273)

Barry, W. A. Marriage research and conflict: An integrative review. *Psychological Bulletin,* 1970, *73,* 41–54.

Barton, K., & Cattell, R. B. Marriage dimensions and personality. *Journal of Personality and Social Psychology,* 1972, *21,* 369–374.

Bartz, K. W., & Nye, F. I. Early marriage: A propositional formulation. *Journal of Marriage and the Family,* 1970, *32,* 258–268.

Bass, B. M. Amount of participation, coalescence and profitability of decision-making discussions. *Journal of Abnormal and Social Psychology,* 1963, *67,* 92–94.

Bate-Boerop, J. L. General systems theory and family therapy in practice. *Family Therapy,* 1975, *2,* 69–77.

Bateson, G. Information and codification: A philosophical approach. In J. Reusch & G. Bateson (Eds.), *Communication: The Social Matrix of Psychiatry.* New York: W. W. Norton, 1951.

Bateson, G. Exchange of information about patterns of human behavior. In W. S. Fields & W. Abbott (Eds.), *Information Storage and Neural Control.* Springfield, IL: Charles C. Thomas, 1963.

Bateson, G. *Steps to an Ecology of Mind.* New York: Ballantine Books, 1972.

Battle, C. C., Imber, S. D., Hoehn-Saric, R., Stone, A. R., Nash, C., & Frank, J. D. Target complaints as criteria of improvement. *American Journal of Psychotherapy,* 1966, *20,* 184–192.

Bavelas, A. Communication patterns in task-oriented groups. *Journal of the Acoustical Society of America,* 1950, *22,* 725–730.

Beach, F. A. Cerebral and hormonal control of reflexive mechanisms involved in copulatory behavior. *Physiological Review,* 1967, *47,* 289–316.

Bean, F. D., & Kerckhoff, A. C. Personality and person perception in husband–wife conflict. *Journal of Marriage and the Family,* 1971, *33,* 351–359.

Beck, A. T. *Depression: Causes and Treatment.* Philadelphia: University of Pennsylvania Press, 1967.

Beck, D. F. Research findings on the outcomes of marital counseling. *Social Casework,* 1975, *56,* 153–181.

Becker, J. *Affective Disorders.* Morristown, NJ: General Learning Press, 1977.

Beer, S. *Decision and Control.* London: John Wiley and Sons, 1966.

Bell, R. R. *Marriage and Family Interaction.* Homewood, IL: Dorsey Press, 1963.

Bellack, A. S., & Hersen, M. Self-report inventories in behavioral assessment. In J. D. Cone & R. P. Hawkins (Eds.), *Behavioral Assessment: New Directions in Clinical Psychology.* New York: Brunner/Mazel, 1977.

Belson, R. The importance of the second interview in marriage counseling. *Counseling Psychologist,* 1975, *5,* 27–31.

Bem, D. J. Self-perception: An alternative interpretation of cognitive dissonance phenomena. *Psychological Review,* 1967, *74,* 183–200.

Bem, D. J., & McConnell, H. K. Testing the self-perception explanation of dissonance phenomena: On the salience of premanipulation attitudes. *Journal of Personality and Social Psychology,* 1970, *14,* 23–31.

Bennis, W. G., Schein, E. H., Steele, F. I., & Berlew, D. E. *Interpersonal Dynamics.* Homewood, IL: Dorsey Press, 1968.

Benson, J. S., & Kennelly, K. J. Learned helplessness: The result of uncontrollable reinforcements or uncontrollable aversive stimuli? *Journal of Personality and Social Psychology,* 1976, *34,* 138–145.

Bent, R. J., Putnam, D. G., Kiesler, D. J., & Nowicki, S. Expectancies and characteristics of outpatient clinics applying for services at a community mental health facility. *Journal of Consulting and Clinical Psychology,* 1975, *43,* 280.

Bentler, P. M., & Newcomb, M. D. Longitudinal study of marital success and failure. *Journal of Consulting and Clinical Psychology,* 1978, *46,* 5, 1053–1070.

Benton, A. A., Kelley, H. H., & Liebling, B. Effects of extremity of offers and concession rate on the outcomes of bargaining. *Journal of Personality and Social Psychology,* 1972, *24,* 73–83.

Bergin, A. E. Some implications of psychotherapy research for therapeutic practice. *Journal of Abnormal Psychology,* 1966, *71,* 235–246.

Bergin, A. E., & Lambert, M. J. The evaluation of therapeutic outcomes. In S. L. Garfield & A. E. Bergin (Eds.), *Handbook of Psychotherapy and Behavior Change: An Empirical Analysis.* New York: John Wiley and Sons, 1978.

Bergner, R. M. The development and evaluation of a training videotape for the resolution of marital conflict. *Dissertation Abstracts International,* 1974, *34,* 3485.

Bernard, J. The adjustments of married mates. In H. T. Christensen (Ed.), *Handbook of Marriage and the Family.* Chicago: Rand McNally, 1964.

Bernard, J. *The Future of Marriage.* New York: Bantam Books, 1972.

Bernard, L. L. *An Introduction to Social Psychology.* New York: Holt, 1924.

Berne, E. *Transactional Analysis in Psychotherapy.* New York: Castle Books, 1961.

Berne, E. *Games People Play.* New York: Grove Press, 1964.

Bernstein, B. E. Lawyer and counselor as an interdisciplinary team: The timely referral. *Journal of Marriage and Family Counseling,* 1976, *2,* 347–354.

Bernstein, D. A., & Borkovec, T. D. *Progressive Relaxation Training: A Manual for the Helping Professions.* Champaign, IL: Research Press, 1973.

Bernstein, I. *Arbitration of Wages.* Berkeley: University of California Press, 1954.

Berscheid, E., Graziano, W., Monson, T., & Dermer, M. Outcome dependency: Attention, attribution, and attraction. *Journal of Personality and Social Psychology,* 1977, *35,* 978–989.

Beutler, L. E., Johnson, P. T., Neville, C. W., & Workman, S. N. "Accurate empathy" and the A-B dichotomy. *Journal of Consulting and Clinical Psychology,* 1972, *38,* 272–275.

Biddle, B. J., & Thomas, E. J. *Role Theory: Concepts and Research.* New York: John Wiley and Sons, 1966.

Bienvenu, M. J. Measurement of marital communication. *The Family Coordinator,* 1970, *19,* 26–31.

Birchler, G. R. *Differential Patterns of Instrumental Affiliative Behavior as a Function of Degree of Marital Distress and Level of Intimacy.* Unpublished doctoral dissertation, University of Oregon, 1972.

Birchler, G. R., Weiss, R. L., & Wampler, L. D. *Differential Patterns of Social Reinforcement as a Function of Degree of Marital Distress and Level of Intimacy.* Paper presented at the annual meeting of the Western Psychological Association, Portland, OR, April 1972.

Birchler, G. R., Weiss, R. L., & Vincent, J. P. A. A multimethod analysis of social reinforcement exchange between maritally distressed and nondistressed spouse and stranger dyads. *Journal of Personality and Social Psychology,* 1975, *31,* 349–360.

Birdwhistell, R. L. *Kinesics and Context: Essays on Body Motion Communication.* Philadelphia: University of Pennsylvania Press, 1970.

Bixenstine, V. E., Potash, H. M., & Wilson, K. V. Effects of levels of cooperative choice by the other player on choices in a Prisoner's Dilemma game, Part 1. *Journal of Abnormal and Social Psychology,* 1963, *66,* 308–313.

Blair, M., & Pasmore, J. Frigid wives: A clinical classification. *Proceedings of the Sixth International Congress of Psychotherapy,* 1964, *4,* 1.

Blakeney, P., Kinder, B. N., & Creson, D. A short-term, intensive workshop approach for the treatment of human sexual inadequacy. *Journal of Sex and Marital Therapy,* 1976, *2,* 124–129.

Blau, P. *Exchange and Power in Social Life.* New York: John Wiley and Sons, 1964.

Blazer, J. A. Married virgins: A study of unconsummated marriages. *Journal of Marriage and the Family,* 1964, *26,* 213.

Blood, R. O. Resolving family conflicts. *Journal of Conflict Resolution,* 1960, *4,* 209–219.

Blood, R. O. *Marriage.* New York: The Free Press, 1969.

Blood, R. O., Jr., & Hamblin, R. L. The effect of wife's employment on the family power structure. *Social Forces,* 1958, *36,* 347–352.

Blood, R. O., & Wolfe, D. M. *Husbands and Wives: The Dynamics of Married Living.* Glencoe, IL: The Free Press, 1960.

Bloom, B. L., Asher, S. J., & White, S. W. Marital disruption as a stressor: A review and analysis. *Psychological Bulletin,* 1978, *85,* 867–894.

Blumenthal, M. D. Mental health among the divorced: A field study of divorced and never divorced persons. *Archives of General Psychiatry,* 1967, *16,* 603–608.

Booth, A., & Welch, S. Spousal consensus and its correlates: A reassessment. *Journal of Marriage and the Family,* 1978, *40,* 23–32.

Bordin, E. S. Inside the therapeutic hour. In E. A. Rubinstein & M. B. Parloff (Eds.), *Research in Psychotherapy.* Washington, DC: American Psychological Association, 1959.

Bott, E. *Family and Social Networks.* London: Tavistock Publications, 1957.

Bott, E. *Family and Social Network: Roles, Norms, and External Relationships in Ordinary Urban Families.* New York: The Free Press, 1971.

Bower, J. L. Group decision making: A report of an experimental study. *Behavioral Science,* 1965, *10,* 277–289.

Bowers, K. S. Situationalism in psychology: An analysis and a critique. *Psychological Review,* 1973, *80,* 307–336.

Bramel, D. A dissonance theory approach to defensive projection. *Journal of Abnormal and Social Psychology,* 1962, *64,* 121–129.

Bramel, D. Selection of a target for defensive projection. *Journal of Abnormal and Social Psychology,* 1963, *66,* 318–324.

Brandwein, R. A., Brown, C. A., & Fox, E. M. Women and children last: The social situation of divorced mothers and their families. *Journal of Marriage and the Family*, 1974, *36*, 498–514.

Brehm, J. W. *A Theory of Psychological Reactance*. New York: Academic Press, 1966.

Brewer, R. E., & Brewer, M. B. Attraction and accuracy of perception in dyads. *Journal of Personality and Social Psychology*, 1968, *8*, 188–193.

Briscoe, C. W., & Smith, J. B. Psychiatric illness—marital units and divorce. *Journal of Nervous and Mental Disease*, 1974, *158*, 440–445.

Brittan, A. *Meanings and Situations*. London: Routledge and Kegan Paul, 1973.

Broderick, C. Power in the governance of families. In R. E. Cromwell & D. H. Olson (Eds.), *Power in Families*. New York: John Wiley and Sons, 1975.

Brown, C. A., Feldberg, R., Fox, E. M., & Kohen, J. Divorce: Chance of a new lifetime. *Journal of Social Issues*, 1976, *32*, 119–133.

Brown, J. S. Gradients of approach and avoidance responses and their relation to motivation. *Journal of Comparative and Physiological Psychology*, 1948, *41*, 450–465.

Brown, P., & Manela, R. Client satisfaction with marital and divorce counseling. *Family Coordinator*, 1977, *26*(3), 294–303.

Bruner, J. S., & Tagiuri, R. The perception of people. In G. Lindzey (Ed.), *Handbook of Social Psychology* (Vol. 2). Reading, MA: Addison-Wesley Publishing Co., 1954.

Buckley, W. *Sociology and Modern Systems Theory*. Englewood Cliffs, NJ: Prentice-Hall, 1967.

Budd, W. G. Prediction of interests between husband and wife. *Journal of Educational Sociology*, 1959, *33*, 37–39.

Bugental, D. B., & Love, L. Nonassertive expression of parental approval and disapproval and its relationship to child disturbance. *Child Development*, 1975, *46*, 747–752.

Bugental, D. B., Love, L. R., Kaswan, J. W., & April, C. Verbal–nonverbal conflict in parental messages to normal and disturbed children. *Journal of Abnormal Psychology*, 1977, *77*, 6–10.

Bumpass, L. L., & Sweet, J. A. Differentials in marital instability, 1970. *American Sociological Review*, 1972, *37*, 754–766.

Burchinal, L., & Bauder, W. Decision-making patterns among Iowa farm and nonfarm families. *Journal of Marriage and the Family*, 1965, *27*, 525–530.

Burgess, E. W., & Locke, H. S. *The Family: From Institution to Companionship*. New York: American Book Company, 1945.

Burgess, E. W., & Wallin, P. *Engagement and Marriage*. Chicago: J. B. Lippincott Co., 1953.

Burtt, E. A. *Right Thinking: A Study of Its Principles and Methods*. New York: Harpers, 1946.

Byrne, D., & Blaylock, B. Similarity and assumed similarity of attitudes between husbands and wives. *Journal of Abnormal and Social Psychology*, 1963, *67*, 636–640.

Byrne, D., & Nelson, D. Attraction as a linear function of proportion of positive reinforcements. *Journal of Personality and Social Psychology*, 1965, *1*, 599–664.

Byrne, D., & Rhamey, R. Magnitude of positive and negative reinforcements as a determinant of attraction. *Journal of Personality and Social Psychology*, 1965, *2*, 884–889.

Byrne, D., Lamberth, J., Palmer, J., & London, O. Sequential effects as a function of implicit and interpolated attraction responses. *Journal of Personality and Social Psychology*, 1969, *13*, 70–78.

Cadwallader, M. Marriage as a wretched institution. *The Atlantic Monthly*, 1966, *218*, 62–66.

Calvo, G. *Marriage Encounter*. St. Paul: Marriage Encounter, Inc., 1975.

Campbell, D. T., & Fiske, D. W. Convergent and discriminant validation by the multitrait–multimethod matrix. *Psychological Bulletin*, 1959, *56*, 81–105.

Canavan-Gumpert, D. Generating reward and cost orientations through praise and criticism. *Journal of Personality and Social Psychology*, 1977, *35*, 501–513.

Cannon, W. Organization for physiological homeostasis. *Physiological Review*, 1929, *9*, 399–431.

Cappon, D. Results of psychotherapy. *British Journal of Psychiatry*, 1964, *110*, 35–45.

Carkhuff, R. R., & Berenson, B. G. *Beyond Counseling and Therapy.* New York: Holt, Rinehart and Winston, 1967.

Carkhuff, R. R., & Bierman, R. Training as a preferred mode of treatment for parents of emotionally disturbed children. *Journal of Counseling Psychology,* 1970, *17,* 151–161.

Carson, R. C. *Interpersonal Concepts of Personality.* Chicago: Aldine, 1969.

Carter, H., & Glick, P. C. *Marriage and Divorce: A Social and Economic Study.* Cambridge, MA: Harvard University Press, 1976.

Carter, R. D., & Thomas, E. J. Modification of problematic marital communication using corrective feedback and instruction. *Behavior Therapy,* 1973, *4,* 100–109.

Cartwright, D. A field theoretical conception of power. In D. Cartwright (Ed.), *Studies in Social Power.* Ann Arbor, MI: Institute for Social Research, 1959.

Cartwright, D. S. Success in psychotherapy as a function of certain actuarial variables. *Journal of Consulting Psychology,* 1955, *19,* 357–363.

Cashdan, S. *Interactional Psychotherapy: Stages and Strategies in Behavioral Change.* New York: Grune and Stratton, 1973.

Casriel, D. *A Scream Away from Happiness.* New York: Grosset and Dunlap, 1974.

Cattell, R. B. *Personality: A Systematic Theoretical and Factual Study.* New York: McGraw-Hill, 1950.

Centers, R., Raven, B. J., & Rodrigues, A. Conjugal power structure: A re-examination. *American Sociological Review,* 1971, *36,* 264–277.

Chadwick, B. A., Albrecht, S. L., & Kunz, P. R. Marital and family role satisfaction. *Journal of Marriage and the Family,* 1976, *38,* 431–440.

Chamow, L. A functional approach to family assessment. *Family Therapy,* 1975, *2,* 259–268.

Chertkoff, J. M., & Conley, M. Opening offer and frequency of concession as bargaining strategies. *Journal of Personality and Social Psychology,* 1967, *7,* 301–306.

Chesterton, G. K. On running after one's hat. In H. Preston (Ed.). *Great Essays.* New York: Washington Square Press, 1960.

Cimbalo, R. S., Faling, V., & Mousaw, P. The course of love: A cross-sectional design. *Psychological Reports,* 1976, *38,* 1292–1294.

Clarke, F. P. Interpersonal communication variables as predictors of marital satisfaction–attraction. *Dissertation Abstracts International,* 1974, *34,* 4458–4459.

Clatworthy, N. M. Living together. In N. Glazer-Malbin (Ed.), *Old Family/New Family: Interpersonal Relationships.* New York: D. Van Nostrand Co., 1975.

Cleghorn, J. M., & Leven, S. Training family therapists by setting learning objectives. *American Journal of Orthopsychiatry,* 1973, *43,* 439–446.

Clements, W. H. Marital interaction and marital stability: A point of view and a descriptive comparison of stable and unstable marriages. *Journal of Marriage and the Family,* 1967, *29,* 697–702.

Clynes, P. J. *Synectics: The Psychology of Emotion.* New York: Vantage, 1978.

Cole, C. M. Barriers to the termination of an intimate relationship: A behavioral analysis of married and living-together couples. *Dissertation Abstracts International,* 1976, *36,* 3594.

Cole, C. M., & Vincent, J. P. *Cognitive and Behavioral Patterns in Cohabitative and Marital Dyads.* Unpublished manuscript, University of Houston, 1975.

Coleman, J. S. Loss of power. *American Sociological Review,* 1973, *38,* 1–17.

Coleman, R. E., & Miller, A. G. The relationship between depression and marital maladjustment in a clinic population: A multitrait–multimethod study. *Journal of Consulting and Clinical Psychology,* 1975, *43,* 647–651.

Collins, J. *The Effects of the Conjugal Relationship Modification Method on Marital Communication and Adjustment.* Unpublished doctoral dissertation, Pennsylvania State University, 1971.

Combs, A. W., Avila, D. L., & Purkey, W. W. *Helping Relationships: Basic Concepts for the Helping Professions.* Boston: Allyn and Bacon, 1971.

Cone, J. D. Social desirability and marital happiness. *Psychological Reports*, 1967, *21*, 770–772.

Conover, P. W. An analysis of communes and intentional communities with particular attention to sexual and genderal relations. *The Family Coordinator*, 1975, *24*, 453–464.

Cooper, A. J. A factual study of male potency disorders. *British Journal of Psychiatry*, 1968, *114*, 719–731.

Cooper, A. J. Disorders of sexual potency in the male: A clinical and statistical study of some factors related to short-term prognosis. *British Journal of Psychiatry*, 1969, *115*, 709–719. (a)

Cooper, A. J. Frigidity, treatment and short-term prognosis. *Journal of Psychosomatic Research*, 1969, *14*, 133. (b)

Cooper, A. J. Outpatient treatment of impotence. *Journal of Nervous and Mental Disease*, 1969, *149*, 360–371. (c)

Corrales, R. G. Power and satisfaction in early marriage. In R. E. Cromwell & D. H. Olson (Eds.), *Power in Families*. New York: John Wiley and Sons, 1975.

Corsini, R. J. Multiple predictors of marital happiness. *Marriage and Family Living*, 1956, *18*, 240–242.

Coser, L. A. The functions of social conflict. In L. A. Coser & B. Rosenberg (Eds.), *Sociological Theory: A Book of Readings*. New York: Macmillan Co., 1969.

Coursey, R. D., Specter, G. A., Murrell, S. A., & Hunt, B. *Program Evaluation for Mental Health: Methods, Strategies, and Participants*. New York: Grune and Stratton, 1977.

Cox, M. *Structuring the Therapeutic Process: Compromise with Chaos*. New York: Pergamon Press, 1978.

Cox, P. R. *Demography*. Cambridge, England: Cambridge University Press, 1970.

Cozby, P. W. Self-disclosure: A literature review. *Psychological Bulletin*, 1973, *79*, 73–91.

Crasilneck, H. B., & Hall, J. A. *Clinical Hypnosis: Principles and Applications*. New York: Grune and Stratton, 1975.

Crenshaw, R. T., & Crenshaw, T. L. Unpublished interview questionnaire, San Diego, 1977.

Crenshaw, R. T., & Crenshaw, T. L. *Expressing Your Own Feelings: The Key to a Successful Relationship*. San Diego: Courseware, 1978.

Croake, J. W., & Lyon, R. S. Research design in marital adjustment studies. *International Journal of Family Therapy*, 1978, *6*, 32–35.

Cromwell, R. E., & Olson, D. H. Multidisciplinary perspectives of power. In R. E. Cromwell & D. H. Olson (Eds.), *Power in Families*. New York: John Wiley and Sons, 1975.

Cromwell, R. E., Klein, D. M., & Wieting, S. G. Family power: A multitrait–multimethod analysis. In R. E. Cromwell & D. H. Olson (Eds.), *Power in Families*. New York: John Wiley and Sons, 1975.

Cronbach, L. J. Proposals leading to analytic treatment of social perception scores. In R. Tagiuri & L. Petrullo (Eds.), *Person Perception and Interpersonal Behavior*. Stanford, CA: Stanford University Press, 1958.

Cronbach, L. J., & Furby, L. How shall we measure "change"—or should we? *Psychological Bulletin*, 1970, *74*, 68–80.

Croome, H. *Introduction to Money*. London: Methune, 1956.

Crowne, D. P., & Marlowe, D. *The Approval Motive: Studies in Evaluative Dependence*. New York: John Wiley and Sons, 1964.

Crutchfield, R. S. Independent thought in a conformist world. In S. M. Farber & R. H. L. Wilson (Eds.) *Conflict and Creativity*. New York: McGraw-Hill, 1963.

Cuber, J. F. Three prerequisite considerations to diagnosis and treatment in marriage counseling. In R. H. Klemer (Ed.), *Counseling in Marital and Sexual Problems: A Physician's Handbook*. Baltimore: Williams and Wilkins, 1965.

Cuber, J. F., & Harroff, P. B. The more total view: Relationships among men and women of the upper middle class. *Marriage and Family Living*, 1963, *25*, 140.

Cuber, J. F., & Harroff, P. B. *Sex and the Significant Americans*. Baltimore: Penguin, 1965.

Cummings, N. A. Prolonged (ideal) versus short-term (realistic) psychotherapy. *Professional Psychology*, 1977, *2*, 491–501.

Cutler, B. R., & Dyer, W. G. Initial adjustment process in young married couples. *Social Forces*, 1965, *44*, 195–201.

Cutright, P. Income and family events: Marital stability. *Journal of Marriage and the Family*, 1971, *33*, 291–306.

Dahlstrom, W. G., Welsh, G. A., & Dahlstrom, L. E. *An MMPI Handbook: Clinical Applications* (Vol. 1). Minneapolis: University of Minnesota Press, 1972.

Davis, J. D. *The Interview as Arena*. Stanford, CA: Stanford University Press, 1971.

Davis, J. H. *Group Performance*. Reading, MA: Addison-Wesley Publishing Co., 1969.

Davison, G. Elimination of a sadistic fantasy by a client-controlled counterconditioning technique: A case study. *Journal of Abnormal Psychology*, 1968, *73*, 84–90.

Davison, G. C. Countercontrol in behavior modification. In L. A. Hamerlynck, L. C. Handy, & E. J. Mash (Eds.), *Behavior Change: Methodology, Concepts and Practice*. Champaign, IL: Research Press, 1973.

Davison, G. C., & Stuart, R. B. Behavior therapy and civil liberties. *American Psychologist*, 1975, *30*, 755–763.

Davison, G. C., & Valins, S. Maintenance of self-attributed and drug-attributed behavior change. *Journal of Personality and Social Psychology*, 1969, *11*, 25–33.

Dawkins, S., & Taylor, R. Non-consummation of marriage: A survey of seventy cases. *The Lancet*, 1961, *22*, 1029–1033.

Day, D. A. The relationship of repression–sensitization to aspects of marital dyad functioning. *Dissertation Abstracts International*, 1973, *34*, 389.

DeBeauvoir, S. *The Second Sex*. New York: Alfred A. Knopf, 1971.

DeBurger, J. E. Marital problems, help-seeking, and emotional orientation as revealed in help-request letters. *Journal of Marriage and the Family*, 1967, *29*, 712–721.

Demarest, D., Sexton, M., & Sexton, J. *Marriage Encounter: A Guide to Sharing*. St. Paul: Carillon Books, 1977.

Demars, E. T. *Improving Our Abilities to Make Decisions*. Salt Lake City: University of Utah Press, 1972.

Derogatis, L. R., Lipman, R. S., & Covi, L. SCL-90: An outpatient psychiatric rating scale (preliminary report). *Psychopharmacology Bulletin*, 1973, *9*, 13–27.

Derogatis, L. R., Lipman, R. S., Rickels, K., Uhlenhuth, E. H., & Covi, L. The Hopkins Symptom Checklist (HSCL): A measure of primary symptom dimensions. In P. Pichot (Ed.), *Psychological Measurements in Psychopharmacology: Modern Problems in Pharmacopsychiatry*. Basel, Switzerland: S. Karger, 1974.

Deutsch, M. Conflicts: Productive and destructive. *Journal of Social Issues*, 1969, *25*, 7–41.

Deutsch, M., & Krauss, R. M. The effect of threat on interpersonal bargaining. *Journal of Abnormal and Social Psychology*, 1960, *61*, 181–189.

Dewey, J. *How We Think*. New York: D. C. Heath, 1910.

Dixon, D. N., & Sciara, A. D. Effectiveness of group reciprocity counseling with married couples. *Journal of Marriage and Family Counseling*, 1977, *3*, 77–83.

Doehrman, M. G. *The Effects of Coercive Communications upon Conflict Resolution in Newlywed Couples*. Unpublished master's thesis, University of Michigan, 1968.

Dollard, J., & Miller, N. E. *Personality and Psychotherapy*. New York: McGraw-Hill, 1950.

Douglas, S. P., & Wind, Y. Examining family role and authority patterns: Two methodological issues. *Journal of Marriage and the Family*, 1978, *40*, 35–47.

Dubble, M. Etiological factors in the unconsummated marriage. *Journal of Psychosomatic Research*, 1977, *21*, 157–160.

Duck, S. W., & Spencer, C. Personal constructs and friendship formation. *Journal of Personality and Social Psychology,* 1972, *23,* 40–45.

Duncan, S. Some signals and rules for taking speaking turns in conversations. *Journal of Personality and Social Psychology,* 1972, *23,* 283–292.

Dunnette, M. D., Campbell, J., & Jaastad, K. The effect of group participation on brainstorming effectiveness for two industrial samples. *Journal of Applied Psychology,* 1963, *47,* 30–37.

Durkheim, E. *Suicide.* New York: The Free Press, 1966.

Dymond, R. Interpersonal perception and marital happiness. *Canadian Journal of Psychology,* 1954, *8,* 164–171.

D'Zurilla, T. J., & Goldfried, M. R. "Problem solving and behavior modification." *Journal of Abnormal Psychology,* 1971, *78,* 107–126.

Eagly, A. H., & Whitehead, G. I. Effect of choice on receptivity to favorable and unfavorable evaluations of oneself. *Journal of Personality and Social Psychology,* 1972, *22,* 223–230.

Edmonds, V. H. Marital conventionalization: Definition and measurement. *Journal of Marriage and the Family,* 1967, *29,* 681–688.

Edmonds, V. H., Withers, G., & Dibatista, B. Adjustment, conservatism, and marital conventionalism. *Journal of Marriage and the Family,* 1972, *34,* 96–103.

Edwards, A. Behavioral decision therapy. *Annual Review of Psychology,* 1961, *12,* 492–493.

Edwards, A. L. *The Social Desirability Variable in Personality Assessment and Research.* New York: Dryden, 1957.

Edwards, A. L. The social desirability variable: A review of the evidence. In I. A. Berg (Ed.), *Response Set in Personality Assessment.* Chicago: Aldine, 1967.

Einstein, A. *Relativity: A Richer Truth.* New York: The Beacon Press, 1950.

Eisler, R. M., Hersen, N., & Agras, W. S. Effects of videotape and instructional feedback on nonverbal marital interaction: An analog study. *Behavior Therapy,* 1973, *4,* 420–425.

Ekman, P., & Friesen, W. V. Nonverbal leakage and clues to deception. *Psychiatry,* 1969, *32,* 88–105.

Elgosin, R. B. Premarital counseling and sexual adjustment in marriage. *Connecticut State Medical Journal,* 1951, *15,* 999–1002.

Elkouri, F. *How Arbitration Works.* Washington, DC: Bureau of National Affairs, 1952.

Elliot, F. A. The neurology of explosive rage: The dyscontrol syndrome. *The Practitioner,* 1976, *217,* 111–119.

Ellis, A. *Reason and Emotion in Psychotherapy.* New York: Lyle Stuart, 1962.

Ellis, A. *The Art and Science of Love.* New York: Bantam Books, 1966.

Ellis, A. *The Sensuous Person.* New York: New American Library, 1974.

Ellis, A. Techniques of handling anger in marriage. *Journal of Marriage and Family Counseling,* 1976, *2,* 305–315.

Ellis, A., & Harper, R. A. *A New Guide to Rational Living.* Englewood Cliffs, NJ: Prentice-Hall, 1975.

Ellis, H. *The Dance of Life.* New York: The Modern Library, 1923.

Ellison, C. Psychosomatic factors in the unconsummated marriage. *Journal of Psychosomatic Research,* 1968, *12,* 61–65.

Ellison, C. Vaginismus. *Medical Aspects of Human Sexuality,* 1972, *6*(8), 34–54.

Ellsworth, R. B. Consumer feedback in measuring the effectiveness of mental health programs. In E. L. Struening & M. Guttentag (Eds.), *Handbook of Evaluation Research.* Beverly Hills, CA: Sage Publications, 1975.

Emerson, R. M. Power–dependence relations. *American Sociological Review,* 1962, *27,* 31–40.

Endler, N. S. The person versus the situation—A pseudo issue? A reply to Alker. *Journal of Personality,* 1973, *41,* 287–303.

Endler, N. S., & Magnusson, D. Toward an interactional psychology of personality. *Psychological Bulletin,* 1976, *83,* 956–974.

Engel, L., & Weiss, R. L. *Behavioral Cues Used by Marital Therapists in Discriminating Distress.*

Paper presented at the Annual Meeting of the Western Psychological Association, Los Angeles, 1976.

Erickson, B., Holmes, J. G., Frey, R., Walker, L., & Thibaut, J. Functions of a third party in the resolution of conflict: The role of the judge in pre-trial conferences. *Journal of Personality and Social Psychology*, 1974, *30*, 293–306.

Eslinger, K. N., Clarke, A. C., & Dynes, R. R. The principle of least interest, dating behavior, and family integration settings. *Journal of Marriage and the Family*, 1972, *34*, 269–272.

Esser, J. K., & Komorita, S. S. Reciprocity and concession making in bargaining. *Journal of Personality and Social Psychology*, 1975, *31*, 864–872.

Etzioni, A. The family: Is it obsolete? What role for the family now? *Journal of Current Social Issues*, 1977, *1*, 4–9.

Ex, J. The nature of the relationship between two persons and the degree of influence on each other. *Acta Psychologica*, 1960, *17*, 39–54.

Fabbri, R. Hypnosis and behavior therapy: A coordinated approach to the treatment of sexual disorders. *The American Journal of Clinical Hypnosis*, 1976, *19*, 4–8.

Farber, B. An index of marital integration. *Sociometry*, 1957, *20*, 117–134.

Feffer, M. A developmental analysis of interpersonal behavior. *Psychological Review*, 1970, *77*, 197–214.

Feidman, L. B. Processes of change in family therapy. *Journal of Family Counseling*, 1976, *4*, 14–22.

Feldman, H. Changes in marriage and parenthood: A methodological design. In E. Peck & J. Senderowitz (Eds.), *Pronatalism: The Myth of Mom and Apple Pie*. New York: Thomas Y. Crowell Co., 1974.

Feldman, H., & Rand, M. E. Egocentrism–altercentrism in the husband–wife relationship. *Journal of Marriage and Family Living*, 1965, *27*, 386–391.

Fenichel, O. Brief psychotherapy. In H. Fenichel & D. Rappaport (Eds.), *The Collected Papers of Otto Fenichel*. New York: W. W. Norton, 1954.

Ferreira, A. J. Family myths. In P. Watzlawick & J. H. Weakland (Eds.), *The Interactional View: Studies at the Mental Research Institute, Palo Alto, 1965–1974*. New York: W. W. Norton, 1977.

Ferreira, A. J., & Winter, W. D. Family interaction and decision-making. *Archives of General Psychiatry*, 1965, *13*, 214–223.

Ferreira, A. J., & Winter, W. D. Stability of interactional variables in family decision-making. *Archives of General Psychiatry*, 1966, *14*, 352–355.

Ferster, C. B. A functional analysis of depression. *American Psychologist*, 1973, *28*, 857–870.

Festinger, L. *A Theory of Cognitive Dissonance*. Evanston, IL: Row, Peterson, 1957.

Festinger, L. *Conflict, Decision, and Dissonance*. Stanford, CA: Stanford University Press, 1964.

Fey, W. F. Doctrine and experience: Their influence upon the psychotherapist. *Journal of Counsling Psychology*, 1958, *22*, 403–409.

Fiedler, F. E. A comparison of therapeutic relationships in psychoanalytic, nondirective, and Adlerian therapy. *Journal of Consulting Psychology*, 1950, *14*, 436–445.

Fiedler, F. E. Quantitative studies on the role of therapists' feelings toward their patients. In O. H. Mowrer (Ed.), *Psychotherapy: Theory and Research*. New York: Roland Press, 1953.

Fiester, A. R., & Rudestam, K. E. A multivariate analysis of the early dropout process. *Journal of Consulting and Clinical Psychology*, 1975, *43*, 528–535.

Filley, A. C. *Interpersonal Conflict Resolution*. Glenview, IL: Scott, Foresman and Co., 1975.

Fisher, B. L., & Sprenkle, D. H. Therapists' perceptions of healthy family functioning. *International Journal of Family Counseling*, 1978, *6*, 9–18.

Fisher, L. Dimensions of family assessment: A critical review. *Journal of Marriage and Family Counseling*, 1976, *2*, 367–376.

Fisher, R. Fractionating conflict. In R. Fisher (Ed.), *International Conflict and Behavioral Science: The Craigville Papers*. New York: Basic Books, 1964.

Fiske, D. W. The shaky evidence is slowly put together. *Journal of Consulting and Clinical Psychology,* 1971, *37,* 314–315.

Fiske, D. W. A source of data is not a measuring instrument. *Journal of Abnormal Psychology,* 1975, *84,* 20–23.

Fitzgerald, M. P. Self-disclosure and expressed self-esteem, social distance and areas of the self revealed. *Journal of Psychology,* 1963, *56,* 405–412.

Flowers, J. V., & Booraem, C. D. Imagination training in the treatment of sexual dysfunction. *The Counseling Psychologist,* 1975, *5*(1), 50–51.

Floyd, W. A. A new look at research in marital and family therapy. *Journal of Family Counseling,* 1976, *4,* 19–23.

Fogarty, T. F. The family emotional self system. *Family Therapy,* 1975, *2,* 79–97.

Foley, V. D. Alcoholism: A family system approach. *Journal of Family Counseling,* 1976, *4,* 12–18.

Ford, D. H., & Urban, H. B. *Systems of Psychotherapy.* New York: John Wiley and Sons, 1963.

Fordney-Settlage, D. S. Heterosexual dysfunction: Evaluation of treatment procedures. *Archives of Sexual Behavior,* 1975, *4,* 367–387.

Frank, J. D. *Persuasion and Healing: A Comparative Study of Psychotherapy.* Baltimore: Johns Hopkins Press, 1961.

Frank, J. D. The role of cognitions in illness and healing. In H. H. Strupp & L. Luborsky (Eds.), *Research in Psychotherapy: Proceedings of a Conference, Chapel Hill, North Carolina,* May 17–20, 1961. Washington, DC: American Psychological Association, 1962.

Frank, E., Anderson, C., & Kupfer, D. Profiles of couples seeking sex therapy and marital therapy. *American Journal of Psychiatry,* 1976, *133,* 559–562.

Frank, E., Anderson, C., & Rubinstein, D. Frequency of sexual dysfunction in "normal" couples. *New England Journal of Medicine,* 1978, *299,* 111–115.

Frederickson, C. G. Life stress and marital conflict: A pilot study. *Journal of Marriage and Family Counseling,* 1977, *3,* 41–47.

Freedman, B. J., & Rice, D. G. Marital therapy in prison: One-partner "couple therapy." *Psychiatry,* 1977, *40,* 175–183.

Freedman, J. L., & Fraser, S. Compliance without pressure: The foot-in-the-door technique. *Journal of Personality and Social Psychology,* 1966, *4,* 195–202.

Freeman, S. J., Leavens, E. J., & McCulloch, D. J. Factors associated with success or failure in marital counseling. *Family Coordinator,* 1969, *18,* 125–128.

French, J. R. P., & Raven, B. H. The bases of social power. In D. Cartwright (Ed.), *Studies in Social Power.* Ann Arbor, MI: Institute for Social Research, 1959.

French, J. R. P., & Snyder, R. Leadership and interpersonal power. In D. Cartwright (Ed.), *Studies in Social Power.* Ann Arbor, MI: Institute for Social Research, 1959.

Freud, S. *Certain Neurotic Mechanisms in Jealousy, Paranoia, and Homosexuality. Collected Papers* (Vol. 11). London: Hogarth, 1922.

Friday, N. *My Secret Garden: Women's Sexual Fantasies.* New York: Trident Press, 1973.

Friedman, D. The treatment of impotence by brietal relaxation therapy. *Behaviour Research and Therapy,* 1968, *6,* 257–261.

Friedman, L. J. *Virgin Wives: A Study of Unconsummated Marriages.* Philadelphia: Lippincott, 1962.

Friedman, M. *Price Theory: A Provisioned Text.* Chicago, IL: Aldine, 1962.

Friedman, R. Techniques for rapid engagement in family therapy. *Child Welfare,* 1977, *56,* 509–517.

Fuchs, K., Hoch, A., Paldi, E., Abramovici, H., Brandes, J. M., Timor-Tritsch, I., & Kleinhaus, M. Hypnodesensitization therapy of vaginismus: Part I. *In vitro* method. Part II. *In vivo* method. *International Journal of Clinical and Experimental Hypnosis,* 1973, *21*(3), 144–156.

Garfield, S. L. Research on client variables in psychotherapy. In A. G. Bergin & S. L. Garfield (Eds.), *Handbook of Psychotherapy and Behavior Change.* New York: John Wiley and Sons, 1971.

Garfield, S. L., & Bergin, A. E. Therapeutic conditions and outcome. *Journal of Abnormal Psychology*, 1971, 77, 108–114.

Garfield, S. L., Prager, R. A., & Bergin, A. E. Evaluation of outcome in psychotherapy. *Journal of Consulting and Clinical Psychology*, 1971, 37, 307–313.

Garfinkel, H. The routine grounds of everyday activities. *Social Problems*, 1964, 11, 225–249.

Garner, H. H. *Psychotherapy: Confrontation Problem-solving Technique*. St. Louis, MO: W. H. Green, 1970.

Garrigan, J. J., & Bambrick, A. E. Short-term family therapy with emotionally disturbed children. *Journal of Marriage and Family Counseling*, 1975, 1, 379–385.

Gebhard, P. H. Factors in marital orgasm. *Journal of Social Issues*, 1966, 22(2), 88–95.

Geiken, K. F. Expectations concerning husband–wife responsibilities in the home. *Marriage and Family Living*, 1964, 26, 349–352.

Geiwitz, P. J. The effects of threats on prisoner's dilemma. *Behavioral Science*, 1967, 12, 232–233.

Gelles, R. J. *The Violent Home: A Study of Physical Aggression between Husbands and Wives*. New York: Sage Publications, 1974.

Gelles, R. J. No place to go: The social dynamics of marital violence. In M. Roy (Ed.), *Battered Women: A Psychosociological Study of Domestic Violence*. New York: Van Nostrand Reinhold, 1977.

Genovese, R. J. Marriage encounter. In S. Miller (Ed.), *Marriages and Families: Enrichment through Communication*. Beverly Hills, CA: Sage Publications, 1975.

Gergen, K. J. *The Psychology of Behavior Exchange*. Reading, MA: Addison-Wesley Publishing Co., 1969.

Gershon, E. S., Dunner, D. L., & Goodwin, F. K. Toward a biology of affective disorders. *Archives of General Psychiatry*, 1971, 25, 1–15.

Gibbs, A. R. Traditional and companionship variation within high and low satisfied black marriages. *Dissertation Abstracts International*, 1977, 37, 5830.

Gibbs, J. P. Marital status and suicide in the United States: A special test of the status integration theory. *American Journal of Sociology*, 1969, 74, 557–572.

Gibson, R. L., Snyder, W. U., & Ray, W. S. A factor analysis of change following client-centered therapy. *Journal of Consulting Psychology*, 1955, 2, 83–90.

Gilbert, S. U., & Horenstein, D. A study of self-disclosure: Level vs. valence. *Journal of Human Communication Research*, 1975, 1, 1–27.

Gilder, G. *Naked Nomads: Unmarried Men in America*. New York: Quadrangle Books, 1974.

Gillespie, D. L. Who has the power? The marital struggle. *Journal of Marriage and the Family*, 1971, 33, 445–458.

Gilman, G. An inquiry into the nature and use of authority. In M. Hare (Ed.), *Organization Theory in Industrial Practice*. New York: John Wiley and Sons, 1962.

Glenn, N. D. The contribution of marriage to the psychological well-being of males and females. *Journal of Marriage and the Family*, 1975, 37, 594–600. (a)

Glenn, N. D. Psychological well-being in the postparental stage: Some evidence from national surveys. *Journal of Marriage and the Family*, 1975, 37, 105–110. (b)

Glenn, N. D., & Weaver, C. N. The marital happiness of remarried divorced persons. *Journal of Marriage and the Family*, 1977, 39, 331–337.

Glenn, N. D., & Weaver, C. N. A multivariate, multisurvey of marital happiness. *Journal of Marriage and the Family*, 1978, 40, 269–282.

Glick, P. C. Demographic analyses of family data. In H. T. Christensen (Ed.), *Handbook of Marriage and the Family*. Chicago: Rand McNally, 1964.

Glick, P. C. A demographer looks at American families. *Journal of Marriage and the Family*, 1975, 37, 15–26.

Glick, P. C., & Norton, A. J. Perspectives on the recent upturn in divorce and remarriage. *Demography*, 1973, 10, 301–314.

Glisson, D. H. A review of behavioral marital counseling: Has practice tuned out theory? *Psychological Record*, 1976, 26(1), 95–104.

Goffman, E. *The Presentation of Self in Everyday Life.* Garden City, NY: Doubleday Anchor Books, 1959.

Goffman, E. *Interaction Rituals: Essays on Face-to-Face Behavior.* Garden City, NY: Doubleday Anchor Books, 1967.

Goldbeck, R. A., Berstein, B. B., Hillix, W. A., & Marx, M. H. Application of the half-split technique to problem-solving tasks. *Journal of Experimental Psychology,* 1957, *53,* 330–338.

Goldfried, M. Behavioral assessment in perspective. In J. D. Cone & R. P. Hawkins (Eds.), *Behavioral Assessment: New Directions in Clinical Psychology.* New York: Bruner/Mazel, 1977.

Goldfried, M. R., & Davison, G. C. *Clinical Behavior Therapy.* New York: Holt, Rinehart and Winston, 1976.

Goldstein, A. P. *Therapist–Patient Expectancies in Psychotherapy.* New York: Macmillan Co., 1962.

Goldstein, A. P. Domains and dilemmas. *International Journal of Psychiatry,* 1969, *7,* 128–134.

Goldstein, A. P., Heller, K., & Sechrest, L. B. *Psychotherapy and the Psychology of Behavior Change.* New York: John Wiley and Sons, 1966.

Golightly, C., & Byrne, D. Attitude statements as positive and negative reinforcements. *Science,* 1964, *146,* 798–799.

Gomes-Schwartz, B. Effective ingredients in psychotherapy: Prediction of outcome from process variables. *Journal of Consulting and Clinical Psychology,* 1978, *46,* 1023–1035.

Goode, W. J. Violence between intimates. In D. J. Mulvihill, M. M. Tumin, & L. A. Cutris (Eds.), *Crimes in Violence.* Washington, DC: U.S. Government Printing Office, 1969.

Goode, W. J. *World Revolution and Family Patterns.* New York: The Free Press, 1970.

Goodman, N., & Ofshe, R. Empathy, communication efficiency and marital status. *Journal of Marriage and the Family,* 1968, *30,* 597–605.

Goodrich, W., Ryder, R. G., & Rausch, H. L. Patterns of newlywed marriage. *Journal of Marriage and the Family,* 1968, *30,* 383–391.

Gordon, C., & Gergen, K. J. (Eds.). *The Self in Social Interaction.* New York: John Wiley and Sons, 1968.

Gordon, R. M. Effects of volunteering and responsibility on the perceived value and effectiveness of a clinical treatment. *Journal of Consulting and Clinical Psychology,* 1976, *44,* 799–801.

Gottman, J., Notarius, C., Gonso, J., & Markman, H. *A Couple's Guide to Communication.* Champaign, IL: Research Press, 1976. (a)

Gottman, J., Notarius, C., Markman, H., Bank, S., Yoppi, B., & Rubin, M. E. Behavior exchange theory and marital decision making. *Journal of Personality and Social Psychology,* 1976, *34,* 14–23. (b)

Gottman, J., Markman, H., & Notarius, C. The topography of marital conflict: A sequential analysis of verbal and nonverbal behavior. *Journal of Marriage and the Family,* 1977, *39,* 461–477.

Gough, H. G. *California Psychological Inventory.* Palo Alto, CA: Consulting Psychologists Press, 1975.

Gouldner, A. The norm of reciprocity: A preliminary statement. *American Sociological Review,* 1960, *25,* 161–179.

Granbois, D., & Willett, R. Equivalence of family role measures based on husband and wife data. *Journal of Marriage and the Family,* 1970, *32,* 68–72.

Green, B. L., Gleser, G. C., Stone, W. N., & Seifert, R. F. Relationships among diverse measures of psychotherapy outcome. *Journal of Consulting and Clinical Psychology,* 1975, *43,* 689–699.

Greenberg, G. S. Conjoint family theory: An entree to a new behavior therapy. *Dissertation Abstracts International,* 1974, *35,* 3878–3879.

Greenberg, G. S. The family interactional perspective: A study and examination of the work of Don D. Jackson. *Family Process,* 1977, *16,* 285–412.

Greenberg, R., Goldstein, A. P., & Perry, M. The influence of referral information upon patient perception in a psychotherapy analogue. *Journal of Nervous and Mental Disease,* 1970, *150,* 31–36.

Greenberg, R. P. Effects of presession information on perception of the therapist and receptivity to influence in a psychotherapy analogue. *Journal of Consulting and Clinical Psychology*, 1969, 33, 425–429.

Greene, B. L. *A Clinical Approach to Marital Problems*, Springfield, IL: Charles C Thomas, 1970.

Greenson, R. *The Technique and Practice of Psychoanalysis*. New York: International Universities Press, 1967.

Greenspoon, J., & Lamal, P. A. Cognitive behavior modification—Who needs it? *The Psychological Record*, 1978, 28, 343–351.

Grinker, R. R. Brief psychotherapy in psychosomatic problems. *Psychosomatic Medicine*, 1947, 9, 78–103.

Grunebaum, H., & Christ, J. (Eds.). *Contemporary Marriage: Structure, Dynamics, and Therapy*. Boston: Little, Brown and Co., 1976.

Grunebaum, H., Christ, J., & Neiberg, N. Diagnosis and treatment planning for couples. *International Journal of Group Psychotherapy*, 1969, 19, 185–202.

Gruver, G. G., & Labadie, S. K. Marital dissatisfaction among college students. *Journal of College Student Personnel*, 1975, 16(6), 454–458.

Guerney, B. Filial therapy: Description and rationale. *Journal of Consulting Psychology*, 1964, 28, 304–310.

Gunter, B. G., & Johnson, D. P. Divorce filing as role behavior: Effect of no-fault law on divorce filing patterns. *Journal of Marriage and the Family*, 1978, 40, 571–574.

Gurin, G., Veroff, J., & Feld, S. *Americans View Their Mental Health: Joint Commission on Mental Illness and Health*, Monograph Series 4. New York: Basic Books, 1960.

Gurman, A. S. The effects and effectiveness of marital therapy: A review of outcome research. *Family Process*, 1973, 12, 145–170.

Gurman, A. S., & Kniskern, D. P. Deterioration in marital and family therapy: Empirical, clinical, and conceptual issues. *Family Process*, 1978, 17, 3–20. (a)

Gurman, A. S., & Kniskern, D. P. Research on marital and family therapy: Progress, perspectives, and prospect. In S. L. Garfield & A. E. Bergin (Eds.), *Handbook of Psychotherapy and Behavior Change: An Empirical Analysis* (2nd ed.). New York: John Wiley and Sons, 1978. (b)

Gutheil, E. A. Psychoanalysis and psychotherapy. *Journal of Clinical Psychopathology and Psychotherapy*, 1944, 6, 207–230.

Guttman, H. A. The new androgyny: Therapy of "liberated" couples. *Journal of the Canadian Psychiatric Association*, 1977, 22, 225–229.

Habermas, J. Toward a theory of communicative competence. In H. P. Dreitzel (Ed.), *Recent Sociology No. 2: Patterns of Communicative Behavior*. New York: Macmillan Co., 1970.

Hadley, T. R., & Jacob, T. Relationship among measures of family power. *Journal of Personality and Social Psychology*, 1973, 27, 6–12.

Haley, J. Family experiments: A new type of experimentation. *Family Process*, 1962, 1, 265–293.

Haley, J. Marriage therapy. *The Archives of General Psychiatry*, 1963, 8, 213–234. (a)

Haley, J. *Strategies of Psychotherapy*. New York: Grune and Stratton, 1963. (b)

Haley, J. Toward a theory of pathological systems. In G. Zuk & I. Boszormenyi-Nagy (Eds.), *Family Therapy and Disturbed Families*. Palo Alto, CA: Science and Behavior Books, 1967.

Haley, J. The art of being a failure as a therapist. In J. Haley (Ed.), *The Power and Tactics of Jesus Christ and Other Essays*. New York: Grossman Publishers, 1969. (a)

Haley, J. Whither family therapy? In J. Haley (Ed.), *The Power and Tactics of Jesus Christ and Other Essays*. New York: Discus Books, 1969. (b)

Haley, J. *Uncommon Therapy: The Psychiatric Techniques of Milton H. Erickson, M.D.* New York: W. W. Norton, 1973.

Haley, J. *Problem-Solving Therapy*. San Francisco: Jossey-Bass, 1977.

Hall, E. T. *The Hidden Dimension*. Garden City, NY: Anchor Books, 1966.

Hall, J. Decisions, decisions, decisions. *Psychology Today*, 1971, 5, 51–58.

Hall, J., & Williams, M. S. A comparison of decision-making performance in established and ad hoc groups. *Journal of Personality and Social Psychology*, 1966, *3*, 214–222.

Hall, S. P. Vaginismus as a cause of dyspareunia: A report of cases and a method of treatment. *Western Journal of Surgery Obstetrics and Gynecology*, 1952, *60*, 117–120.

Hall, W. M., & Valine, W. J. The relationship between self-concept and marital adjustment for commuter college students. *Journal of College Student Personnel*, 1977, *18*, 298–300.

Hamilton, M. A rating scale for depression. *Journal of Neurology, Neurosurgery and Psychiatry*, 1960, *23*, 56–62.

Hammond, D. C., & Stanfield, K. *Multidimensional Psychotherapy: A Counselor's Guide for the MAP Form*. Champaign, IL: Institute for Personality and Ability Testing, 1977.

Hammond, D. C., Hepworth, D. H., & Smith, V. G. *Improving Therapeutic Communication: A Guide for Developing Effective Techniques*. San Francisco: Jossey-Bass, 1977.

Hamner, W. C. Effects of bargaining strategy and pressure to reach agreement in a stalemated negotiation. *Journal of Personality and Social Psychology*, 1974, *30*, 458–467.

Hansen, R. D., & Donoghue, J. M. Evolving sources of happiness for men over the life cycle: Structural analysis. *Journal of Personality and Social Psychology*, 1977, *35*(5), 294–302.

Hargreaves, W. A., Attkisson, C. C., & Sorensen, J. E. *Resource Materials for Community Mental Health Program Evaluation*. Rockville, MD: U.S. Dept. of Health, Education and Welfare Publication No. (ADM) 77-328, 1977.

Harper, R. A. *Psychoanalysis and Psychotherapy*. Englewood Cliffs, NJ: Prentice-Hall, 1959.

Harrell, J., & Guerney, B. Training married couples in conflict negotiation skills. In D. H. L. Olson (Ed.), *Treating Relationships*. Lake Mills, IA: Graphic Publishing Co., 1976.

Harry, J. Evolving sources of happiness for men over the life cycle: A structural analysis. *Journal of Marriage and the Family*, 1976, *38*, 289–296.

Harsanyi, J. C. Measurement of social power, opportunity costs, and the theory of two person bargaining games. *Behavioral Science*, 1962, *7*, 67–80.

Harvey, J. H., Ickes, W. J., & Kidd, R. F. *New Directions in Attribution Research*. Hillsdale, NJ: Erlbaum, 1976.

Hastings, D. W. *A Doctor Speaks on Sexual Expression in Marriage*. New York: Bantam Books, 1972.

Hawkins, J. L. Associations between companionship, hostility and marital satisfaction. *Journal of Marriage and the Family*, 1968, *30*, 647–650.

Hays, W. L. An approach to the study of trait implication and trait similarity. In R. Tagiuri & L. Petrullo (Eds.), *Person Perception and Interpersonal Behavior*. Stanford, CA: Stanford University Press, 1958.

Heer, D. M. Dominance and the working wife. *Social Forces*, 1958, *36*, 341–347.

Heer, D. M. Husband and wife perceptions of family power structure. *Marriage and Family Living*, 1962, *24*, 65–67.

Heer, D. M. The measurement and bases of family power: An overview. *Marriage and Family Living*, 1963, *25*, 133–139.

Heer, D. M. The prevalence of black–white marriages in the United States, 1960 and 1970. *Journal of Marriage and the Family*, 1974, *36*, 246–258.

Heider, F. *The Psychology of Interpersonal Relations*. New York: John Wiley and Sons, 1958.

Heiman, J. R., LoPiccolo, L., & LoPiccolo, J. *Becoming Orgasmic: A Sexual Growth Program for Women*. Englewood Cliffs, NJ: Prentice-Hall, 1976.

Heitler, J. B. Preparatory techniques in initiating expressive psychotherapy with lower-class, unsophisticated patients. *Psychological Bulletin*, 1976, *83*, 339–352.

Heller, P. L. Familism scale: Revalidation and revision. *Journal of Marriage and the Family*, 1976, *38*, 423–429.

Helson, H. (Ed.). *Theoretical Foundations of Psychology*. Princeton, NJ: Van Nostrand, 1951.

Helson, H. Adaptation level theory. In S. Koch (Ed.), *Psychology: A Study of a Science* (Vol. 1). New York: McGraw-Hill, 1959.

Helson, H. *Adaptation-Level Theory: An Experimental and Systematic Approach to Behavior*. New York: Harcourt, Brace, 1964.

Henshel, A. M. Swinging: A study of decision making in marriage. In J. Huber (Ed.), *Changing Women in a Changing Society*. Chicago: University of Chicago Press, 1973.

Hepker, W., & Cloyd, J. S. Role relationships and role performance: The male married student. *Journal of Marriage and the Family*, 1974, *36*, 688–695.

Hersen, M., & Barlow, D. (Eds.). *Single Subject Designs*. New York: Pergamon Press, 1976.

Herzog, E., & Sudia, C. E. *Boys in Fatherless Families*. Washington, DC: Children's Bureau Publication No. 72-33, 1971.

Hetherington, E. M. Effects of father absence on personality development in adolescent daughters. *Developmental Psychology*, 1972, *7*, 313–326.

Hetherington, E. M., Cox, M., & Cox, R. Divorced fathers. *Family Coordinator*, 1976, *25*, 417–428.

Hetherington, E. M., Cox, M., & Cox, R. The aftermath of divorce. In J. H. Stevens & M. Mathews (Eds.), *Mother–Child, Father–Child Relations*. Washington, DC: National Association for Education of Young Children, 1977.

Hewitt, J. Liking and the proportion of favorable evaluations. *Journal of Personality and Social Psychology*, 1972, *22*, 231–235.

Hickok, J. E., & Komechak, M. G. Behavior modification in marital conflict: A case report. *Family Process*, 1974, *13*, 111–119.

Hicks, D. J. Imitation and retention of film-mediated aggressive peer and adult models. *Journal of Personality and Social Psychology*, 1965, *2*, 97–100.

Hicks, M. S., & Platt, M. Marital happiness and stability: A review of the research in the sixties. *Journal of Marriage and the Family*, 1970, *32*, 553–574.

Hill, R. Decision making and the family life cycle. In E. Shanas & G. F. Streib (Eds.), *Social Structure and the Family: Generational Relations*. Englewood Cliffs, NJ: Prentice-Hall, 1965.

Hill, R. Modern systems theory and the family: A confrontation. *Social Science Information*, 1971, *10*, 7–26.

Hilliard, A. L. *The Forms of Value: The Extension of a Hedonistic Axiology*. New York: Columbia University Press, 1950.

Hite, S. *The Hite Report*. Boston: Macmillan Co., 1976.

Hobart, C. W., & Klausner, W. J. Some social integration correlates of marital role disagreements, and marital adjustment. *Marriage and Family Living*, 1959, *21*, 256–263.

Hoehn-Saric, R., Frank, J. D., Imber, S. D., Nash, E. H., Stone, A. R., & Battle, C. C. Systematic preparation of patients for psychotherapy. I. Effects of therapy behavior and outcome. *Journal of Psychiatric Research*, 1964, *2*, 267–281.

Hoffman, L. R. Group problem solving, In L. Berkowitz (Ed.), *Advances in Experimental Social Psychology*, New York: Academic Press, 1965.

Hoffman, M. L. Power assertion by the parent and its impact on the child. *Child Development*, 1960, *31*, 129–143.

Hollander, E. P. Competence and conformity in the acceptance of influence. *Journal of Abnormal and Social Psychology*, 1960, *61*, 365–369. (a)

Hollander, E. P. Reconsidering the issue of conformity in personality. In H. P. David & J. C. Brengelmann (Eds.), *Perspectives in Personality Research*. New York: Springfield, 1960. (b)

Holmes, T. H., & Rahe, R. H. The social readjustment rating scale. *Journal of Psychosomatic Research*, 1967, *11*, 213–218.

Homan, P. T., Hart, A. G., & Sametz, A. W. *The Economic Order*. New York: Harcourt, Brace, 1961.

Homans, C. G. *Social Behavior: Its Elementary Forms*. New York: Harcourt, Brace and World, 1961.

Hora, T. Tao, Zen and existential psychotherapy. *Psychologia*, 1959, *2*, 236–242.

Horai, J., & Tedeschi, J. T. The effects of threat credibility and magnitude of punishment upon compliance. *Journal of Personality and Social Psychology*, 1969, *12*, 164–169.

Horowitz, M. J. A study of clinician's judgments from projective test protocols. *Journal of Consulting Psychology*, 1962, *26*, 251–256.

Huber, J. *Changing Women in a Changing Society*. Chicago: University of Chicago Press, 1973.

Huesmann, L. H., & Levinger, G. *Incremental Exchange Theory: A Formal Model for Progression in Dyadic Social Interactions*. Paper presented at the Annual Meeting of the American Psychological Association, Honolulu, September 2, 1972.

Hull, C. L. *Principles of Behavior*. New York: Appleton-Century-Crofts, 1943.

Human Development Institute. *Improving Communication in Marriage*. Atlanta: Human Development Institute, 1967.

Hunt, M., & Hunt, B. *The Divorce Experience: A New Look at the World of the Formerly Married*. New York: McGraw-Hill, 1978.

Hunt, R. A. The effect of item weighting on the Locke–Wallace Marital Adjustment Scale. *Journal of Marriage and the Family*, 1978, *40*, 249–256.

Hurley, J. R., & Palones, D. P. Marital satisfaction and child density among university student parents. *Journal of Marriage and the Family*, 1967, *29*, 483–484.

Hursch, C. J., Karacan, I., & Williams, R. L. Some characteristics of nocturnal penile tumescence in early middle aged males. *Comprehensive Psychiatry*, 1972, *13*, 539–548.

Hurvitz, N. *Marital Roles Inventory*. Los Angeles: Western Psychological Services, 1961.

Hurvitz, N. Control roles, marital strain, role deviation, and marital adjustment. *Journal of Marriage and the Family*, 1965, *27*, 29–31.

Hurvitz, N. Interaction hypotheses in marriage counseling. *The Family Coordinator*, 1970, *19*, 64–75.

Hurvitz, N. The family therapist as intermediary. *The Family Coordinator*, 1974, *23*, 145–158.

Husted, J. R. Desensitization procedures in dealing with female sexual dysfunction. *The Counseling Psychologist*, 1975, *5*(1), 30–37.

Insko, C. A., & Wilson, M. Interpersonal attraction as a function of social interaction. *Journal of Personality and Social Psychology*, 1977, *35*, 903–911.

Institute of Social Research. Measuring the quality of life in America. *ISR Newsletter*, 1974, *2*, 1–4.

Jackson, D. D. The question of family homeostasis. *Psychiatric Quarterly Supplement*, 1957, *31*, 79–90.

Jackson, D. D. Family rules—Marital quid pro quo. *Achives of General Psychiatry*, 1965, *12*, 589–594. (a)

Jackson, D. D. The study of the family. *Family Process*, 1965, *4*, 1–20. (b)

Jackson, D. D. *Therapy, Communication, and Change: Human Communication* (Vol. 1). Palo Alto, CA: Science and Behavior Books, 1968. (a)

Jackson, D. D. *Therapy, Communication, and Change: Human Communication* (Vol. 2). Palo Alto, CA: Science and Behavior Books, 1968. (b)

Jaco, D. E., & Shepard, J. M. Demographic homogeneity and spousal consensus: A methodological perspective. *Journal of Marriage and the Family*, 1975, *37*, 161–169.

Jacob, T. Assessment of marital dysfunction. In M. Hersen & A. S. Bellack (Eds.), *Behavioral Assessment: A Practical Handbook*. New York: Pergamon Press, 1976.

Jacob, T., Kornblith, S., Anderson, C., & Hartz, M. Role expectation and role performance in distressed and normal couples. *Journal of Abnormal Psychology*, 1978, *87*, 286–290.

Jacobson, G. F. The scope and practice of an early-access brief treatment psychiatric center. In H. H. Barten (Ed.), *Brief Therapies*. New York: Behavioral Publications, 1971.

Jacobson, N., & Margolin, G. *Marital Therapy: Strategies Based on Social Learning and Behavior Exchange Principles*. New York: Brunner/Mazel, 1979.

Jacobson, N. S. Training couples to solve their marital problems: A behavioral approach to relationship discord. *International Journal of Family Counseling*, 1977, *4*, 22–31.

Jacobson, N. S. Specific and nonspecific factors in the effectiveness of a behavioral approach to the treatment of marital discord. *Journal of Consulting and Clinical Psychology*, 1978, *46*, 442–452.

Jacobson, P. H. *American Marriage and Divorce*. New York: Rinehart, 1959.

Jacobson, W. D. *Power and Interpersonal Relations*. Bellmont, CA: Wadsworth Publishing Co., 1972.

Jakobovits, T. The treatment of impotence with methyltestosterone thyroid. *Fertility and Sterility*, 1970, *21*, 32–35.

James, W. *Essays in Pragmatism*. New York: Hafner Publishing Co., 1948.

Jankovich, R., & Miller, P. R. Response of women with primary orgasmic dysfunction to audiovisual education. *Journal of Sex and Marital Therapy*, 1978, *4*, 16–19.

Jayaratne, S., & Levy, P. *Empirical Clinical Practice*. New York: Columbia University Press, 1979.

Jayaratne, S., Stuart, R. B., & Tripodi, T. Methods for assessing the effectiveness of services for delinquents. In P. O. Davidson, F. Clark, & L. A. Hamerlynck (Eds.), *Evaluative Research in the Behavioral Sciences*. Champaign, IL: Research Press, 1974.

Jenkins, M. A. The influence of verbal information, models and behavioral rehearsal on the acquisition of appropriate "mate" behaviors. *Dissertation Abstracts International*, 1976, *37*, 1436.

Johannis, T. B., Jr., & Rollins, J. M. Teenager perceptions of family decision making. *Family Life Coordinator*, 1959, *7*, 70–74.

Johnson, D. F., & Pruitt, D. G. Preintervention effects of mediation versus arbitration. *Journal of Applied Psychology*, 1972, *56*, 1–10.

Johnson, J. Prognosis of disorders of sexual potency in the male. *Journal of Psychosomatic Research*, 1965, *9*, 195–200.

Johnson, S. M., & Labitz, G. K. The personal and marital adjustment of parents as related to observed child deviance and parenting behaviors. *Journal of Abnormal Child Psychology*, 1974, *2*, 193–207.

Jones, E. E. *Ingratiation*. New York: Appleton-Century-Crofts, 1964.

Jones, E. E., & Davis, K. E. From arts to dispositions: The attribution process in person perception. In L. Berkowitz (Ed.), *Advances in Experimental Social Psychology*, (Vol. 2). New York: Academic Press, 1965.

Jones, E. E., & Gerard, H. B. *Foundations of Social Psychology*. New York: John Wiley and Sons, 1967.

Jones, E. E., Gergen, K. J., & Davis, K. E. Some determinants of reactions to being approved or disproved as a person. *Psychological Monographs*, 1962, *76* (Whole No. 521).

Jones, E. E., & Nisbett, R. E. The actor and the observer: Divergent perceptions of the causes of behavior. Morristown, NJ: General Learning Press, 1971.

Jones, R. A. *Self-fulfilling Prophesies: Social, Psychological, and Physiological Effects of Experiences*. Hillsdale, NJ: Lawrence Erlbaum Associates, 1977.

Jones, W. J., & Park, P. M. Treatment of single-partner sexual dysfunction by systematic desensitization. *Obstetrics and Gynecology*, 1972, *39*(3), 411–417.

Jones, W. P. Some implications of the Sixteen Personality Factor Questionnaire for marital guidance. *Family Coordinator*, 1976, *25*, 189–192.

Jones, W. T. *The Twentieth Century to Wittgenstein and Sartre*. New York: Hartcourt Brace Jovanovich, 1975.

Jourard, S. M. Self-disclosure and other-cathesis. *Journal of Abnormal and Social Psychology*, 1959, *59*, 428–431.

Jourard, S. M. *The Transparent Self*. New York: Van Nostrand, 1971.

Jourard, S. M., & Jaffe, P. E. Influence of an interviewer's disclosure on the self-disclosing behavior of interviewees. *Journal of Counseling Psychology*, 1970, *17*, 252–257.

Jung, C. G. *Modern Man in Search of a Soul*. New York: Harcourt, 1933.

Kanfer, F. H., & Grimm, L. G. Freedom of choice and behavioral change. *Journal of Consulting and Clinical Psychology*, 1978, *46*, 873–878.

Kanfer, F. H., & Phillips, J. S. A survey of current behavior therapies and a proposal for classification. In C. M. Franks (Ed.), *Behavior Therapy: Appraisal and Status.* New York: McGraw-Hill, 1969.

Kanfer, F. H., & Seidner, M. Self-control: Factors enhancing the tolerance of noxious stimulation. *Journal of Personality and Social Psychology,* 1973, *25,* 381–389.

Kanouse, D. E., & Hanson, L. R. *Negativity in Evaluations.* Morristown, NJ: General Learning Press, 1972.

Kantor, D., & Lehr, W. *Inside the Family: Toward a Theory of Family Process.* San Francisco: Jossey-Bass, 1975.

Kaplan, A. G., & Bean, J. P. *Beyond Sex-Role Stereotypes: Readings toward a Psychology of Androgyny.* Boston: Little, Brown and Co., 1977.

Kaplan, H. S. *The New Sex Therapy.* New York: Brunner/Mazel, 1974.

Kaplan, H. S. Hypoactive sexual desire. *Journal of Sex and Marital Therapy,* 1977, *3,* 3–9.

Kaplan, H. S. *Disorders of Sexual Desire.* New York: Brunner/Mazel, 1979.

Kaplan, H. S., & Kohl, R. N. Adverse reactions to the rapid treatment of sexual problems. *Psychosomatics,* 1972, *13,* 185–190.

Kaplan, H. S., Kohl, R. N., Pomeroy, W. B., Offit, A. K., & Hogan, B. Group treatment of premature ejaculation. *Archives of Sexual Behavior,* 1974, *3,* 443–451.

Kaplan, M. F., & Anderson, N. H. Information integration theory and reinforcement theory as approaches to interpersonal attraction. *Journal of Personality and Social Psychology,* 1973, *28,* 301–312.

Karacan, I. The developmental aspect and the effect of certain clinical conditions upon penile erection during sleep. *Excerpta Medica International Congress Series,* 1968, *150,* 2356–2359.

Karacan, I., Williams, R. L., Thornby, J. I., & Salis, P. J. Sleep-related penile tumescence as a function of age. *American Journal of Psychiatry,* 1975, *132*(9), 932–937.

Kargman, M. W. The clinical use of social system theory in marriage counseling. *Marriage and Family Living,* 1957, *19,* 263–269.

Karlsson, G. *Adaptability and Communication in Marriage.* New Brunswick, NJ: Bedminister Press, 1963.

Karrass, C. L. *The Negotiating Game.* New York: World Publishing Co., 1970.

Katz, A. J., de Krasinski, M., Philip, E., & Wieser, C. Change in interactions as a measure of effectiveness in short term family therapy. *Family Therapy,* 1975, *2,* 31–56.

Katz, D. Psychological barriers to communication. *The Annals of the Academy of Political and Social Science,* 1947, *250,* 17–25.

Katz, M. M., & Lyerly, S. B. Methods for measuring adjustment and social behavior in the community: I. Rationale, description, discriminative validity and scale development. *Psychological Reports,* 1963, *13,* 1503–1555.

Katz, M. M., Cole, J. O., & Lowery, H. A. Studies of the diagnostic process: The influence of symptom perception, past experiences, and ethnic background on diagnostic decisions. *American Journal of Psychiatry,* 1969, *125,* 937–947.

Kazdin, A. E. *Behavior Modification in Applied Settings.* Homewood, IL: Dorsey Press, 1975.

Kedia, K., & Markland, C. The effect of pharmacological agents on ejaculation. *The Journal of Urology,* 1975, *114,* 569–573.

Kegel, A. H. Sexual functions of the pubococcygeus muscle. *Western Journal of Surgery, Obstetrics and Gynecology,* 1952, *60,* 521–524.

Kell, B. L., & Mueller, W. J. *Impact and Change: A Study of Counseling Relationships.* New York: Appleton-Century-Crofts, 1966.

Kelley, E. L. The reassessment of specific attitudes after twenty. *Journal of Social Issues,* 1961, *27,* 29–37.

Kelley, H. H. *Threats in Interpersonal Negotiations.* Paper presented at the Pittsburgh Seminar on Social Sciences of Organization, University of Pittsburgh, 1962.

Kelley, H. H. Experimental studies of threats in interpersonal negotiations. *Journal of Conflict Resolution,* 1965, *9,* 79–105.

Kelley, H. H., & Thibaut, J. W. *Interpersonal Relations.* New York: John Wiley and Sons, 1978.

Kelley, H. H., Thibaut, J. W., Radloff, R., & Mundy, D. The development of cooperation in the "minimal social situation." *Psychological Monographs: General and Applied,* 1962, *76,* Whole No. 538.

Kelly, C. M. Mental ability and personality factors in listening. *Quarterly Journal of Speech,* 1963, *49,* 152–156.

Kelly, C. M. Listening: Complex of activities—and a unitary skill? *Speech Monographs,* 1967, *34,* 455–466.

Kelly, C. M. Empathic listening. In R. S. Cathcart & L. A. Samovar (Eds.), *Small Group Communication.* Dubuque, IA: William C. Brown, 1970.

Kelly, G. *The Psychology of Personal Constructs.* New York: W. W. Norton, 1955.

Kenkel, W. F. Influence differentiation in family decision-making. *Sociology and Social Research,* 1957, *42,* 18–25.

Kenkel, W. F. Observational studies of husband–wife interaction in family decision making. In M. B. Sussman (Ed.), *Sourcebook in Marriage and the Family.* Boston: Houghton Mifflin Co., 1963.

Kenney, D. T. *An Experimental Test of the Cathartic Theory of Aggression.* Unpublished Ph.D. dissertation, University of Washington, 1952.

Kerckhoff, A. C. Patterns of marriage and family formulation and dissolution. *Journal of Consumer Research,* 1976, *2,* 261–275.

Kieren, D., & Tallman, I. Spousal adaptability: An assessment of marital competence. *Journal of Marriage and the Family,* 1972, *34,* 247–256.

Kiesler, D. J. *Use of Individualized Measures in Psychotherapy and Mental Health Program Evaluation Research: A Review of Target Complaints, Problem Oriented Record and Goal Attainment Scaling.* Rockville, MD: Clinical Research Branch, National Institute of Mental Health, 1977.

Kimmel, P. R., & Wavens, J. W. Game theory versus mutual identification: Two criteria for assessing marital relationships. *Journal of Marriage and Family,* 1966, *28,* 460–465.

King, J. A. Parameters relevant to determining the effect of early experience upon the adult behavior of animals. *Psychological Bulletin,* 1958, *55,* 46–58.

Kinsey, A., Pomeroy, W., Martin, C., & Gebhard, P. *Sexual Behavior in the Human Female.* Philadelphia: Saunders, 1953.

Kipnis, D. Does power corrupt? *Journal of Personality and Social Psychology,* 1972, *24,* 33–41.

Kiresuk, T. J., & Lund, S. H. Goal attainment scaling: Research, evaluation and utilization. In H. C. Schulberg & F. Baker (Eds.), *Program Evaluation in the Health Fields* (Vol. 2). New York: Behavioral Publications, 1977.

Kiresuk, T. J., & Sherman, R. E. Goal attainment scaling: A general method for evaluating comprehensive community mental health programs. *Community Mental Health Journal,* 1968, *4,* 443–453.

Kirkpatrick, C. *The Family as Process and Institution.* New York: Roland, 1955.

Kline-Graber, G., & Graber, B. Diagnosis and treatment procedures of pubococcygeal deficiencies in women. In J. LoPiccolo & L. LoPiccolo (Eds.), *Handbook of Sex Therapy.* New York: Plenum Press, 1978.

Klir, G. J. *An Approach to General Systems Theory.* New York: Van Nostrand, 1969.

Kluckhohn, F., & Strodtbeck, F. L. *Variations in Value Orientation.* Evanston, IL: Row, Peterson, 1961.

Knapp, J. J. Some non-monogamous marriage styles and related attitudes and practices of marriage counselors. *The Family Coordinator,* 1975, *24,* 505–514.

Knapp, J. An exploratory study of seventeen sexually open marriages. *Journal of Sex Research,* 1976, *12,* 206–219.

Knesevich, J. W., Biggs, J. T., Clayton, P. J., & Ziegler, V. W. Validity of the Hamilton Rating Scale for Depression. *British Journal of Psychiatry,* 1977, *131,* 49–52.

Knott, P. D., & Drost, B. A. Effects of varying intensity of attack and fear arousal on the intensity of counter aggression. *Journal of Personality,* 1972, *40,* 27–37.

Kockott, G., Dittmar, F., & Nusult, L. Systematic desensitization of erectile impotence: A controlled study. *Archives of Sexual Behavior*, 1975, *4*, 493–501.

Koegler, R. R., & Brill, N. Q. *Treatment of Psychiatric Outpatients.* New York: Appleton-Century-Crofts, 1967.

Kolb, T. M., & Straus, M. A. Marital power and marital happiness in relation to problem-solving. *Journal of Marriage and the Family*, 1974, *36*, 756–766.

Komarovsky, M. Class differences in family decision-making on expenditures. In N. F. Nelson (Ed.), *Household Decision-Making.* New York: NYU Press, 1961.

Komarovsky, M. *Blue-Collar Marriage.* New York: Vantage Books, 1967.

Komorita, S. S., & Brenner, A. R. Bargaining and concession making under bilateral monopoly. *Journal of Personality and Social Psychology*, 1968, *9*, 15–20.

Komorita, S. S., Sheposh, J. P., & Braver, S. L. Power, the use of power, and co-operative choice in a two-person game. *Journal of Personality and Social Psychology*, 1968, *8*, 134–142.

Kopel, S., & Arkowitz, H. The role of attribution and self-perception in behavior change: Implications for behavior therapy. *Genetic Psychology Monographs*, 1975, *92*, 175–212.

Kostlan, A. A. A method for the empirical study of psychodiagnosis. *Journal of Consulting Psychology*, 1954, *18*, 83–88.

Kotlar, S. L. Role theory in marriage counseling. *Sociology and Social Research*, 1967–1968, *52*, 50–62.

Kraft, T., & Al-Issa, I. The use of methohexitone sodium in the systematic desensitization of premature ejaculation. *British Journal of Psychiatry*, 1968, *114*, 351–352.

Kraus, A. S., & Lillienfeld, A. M. Some epidemiologic aspects of the high mortality rate in the young widowed group. *Journal of Chronic Diseases*, 1959, *10*, 207–217.

Krech, D., Crutchfield, R. S., & Y Ballachey, E. L. *Individual in Society.* New York: McGraw-Hill, 1962.

Krell, R., & Miles, J. E. Marital therapy of couples in which the husband is a physician. *American Journal of Psychotherapy*, 1976, *30*, 267–275.

Kursh, C. O. The benefits of poor communication. *The Psychoanalytic Review*, 1971, *58*, 189–208.

L'Abate, L., Wildman, R. W., O'Callaghan, J. B., Simon, S. J., Allison, M., Kahn, G., & Rainwater, N. The laboratory evaluation and enrichment of couples: Applications and some preliminary results. *Journal of Marriage and Family Counseling*, 1975, *1*, 351–357.

Laing, R. D., & Esterson, A. *Sanity, Madness and the Family.* Baltimore: Penguin Books, 1970.

Laing, R. D., Phillipson, H., & Lee, A. R. *Interpersonal Perception: A Theory and a Method of Research.* New York: Harper and Row, 1972.

Lambert, M. J., Bergin, A. E., & Collins, J. L. Therapist-induced deterioration in psycho-therapy. In A. S. Gurman & A. M. Razin (Eds.), *The Therapist's Contribution to Effective Psychotherapy: An Empirical Assessment.* New York: Pergamon Press, 1976.

Lambert, M. J., Bergin, A. E., & Collins, J. L. Therapist-induced deterioration in psycho-therapy. In A. S. Gurman & A. M. Razin (Eds.), *Effective Psychotherapy: A Handbook of Research.* New York: Pergamon Press, 1977.

Lamont, C. *Humanism as a Philosophy.* New York: Philosophical Library, 1949.

Lamont, J. A. Vaginismus. In R. Gemme & C. C. Wheeler (Eds.), *Progress in Sexology.* New York: Plenum Press, 1977.

Landfield, A. W., O'Donovan, D., & Narvas, M. M. Improvement ratings by external judges and psychotherapists. *Psychological Reports*, 1962, *11*, 747–748.

Laner, M. R. The medical model, mental illness, and metaphoric mystification among marriage and family counselors. *Family Coordinator*, 1976, *25*, 175–181.

Laner, M. R. Love's labors lost: A theory of marital dissolution. *Journal of Divorce*, 1978, *1*, 213–232.

Lange, A. J., & Jakubowski, P. *Responsible Assertive Behavior.* Champaign, IL: Research Press, 1976.

Langer, E., & Rodin, J. The effects of choice and enhanced personal responsibility for the aged: A field experiment in an institutional setting. *Journal of Personality and Social Psychology*, 1976, *34*, 191–198.

Langer, E. J., Janis, I. L., & Wolfer, J. A. Reduction of psychological stress in surgical patients. *Journal of Experimental Social Psychology*, 1975, *11*, 155–165.

Lansky, M. R., & Davenport, A. E. Difficulties in brief conjoint treatment of sexual dysfunction. *American Journal of Psychiatry*, 1975, *132*(2), 177–179.

Larson, L. E. System and sub-system perception of family roles. *Journal of Marriage and the Family*, 1974, *36*, 123–128.

Laszlo, C. A., Levine, M. D., & Milsun, J. H. A general system framework for social systems. *Behavioral Science*, 1974, *19*, 79–92.

Latane, B., Meitzer, J., Joy, V., Lubell, B., & Cappell, H. Stimulus determinants of social attraction in rats. *Journal of Comparative and Physiological Psychology*, 1972, *79*, 12–21.

Laws, J. L. A feminist view of marital adjustment literature. *Journal of Marriage and the Family*, 1971, *33*, 483–516.

Lazarus, A. A. Group therapy of phobic disorders by systematic desensitization. *Journal of Abnormal and Social Psychology*, 1961, *63*, 504–510.

Lazarus, A. A. The treatment of chronic frigidity by systematic desensitization. *Journal of Nervous and Mental Disease*, 1963, *136*, 272–278.

Lazarus, A. A. Multimodal behavior therapy: Treating the "BASIC ID." *Journal of Nervous and Mental Disease*, 1973, *156*, 404–411.

Lazarus, A. A. *Multimodal Behavior Therapy*. New York: Springer, 1976.

Lazarus, A. A. *Personal communication*, November 26, 1978.

Leary, T. *Multilevel Measurement of Interpersonal Behavior: A Manual for the Use of the Interpersonal System of Personality*. Berkeley: Psychological Consultation Service, 1956.

Leavitt, H. J. Some effects of certain communication patterns on group performance. *Journal of Abnormal Social Psychology*, 1951, *46*, 38–50.

Leckie, F. H. Hypnotherapy in gynecological disorders. *International Journal of Clinical and Experimental Hypnosis*, 1964, *12*, 121–146.

Lederer, W. J., & Jackson, D. D. *Mirages of Marriage*. New York: W. W. Norton, 1968.

Ledwidge, B. Cognitive behavior modification: A step in the wrong direction? *Psychological Bulletin*, 1978, *85*(2), 353–375.

Lee, G. R. Age at marriage and marital satisfaction: A multivariate analysis with implications for marital stability. *Journal of Marriage and the Family*, 1977, *39*, 493–504.

Lefkowitz, M. B. Statistical and clinical approaches to the identification of couples at risk in marriage. *Dissertation Abstracts International*, 1974, *34*, 5199.

Leiblum, S. R., & Kopel, S. A. Screening and prognosis in sex therapy: To treat or not to treat. *Behavior Therapy*, 1977, *8*, 480–486.

Leiblum, S. R., Rosen, R. C., & Pierce, D. Group treatment format: Mixed sexual dysfunctions. *Archives of Sexual Behavior*, 1976, *5*, 313–322.

Leik, R. K. Instrumentality and emotionality in family interaction. *Sociometry*, 1963, *26*, 131–145.

LeMasters, E. E. Parenthood as crisis. *Marriage and Family Living*, 1957, *19*, 352–355.

Lempert, R. Norm-making in social exchange: A contract law model. *Law and Society*, 1972, *4*, 1–32.

Lennard, H. L., & Bernstein, A. *The Anatomy of Psychotherapy*. New York: Columbia University Press, 1960.

Lenthall, G. Marital satisfaction and marital stability. *Journal of Marriage and Family Counseling*, 1977, *3*, 25–31.

Leslie, G. R. Should the partners be seen together or separately? In R. H. Klemer (Ed.), *Counseling in Marital and Sexual Problems: A Physician's Handbook*. Baltimore: Williams and Wilkins Co., 1965.

Leslie, G. R. Family breakdown. In J. B. Turner (Ed.-in-Chief), *Encyclopedia of Social Work*,

Seventeenth Issue (Vol. 1). Washington, DC: National Association of Social Workers, 1977.

Lester, D., & Lester, G. Suicide: The Gamble with Death. Englewood Cliffs, NJ: Prentice-Hall, 1972.

Lett, E. E., Clark, W., & Altman, I. A Propositional Inventory of Research on Interpersonal Distance. Bethesda, MD: Naval Medical Research Institute, 1969.

Levinger, G. Task and social behavior in marriage. Sociometry, 1964, 27, 433–448.

Levinger, G. Altruism in marriage: A test of Buerkle–Badgley Battery. Journal of Marriage and the Family, 1965, 27, 32–33.

Levinger, G. Sources of marital dissatisfaction among applicants for divorce. American Journal of Orthopsychiatry, 1966, 36, 803–807.

Levinger, G. A social psychological perspective on marital dissolution. Journal of Social Issues, 1976, 32, 21–47.

Levinger, G., & Breedlove, J. Interpersonal attraction and agreement: A study of marriage partners. Journal of Personality and Social Psychology, 1966, 3, 367–372.

Levinger, G., & Moles, O. C. In conclusion: Threads in the fabric. Journal of Social Issues, 1976, 32, 193–207.

Levinger, G., & Senn, D. J. Disclosure of feelings in marriage. Merrill-Palmer Quarterly of Behavior and Development, 1967, 13, 237–249.

Levinson, P. J. The Seasons of a Man's Life. New York: Alfred A. Knopf, 1978.

Lévi-Strauss, C. Reciprocity, the essence of social life. In L. Coser & M. Rosenberg (Eds.), Sociological Theory. New York: Macmillan Co., 1957.

Levitsky, A., & Perls, F. S. The rules and games of gestalt therapy. In J. Fagan & I. L. Shepherd (Eds.), Gestalt Therapy Now: Theories, Techniques, Applications. New York: Harper Colophon Books, 1970.

Levy, R. L. Relationship of an overt commitment to task compliance in behavior therapy. Journal of Behavior Therapy and Experimental Psychiatry, 1977, 8, 22–29.

Lewin, K. Resolving Social Conflicts. New York: Harper and Row, 1948.

Lewin, K. Field Theory in Social Science. New York: Harper and Row, 1951.

Lewinsohn, P. M. Clinical and theoretical aspects of depression. In K. S. Calhoun, H. E. Adams, & K. M. Mitchell (Eds.), Innovative Treatment Methods in Psychopathology. New York: John Wiley and Sons, 1974.

Lewinsohn, P. M., & Nichols, R. C. Dimensions of change in mental hospital patients. Journal of Clinical Psychology, 1967, 23, 498–503.

Lewis, J. M., Beavers, W. R., Gossett, J. T., & Phillips, V. A. No Single Thread: Psychological Health in Family Systems. New York: Brunner/Mazel, 1976.

Lewis, R. A. Satisfaction with Conjugal Power over the Family Life Cycle. Paper presented at the Annual Meeting of the National Council on Family Relations, Portland, OR, October 31, 1972.

Lewis, S. A., & Pruitt, D. G. Orientation, aspiration level and communication freedom in integrative bargaining. Proceedings, 79th Annual Convention, American Psychological Association, 1971, Washington, DC.

Liberman, B. L., Frank, J. D., Hoehn-Saric, R., Stone, A. R., Imber, S. D., & Pande, S. K. Patterns of change in treated psychoneurotic patients: A five-year follow-up investigation of the systematic preparation of patients for psychotherapy. Journal of Consulting and Clinical Psychology, 1972, 38, 36–41.

Liberman, R. P., & Raskin, D. E. Depression: A behavioral formulation. Archives of General Psychiatry, 1971, 24, 515–523.

Liberman, R. P., Levine, J., Wheeler, E., Sanders, N., & Wallace, C. J. Marital therapy in groups: A comparative evaluation of behavioral and interactional formats. Acta Psychiatrica Scandinavica, 1976, Supplement 226, 3–34. (a)

Liberman, R. P., Wheeler, E., & Sanders, N. Behavioral therapy for marital disharmony: An educational approach. Journal of Marriage and Family Counseling, 1976, 2, 383–395. (b)

Lieberman, M. A., Yolom, I. D., & Miles, M. B. *Encounter Groups: First Facts.* New York: Basic Books, 1973.

Liem, G. R. Performance and satisfaction as affected by personal control over salient decisions. *Journal of Personality and Social Psychology, 1975, 31,* 232–240.

Lindley, D. V. *Making Decisions.* New York: Wiley Interscience, 1971.

Lindner, B. J. Patterning of psychological type, interpersonal understanding, and marital happiness. *Dissertation Abstracts International,* 1973, *34,* 417–418.

Lobitz, W. C., & Baker, E. L. Group treatment of sexual dysfunction: Coping skill training for single males. In D. Upper & S. M. Ross (Eds.), *Behavioral Group Therapy: Annual Review.* Champaign, IL: Research Press, 1979.

Lobitz, W. C., & Lobitz, G. K. Clinical assessment in the treatment of sexual dysfunction. In J. LoPiccolo & L. LoPiccolo (Eds.), *Handbook of Sex Therapy.* New York: Plenum Press, 1978.

Lobitz, W. C., & LoPiccolo, J. New methods in the behavioral treatment of sexual dysfunction. *Journal of Behavior Therapy and Experimental Psychiatry,* 1972, *3,* 265–271.

Locke, H. *Predicting Adjustment in Marriage.* New York: Holt, Rinehart and Winston, 1951.

Locke, H. J., & Wallace, K. M. Short marital adjustment and prediction tests: Their reliability and validity. *Marriage and Family Living,* 1959, *21,* 251–255.

Locke, H. J., & Williamson, R. C. Marital adjustment: A factor analysis study. *American Sociological Review,* 1958, *23,* 562–569.

Locke, H. J., Sabagh, G., & Thomes, M. M. Correlates of primary communication and empathy. *Research Studies of the State College of Washington,* 1956, *24,* 116–124.

Lombardo, J. P., Weiss, R. F., & Buchanan, W. Reinforcing and attracting functions of yielding. *Journal of Personality and Social Psychology,* 1972, *21,* 350–368.

Lombrillo, J., Kiresuk, T., & Sherman, R. Evaluating a community mental health program: Contract fulfillment analysis. *Hospital and Community Psychiatry,* 1973, *24,* 760–762.

Long, T. J. The effects of pretraining procedures on client behavior during initial counseling interviews. *Dissertation Abstracts,* 1968, *29,* 1784A.

Longabaugh, R., Eldred, S., Bell, N. W., & Sherman, L. J. The interactional world of the chronic schizophrenic. *Psychiatry,* 1966, *29,* 78–99.

LoPiccolo, J. Direct treatment of sexual dysfunction. In J. Money & H. Musaph (Eds.), *Handbook of Sexology.* Amsterdam: ASP Biological and Medical Press B. V., 1977.

LoPiccolo, J., & Lobitz, W. C. Behavior therapy of sexual dysfunction. In L. A. Hamerlynck, L. C. Handy, & E. J. Mash (Eds.), *Behavior Change: Methodology, Concepts and Practice.* Champaign, IL: Research Press, 1973.

LoPiccolo, L., & Heiman, J. R. Sexual assessment and history interview. In J. LoPiccolo & L. LoPiccolo (Eds.), *Handbook of Sex Therapy.* New York: Plenum Press, 1978.

Lorenz, K. *On Aggression.* New York: Harcourt, Brace and World, 1966.

Lorr, M., & McNair, D. M. Methods relating to evaluation of therapeutic outcome. In L. A. Gottschalk & A. H. Auerbach (Eds.), *Methods of Research in Psychotherapy.* New York: Appleton-Century-Crofts, 1966.

Lorr, M., McNair, D. M., Michaux, W. W., & Raskin, A. Frequency of treatment and change in psychotherapy. *Journal of Abnormal and Social Psychology,* 1962, *64,* 281–292.

Lott, A. J., & Lott, B. E. A learning theory approach to interpersonal attitudes. In A. G. Greenwald, T. C. Brock, & T. M. Ostrom (Eds.), *Psychological Foundations of Attitudes.* New York: Academic Press, 1968.

Lovejoy, D. D. College student conceptions of the roles of husband and wife in family decision-making. *The Family Coordinator,* 1961, *10,* 43–46.

Lowe, J. C., & Milulas, W. L. Use of written material in learning self-control of premature ejaculation. *Psychological Reports,* 1975, *37,* 295–298.

Lu, Y. Marital roles and marriage adjustment. *Sociology and Social Research,* 1952, *34,* 364–368.

Luckey, E. B. Marital interaction and perceptual congruence of self and family concepts. *Sociometry,* 1961, *24,* 234–250.

Luckey, E. B., & Bain, J. K. Children: A factor in marital satisfaction. *Journal of Marriage and the Family*, 1970, *32*, 43–44.

Lunghi, M. E. The stability of mood and social perception measures in a sample of depressive in-patients. *British Journal of Psychiatry*, 1977, *130*, 598–604.

Luria, A. *The Nature of Human Conflicts*. New York: Liveright, 1932.

Lynch, J. J. *The Broken Heart: The Medical Consequences of Loneliness*. New York: Basic Books, 1977.

MacAndrew, C. The differentiation of male alcoholic outpatients from nonalcoholic psychiatric outpatients by means of the MMPI. *Quarterly Journal of Studies on Alcohol*, 1965, *26*, 238–246.

Mace, D. R. Marital intimacy and the deadly love–anger cycle. *Journal of Marriage and Family Counseling*, 1976, *2*, 131–137.

Mack, D. E. The power relation in black families and white families. *Journal of Personality and Social Psychology*, 1974, *30*, 409–413.

MacPhillamy, D. J., & Lewinsohn, P. M. Depression as a function of levels of desired and obtained pleasure. *Journal of Abnormal Psychology*, 1973, *81*, 259–295.

Magnus, E. C. Measurement of counselor bias in assessment of marital couples with traditional and nontraditional interaction patterns. *Dissertation Abstracts International*, 1975, *36*, 2635.

Mahoney, J. J., & Thoresen, C. E. (Eds.). *Self-control: Power to the Person*. Monterey, CA: Brooks/Cole, 1974.

Mahoney, M. J. Some applied issues in self-monitoring. In J. D. Cone & R. P. Hawkins (Eds.), *Behavioral Assessment: New Directions in Clinical Psychology*. New York: Brunner/Mazel, 1977.

Maier, N. *Problem-solving Discussions and Conferences: Leadership Methods and Skills*. New York: McGraw-Hill, 1963.

Maier, N. R. F., & Hoffman, L. R. Using trained developmental discussion leaders to improve further the quality of group decision. *Journal of Applied Psychology*, 1960, *44*, 247–251.

Malan, D. On assessing the results of psychotherapy. *British Journal of Medical Psychology*, 1959, *32*, 86–105.

Malan, D. H. *A Study of Brief Psychotherapy*. New York: Plenum Press, 1963.

Malan, D., Heath, E. S., Bacal, H. A., & Balfour, F. H. G. Psychodynamic changes in untreated neurotic patients. *Archives of General Psychiatry*, 1975, *32*, 110–126.

Malinowski, B. The problem of meaning in primitive languages. In C. K. Ogden & I. A. Richards (Eds.), *The Meaning of Meaning*. New York: Harcourt Brace Jovanovich, 1923.

Mangus, A. Relation between the young woman's conceptions of her intimate male associates and of her ideal husband. *Journal of Social Psychology*, 1936, *7*, 403–420.

Manning, W. H., & DuBois, P. H. Correlational methods in research and human learning. *Perceptual and Motor Skills*, 1962, *15*, 287–321.

March, J. G. An introduction to the theory and measurement of influence. *American Political Science Review*, 1955, *49*, 431–451.

Margolin, G. A multilevel approach to the assessment of communication positiveness in distressed marital couples. *International Journal of Family Counseling*, 1977, *6*, 81–89.

Margolin, G. Relationships among marital assessment procedures: A correlational study. *Journal of Consulting and Clinical Psychology*, 1978, *46*, 1476–1486.

Margolis, R., & Leslie, C. H. Review of studies on a mixture of methyltestosterone in the treatment of impotence. *Current Therapeutic Research*, 1966, *8*, 280–284.

Margolis, R., Sangree, H., Prieto, P., Stein, L., & Chinn, S. Clinical studies on the use of afrodex in treatment of impotence: Statistical study of 4,000 cases. *Current Therapeutic Reasearch*, 1967, *9*, 213–219.

Marini, M. M. Dimensions of marriage happiness: A research note. *Journal of Marriage and the Family*, 1976, *38*, 443–447.

Maris, R. W. *Social Forces in Urban Suicide*. Homewood, IL: Dorsey Press, 1969.

Marmor, J. Common operational factors in diverse approaches to behavior change. In A. Burton (Ed.), *What Makes Behavior Change Possible?* New York: Brunner/Mazel, 1976.

Marquis, J. N. Orgasmic reconditioning: Changing sexual object choice through controlling masturbation fantasies. *Journal of Behavior Therapy and Experimental Psychiatry,* 1970, *1,* 263–271.

Martin, P. J., & Sterne, A. L. Prognostic expectations and treatment outcome. *Journal of Consulting and Clinical Psychology,* 1975, *43,* 572–576.

Martin, W. T. Status integration, social stress, and mental illness: Accounting for marital status variations in mental hospitalization rates. *Journal of Health and Social Behavior,* 1976, *17,* 280–294.

Maslow, A. H. *New Knowledge in Human Values.* New York: Harper and Row, 1959.

Masters, W. H., & Johnson, V. E. *Human Sexual Inadequacy.* Boston: Little, Brown and Co., 1970.

Masters, W. H., & Johnson, V. E. A pictorial review of the stages of sexual response in men. *Medical Aspects of Human Sexuality,* 1972, *6,* 78–83.

Masters, W. H. Johnson, V. E., & Kolodny, R. C. *Post-graduate Workshop on Human Sexual Function and Dysfunction.* St. Louis: Reproductive Biology Research Foundation, 1978.

Mathews, V. C., & Milhanovich, C. S. New orientations on marital adjustment. *Marriage and Family Living,* 1963, *25,* 300–305.

Mayer, J. E., & Zander, M. *The Disclosure of Marital Problems: An Exploratory Study of Lower and Middle Class Wives.* New York: Community Service Society, 1966.

McCain, H. B. The social network and wife as companion. *Dissertation Abstracts International,* 1974, *34,* 7348.

McCall, G. J., & Simmons, J. L. *Identities and Interactions.* New York: The Free Press, 1966.

McCary, J. L. *McCary's Human Sexuality* (3rd ed.). New York: D. Van Nostrand, 1978.

McClintock, C. G., & McNeel, S. P. Prior dyadic experience and monetary reward as determinants of cooperative and competitive game behavior. *Journal of Personality and Social Psychology,* 1967, *5,* 282–294.

McDermott, J. F. Divorce and its psychiatric sequelae in children. *Archives of General Psychiatry,* 1970, *23,* 421–427.

McDonald, D. *The Language of Argument.* Scranton, PA: Chandler Publishing Company, 1971.

McDonald, G. W. Coalition formation in marital therapy triads. *Family Therapy,* 1975, *2,* 141–148.

McGovern, K., Kirkpatrick, C., & LoPiccolo, J. A behavioral group treatment program for sexually dysfunctional couples. *Journal of Marriage and Family Counseling,* 1976, *2,* 397–404.

McGovern, K. B., McMullen, R. S., & LoPiccolo, J. Secondary orgasmic dysfunction: I. Analysis and strategies for treatment. *Archives of Sexual Behavior,* 1975, *4*(3), 265–275.

McLean, P. Therapeutic decision making in the behavioral treatment of depression. In P. O. Davidson (Ed.), *The Behavioral Management of Anxiety, Depression and Pain.* New York: Brunner/Mazel, 1976.

McMillan, E. L. Problem build-up: A description of couples in marriage counseling. *The Family Coordinator,* 1969, *18,* 260–267.

McMullen, S. J. Automated procedures for treatment of primary orgasmic dysfunction. *Dissertation Abstracts International,* 1976, *37*(10B), 5364.

McPherson, S. Communication of intents among parents and their disturbed adolescent child. *Journal of Abnormal Psychology,* 1970, *76,* 98–105.

Mead, G. H. *Mind, Self and Society.* Chicago: University of Chicago Press, 1934.

Mead, G. H. *The Philosophy of the Act.* Chicago: University of Chicago Press, 1938.

Mead, M. *Male and Female: A Study of the Sexes in a Changing World.* New York: William Morrow and Co., 1949.

Meck, D. S., & Leunes, A. Perceived similarity and the marital dyad. *Family Therapy,* 1976, *3,* 229–234.

Meck, D. S., & Leunes, A. Marital instability in a semirural setting: Personality considerations. *Journal of Community Psychology*, 1977, *5*, 278–281. (a)

Meck, D. S., & Leunes, A. Personality similarity–dissimilarity and underlying psychopathology in couples seeking marital counseling. *Journal of Marriage and Family Counseling*, 1977, *3*, 63–66. (b)

Meehl, P. E. Some ruminations on the validation of clinical procedures. *Canadian Journal of Psychology*, 1959, *13*, 102–128.

Mehrabian, A. Significance of posture and position in the communication of attitude and status relationships. *Psychological Bulletin*, 1969, *71*, 359–372.

Mehrabian, A. *Tactics of Social Influence*. Englewood Cliffs, NJ: Prentice-Hall, 1970.

Mehrabian, A. *Nonverbal Communication*. Chicago: Aldine Atherton, 1972.

Mehrabian, A., & Williams, M. Nonverbal concomitants of perceived and intended persuasiveness. *Journal of Personality and Social Psychology*, 1969, *13*, 37–58.

Meichenbaum, D. *Cognitive-Behavior Modification*. New York: Plenum Press, 1977.

Meisel, S. S. The treatment of sexual problems in marital and family therapy. *Clinical Social Work Journal*, 1977, *5*, 200–209.

Meltzoff, J., & Kornreich, M. *Research in Psychotherapy*. New York: Atherton Press, 1970.

Merrill, F. E. *Courtship and Marriage*. New York: Henry Holt, 1959.

Merton, R. *Social Theory and Social Structure*. New York: The Free Press, 1957.

Messinger, L. Remarriage between divorced people with children from previous marriages: A proposal for preparation for remarriage. *Journal of Marriage and Family Counseling*, 1977, *2*, 193–200.

Mettee, D. R. Changes in liking as a function of the magnitude and effect of sequential evaluations. *Journal of Experimental Social Psychology*, 1971, *7*, 157–172.

Meyer, J. K., Schmidt, C. W., Lucas, M. J., & Smith, E. Short-term treatment of sexual problems: Interim report. *American Journal of Psychiatry*, 1975, *132*(2), 172–176.

Meyer, J. P., & Pepper, S. Need compatibility and marital adjustment in young married couples. *Journal of Personality and Social Psychology*, 1977, *35*(5), 331–342.

Miaoulis, C. N. A study of the innovative use of time and planned short-term treatment in conjoint marital counseling. *Dissertation Abstracts International*, 1976, *37*(4-A), 1993–1994.

Middleton, R., & Putney, S. Dominance in decisions in the family race and class differences. *American Journal of Sociology*, 1960, *65*, 605–609.

Milburn, T. W. *Some Conditions When Perceived Threats Do and Do Not Provoke Violent Responses*. Paper presented at the 72nd annual meeting of the American Psychological Association, New Orleans, 1974.

Miles, J. E., Krell, R., & Tsung-yi, L. The doctor's wife: Mental illness and marital pattern. *International Journal of Psychiatry in Medicine*, 1975, *6*(4), 481–487.

Millenson, J. R. *Principles of Behavioral Analysis*. New York: Macmillan Co., 1967.

Miller, B. C. A multivariate developmental model of marital satisfaction. *Journal of Marriage and the Family*, 1976, *38*, 643–657.

Miller, G. A., Heise, G. A., & Lichten, W. The intelligibility of speech as a function of the test materials. *Journal of Experimental Psychology*, 1951, *41*, 329–335.

Miller, G. A., Galanter, E., & Pribram, K. H. *Plans and Structure of Behavior*. New York: Holt, Rinehart & Winston, 1960.

Miller, H., &. Geller, D. Structural balance in dyads. *Journal of Personality and Social Psychology*, 1972, *21*, 135–138.

Miller, N. E. Experimental studies of conflict. In J. M. Hunt (Ed.), *Personality and the Behavior Disorders*. New York: Roland, 1944.

Miller, N. E. Some implications of modern behavior therapy for personality change and psychotherapy. In P. Worchel & D. Byrne (Eds.), *Personality Change*. New York: John Wiley and Sons, 1964.

Miller, N. E., & Dollard, J. *Social Learning and Imitation*. New Haven, CT: Yale University Press, 1941.

Miller, S. *Marriages and Families: Enrichment through Communication.* Beverly Hills, CA: Sage Publications, 1975.

Miller, S., Nunnally, E. W., & Wackman, D. B. *Alive and Aware: Improving Communication in Relationships.* Minneapolis: Interpersonal Communications Programs, 1975.

Miller, S., Nunnally, E. W., Wackman, D. B., & Ferris, R. H. *Couple Workbook: Increasing Awareness and Communication Skills.* Minneapolis: Interpersonal Communication Programs, 1976.

Miller, W. R., & Seligman, M. E. P. Depression and learned helplessness in man. *Journal of Abnormal Psychology,* 1975, *84,* 228–238.

Mills, T. M. Power relations in three-person groups. *American Sociological Review,* 1953, *18,* 351–357.

Mintz, J. What is "success" in psychotherapy? *Journal of Abnormal Psychology,* 1972, *80,* 11–19.

Minuchin, S., Averswald, E., & King, C. H. *The Study and Treatment of Families Who Produce Multiple Acting-Out Boys.* Paper presented at American Orthopsychiatric Association, March 1963.

Mirowitz, J. M. Utilization of hypnosis in psychic impotence. *British Journal of Medical Hypnosis,* 1966, *17,* 25–32.

Mischel, W. *Personality and Assessment.* New York: John Wiley and Sons, 1968.

Mischel, W. Toward a cognitive social learning reconceptualization of personality. *Psychological Review,* 1973, *80,* 252–283.

Mishler, E. G., & Waxler, N. E. *Interaction in Families.* New York: John Wiley and Sons, 1968.

Monahan, T. P. Family status and the delinquent child: A reappraisal and some new findings. *Social Forces,* 1957, *35,* 250–258.

Montague, E. K., & Taylor, E. N. Preliminary handbook on procedures for evaluating mental health indirect service programs in schools. *Technical Report No. 71-18.* Alexandria, VA: Human Resources Research Organization, 1971.

Moore, O. K., & Anderson, A. R. Some principles for the design of clarifying educational environments. In J. Aldous, T. Condon, R. Hill, M. Straus, & I. Tallman (Eds.), *Family Problem-Solving.* Hinsdale, IL: The Dryden Press, 1971.

Moore, W. E., & Tumin, M. M. Some social functions of ignorance. *American Sociological Review,* 1949, *14,* 787–795.

Moos, R. H. *Family Environment Scale.* Palo Alto; CA: Consulting Psychologists Press, 1974.

Morgan, J. N. *Five Thousand American Families: Patterns of Economic Progress.* Ann Arbor, MI: Institute for Social Research, 1973.

Morris, R. J., & Suckerman, K. R. Therapist warmth as a factor in automated systematic desensitization. *Journal of Consulting and Clinical Psychology,* 1974, *42,* 244–250.

Morse, B. L. An investigation of the relationship between marital adjustment and marital interaction. *Dissertation Abstracts International,* 1973, *34*(1B), 420.

Moscovici, S., & Doise, W. Decision making in groups. In C. Nemeth (Ed.), *Social Psychology: Classic and Contemporary Integrations.* Chicago: Rand McNally College Publishing Company, 1974.

Mouton, J. S., & Blake, R. R. *The Marriage Grid.* New York: McGraw-Hill, 1971.

Mowrer, O. H., & Ullman, A. D. Time as a determinant in integrative learning. *Psychological Review,* 1945, *52,* 61–90.

Mueller, P. S., & Orfanidis, M. M. A method of co-therapy for schizophrenic families. *Family Process,* 1976, *15,* 179–191.

Mueller, W. J. Patterns of behavior and their reciprocal impact in the family and in psychotherapy. *Journal of Counseling Psychology,* 1969, *16,* Whole No. 2, Part 2, 1–25.

Muench, G. A. An investigation of time-limited psychotherapy. *American Psychologist,* 1964, *19,* 317–318. (Abstract)

Mulder, M. Communication structure, decision structure and group performance. *Sociometry,* 1960, *23,* 1–14.

Mullen, J., & Abeles, N. Relationship of liking, empathy, and therapist's experience to outcome of therapy. *Journal of Consulting Psychology*, 1971, *18*, 39–43.

Munjack, D., Cristol, A., Goldstein, A., Phillips, D., Goldberg, A., Whipple, K., Staples, F., & Kanno, P. Behavioral treatment of orgasmic dysfunction: A controlled study. *British Journal of Psychiatry*, 1976, *129*, 497–502.

Munjack, D. J., & Oziel, L. J. Resistance in the behavioral treatment of sexual dysfunction. *Journal of Sex and Marital Therapy*, 1978, 4, 122–138.

Murray, H. A. *Explorations in Personality*. New York: Oxford, 1938.

Murray, H. A. Preparations for the scaffold of a comprehensive system. In S. Koch (Ed.), *Psychology: A Study of a Science* (Vol. 3). *Formulations of the Person and the Social Context*. New York: McGraw-Hill, 1959.

Murray, M. E. A model for family therapy integrating system and subsystem dynamics. *Family Therapy*, 1975, *2*, 187–197.

Murrell, S. A., & Stachowiak, J. G. Consistency, rigidity, and power in the interaction patterns of clinic and nonclinic families. *Journal of Abnormal Psychology*. 1976, *72*, 265–272.

Murstein, B. I. *Current and Future Intimate Lifestyles*. New York: Springer, 1977.

Murstein, B. I., & Christy, P. Physical attractiveness and marriage adjustment in middle-aged couples. *Journal of Personality and Social Psychology*, 1976, *34*, 537–542.

Murstein, B. I., Cerreto, M., & MacDonald, M. G. A theory and investigation of the effect of exchange-orientation on marriage and friendship. *Journal of Marriage and the Family*, 1977, *40*, 543–548.

Nagel, J. H. Some questions about the concept of power. *Behavioral Science*, 1968, *13*, 129–137.

National Center for Health Statistics. Increases in divorces: United States, 1967. Vital and Health Statistics, Series 21, Number 20. Rockville, MD: Public Health Service, 1970.

National Center for Health Statistics. Divorces: Analysis of changes: United States, 1969. Vital and Health Statistics, Series 21, Number 22. Rockville, MD: DHEW Publication No. (HSM) 73:1900, 1973. (a)

National Center for Health Statistics. 100 years of marriage and divorce statistics, United States, 1867–1967. Rockville, MD: DHEW Publication No. (HRA) 74-1902, 1973. (b)

National Center for Health Statistics, Unpublished data. Cited by H. Carter & P. C. Glick, *Marriage and Divorce: A Social and Economic Study*. Cambridge, MA: Harvard University Press, 1976.

National Center for Health Statistics. Divorces and divorce rates: United States. Hyattsville, MD: DHEW Publication No. (PHS) 78-1907, 1978. (a)

National Center for Health Statistics. Divorces and divorce rates: United States. Vital and Health Statistics, Series 21, Number 29. Hyattsville, MD: DHEW Publication No. (PHS) 78-1907, 1978. (b)

National Center for Health Statistics. Facts of life and death. Hyattsville, MD: DHEW Publication No. (PHS) 79-1222, 1978. (c)

National Center for Health Statistics. Monthly Vital Statistics Report: Provisional statistics. DHEW Publication No. (PHS) 79-1120, *26*(13), December 7, 1978. (d)

National Center for Health Statistics. Divorces by marriage cohort. Hyattsyville, MD: DHEW Publication No. (PHS) 79-1912, 1979. (a)

National Center for Health Statistics. First marriages: United States, 1968–1976. Hyattsville, MD: DHEW Publication No. (PHS) 79-1913, 1979. (b)

National Center for Health Statistics. Births, marriages, divorces and deaths for January, 1980. Monthly Vital Statistics Report, 1980, *29*(1), April 9, 1980.

Navran, L. Communication and adjustment in marriage. *Family Process*, 1967, *6*, 173–184.

Negele, R. A. A study of the effectiveness of brief time-limited psychotherapy with children and their parents. *Dissertation Abstracts International*, 1976, *36*, 4172.

Nelson, R. E., & Craighead, W. E. Selective recall of positive and negative feedback, self-control behaviors, and depression. *Journal of Abnormal Psychology*, 1977, *86*, 379–388.

Nelson, R. O. Methodological issues in assessment via self-monitoring. In J. D. Cone & R. P. Hawkins (Eds.), *Behavioral Assessment: New Directions in Clinical Psychology*. New York: Brunner/Mazel, 1977.

Nemeth, C. Bargaining and reciprocity. *Psychological Bulletin*, 1970, 74, 297–308.

Neugarten, B. L., & Gutmann, D. L. Age–sex roles and personality in middle age: A thematic apperception study. In B. L. Neugarten (Ed.), *Middle Age and Aging*. Chicago: University of Chicago Press, 1968.

Newcomb, T. M. An approach to the study of communicative acts. *Psychological Review*, 1953, 60, 393–404.

Newcomb, T. M. The prediction of interpersonal attraction. *American Psychologists*, 1956, 11, 575–586.

Newcomb, T. M. *The Acquaintance Process*. New York: Holt, Rinehart and Winston, 1961.

Newell, A. G. A case of ejaculatory incompetence treated with a mechanical aid. *Journal of Behavior Therapy and Experimental Psychiatry*, 1976, 7, 193–194.

Nichols, R. C., & Beck, K. W. Factors in psychotherapy change. *Journal of Consulting Psychology*, 1960, 24, 388–399.

Nierenberg, G. I. *The Art of Negotiations: Psychological Strategies for Gaining Advantageous Bargains*. New York: Hawthorn Books, 1968.

Nierenberg, G. I., & Calero, H. H. *Meta-talk: Guide to Hidden Meanings in Conversations*. New York: Simon and Schuster, 1973.

Nisbett, R. E., & Valins, S. *Perceiving the Causes of One's Own Behavior*. New York: General Learning Press, 1971.

Nisbett, R. E., Caputo, C., Legant, P., & Marecek, J. Behavior as seen by the actor and as seen by the observer. *Journal of Personality and Social Psychology*, 1973, 27, 154–164.

Noonan, J. R. A follow-up of pretherapy dropouts, *Journal of Community Psychology*, 1973, 1, 43–45.

Nord, W. R. Social exchange theory: An integrative approach to social conformity. *Psychological Bulletin*, 1969, 71, 174–208.

Norton, A. J., & Glick, P. C. Marital instability: Past, present, and future. *Journal of Social Issues*, 1976, 32, 5–20.

Nunnally, E. W., Miller, S., & Wackman, D. B. The Minnesota Couples' Communication Program. *Small Group Behavior*, 1975, 6, 57–71.

Nye, F. I. Child adjustment in broken and in unhappy unbroken homes. *Marriage and Family Living*, 1957, 19, 356–361.

Nye, F. I. Field research. In H. T. Christensen (Ed.), *Handbook of Marriage and the Family*. Chicago: Rand McNally, 1964.

Nye, F. I. *Role Structure and Analysis of the Family*. Beverly Hills, CA: Sage Publications, 1976.

Nye, F. I., & Berardo, F. On the causes of divorce. In F. I. Nye & F. Berardo (Eds.), *The Family: Its Structure and Interaction*. New York: Macmillan Co., 1973.

Nye, F. I., & McLaughlin, S. Role competence and marital satisfaction. In F. I. Nye (Ed.), *Role Structure and Analysis of the Family*. Beverly Hills, CA: Sage Publications, 1976.

Obler, M. Systematic desensitization in sexual disorders. *Journal of Behavior Therapy and Experimental Psychiatry*, 1973, 4, 93–101.

O'Connor, J. F. Sexual problems, therapy and prognostic factors. In J. K. Meyer (Ed.), *Clinical Management of Sexual Disorders*. Baltimore: Williams and Wilkins, 1976.

O'Connor, J. F., & Stern, L. O. Results of treatment in functional sexual disorders. *New York State Journal of Medicine*, August 1972, 72, 1927–1934.

Odita, F. C., & Janssens, M. A. Family stability in the context of economic deprivation. *The Family Coordinator*, 1977, 26, 252–258.

Oldz, J. S. The effects of a time limited and non-time limited mode of counseling on producing therapeutic change. *Dissertation Abstracts International*, 1977, 1450B.

Olson, D. H. The measurement of family power by self-report and behavioral methods. *Journal of Marriage and the Family*, 1969, 31, 545–550.

Olson, D. H. Marital and family therapy: Integrative review and critique. *Journal of Marriage and the Family*, 1970, *32*, 501–538.

Olson, D. H. The powerlessness of family power: Empirical and clinical considerations. *Science and Psychoanalysis*, 1972, *20*, 139.

Olson, D. H., & Cromwell, R. E. Methodological issues in family power. In R. E. Cromwell & D. H. Olson, (Eds.), *Power in Families*. New York: John Wiley and Sons, 1975.

Olson, D. H., & Rabunsky, C. Validity of four measures of family power. *Journal of Marriage and the Family*, 1972, *34*, 224–234.

Olson, D. H., & Sprenkle, D. H. Emerging trends in treating relationships. *Journal of Marriage and Family Counseling*, 1976, *2*(4), 317–329.

Oltmans, T. F., Broderick, J. E., & O'Leary, D. K. Marital adjustment and the efficacy of behavior therapy with children. *Journal of Consulting and Clinical Psychology*, 1977, *45*, 724–729.

O'Neill, N., & O'Neill, G. *Open Marriage: A New Life Style for Couples*. New York: J. B. Lippincott, 1972.

Orden, S. R., & Bradburn, N. A. Dimensions of marriage happiness. *American Journal of Sociology*, 1968, *73*, 715–731.

Orford, J. A study of the personalities of excessive drinkers and their wives, using the approaches of Leary and Eysenck. *Journal of Consulting and Clinical Psychology*, 1976, *44*, 534–545.

Orlansky, H. Infant care and personality. *Psychological Bulletin*, 1949, *46*, 1–48.

Orne, M., & Wender, P. Anticipatory socialization for psychotherapy: Method and rationale. *American Journal of Psychiatry*, 1968, *124*, 88–98.

Ort, R. S. A study of role-conflicts as related to happiness in marriage. *Journal of Abnormal and Social Psychology*, 1950, *45*, 691–699.

Osgood, C. E. Suggestions for winning the real war with communism. *Journal of Conflict Resolution*, 1959, *3*, 295–325.

Osgood, C. E. *An Alternative to War or Surrender*. Urbana, IL: University of Illinois Press, 1962.

Osgood, C. E., Suci, G. J., & Tannenbaum, P. H. *The Measurement of Meaning*. Urbana, IL: University of Illinois Press, 1967.

Oskamp, S. Effects of programmed strategies on cooperation in the Prisoner's Dilemma and other mixed-motive games. *Journal of Conflict Resolution*, 1971, *15*, 225–259.

Osmond, M. W. Reciprocity: A dynamic model and a method to study family power. *Journal of Marriage and the Family*, 1978, *40*, 49–61.

Osmond, M. W., & Martin, P. Y. A contingency model of marital organization in low income families. *Journal of Marriage and the Family*, 1978, *40*, 315–329.

Otto, H. The personal and family resource development programmes: A preliminary report. *International Journal of Social Psychiatry*, 1962, *2*, 329–338.

Overall, J. E., Henry, B. W., & Woodward, A. Dependence of marital problems on parental family history. *Journal of Abnormal Psychology*, 1974, *83*, 446–450.

Paquin, M. J. The status of family and marital therapy outcomes: Methodological and substantive considerations. *Canadian Psychological Review*, 1977, *18*, 221–232.

Parham, T. M. The culture of poverty. *Public Welfare*, 1968, *26*, 193–199.

Parke, R. D., Ewall, W., & Slaby, R. G. Hostile and helpful verbalizations as regulators of nonverbal aggression. *Journal of Personality and Social Psychology*, 1972, *23*, 243–248.

Parsons, T. The social structure of the family. *Essays in Sociological Theory, Pure and Applied*. Glencoe, IL: The Free Press, 1949.

Parsons, T. *The Social System*. Glencoe, IL: The Free Press, 1951.

Parsons, T., & Bales, R. F. *Family, Socialization and Interaction Process*. Glencoe, IL: The Free Press, 1955.

Pascal, G. R., & Zax, M. Psychotherapeutics: Success or failure? *Journal of Consulting Psychology*, 1956, *20*, 325–331.

Pascal, H. J. Need interaction as a factor in marital adjustment. *Dissertation Abstracts International*, 1974, *35*, 2056–2057.

Patterson, C. H. *Theories of Counseling and Psychotherapy.* New York: Harper and Row. 1973.

Patterson, G. R. *Families: Applications of Social Learning to Family Life.* Champaign, IL: Research Press, 1971.

Patterson, G. R. Naturalistic observation in clinical assessment. *Journal of Abnormal Child Psychology,* 1977, 5, 309–322.

Patterson, G. R., & Hops, H. Coercion, a game for two: Intervention techniques for marital conflict. In R. E. Ulrich & P. Montjoy (Eds.), *The Experimental Analysis of Social Behavior.* New York: Appleton-Century-Crofts, 1972.

Patterson, G. R., & Reid, J. B. Reciprocity and coercion: Two facets of social systems. In C. Neuringer & J. Michael (Eds.), *Behavior Modification in Clinical Psychology.* New York: Appleton-Century-Crofts, 1970.

Patterson, G. R., Hops, H., & Weiss, R. L. Interpersonal skills training for couples in early stages of conflict. *Journal of Marriage and the Family,* 1975, 37, 295–303.

Patterson, G. R., Weiss, R. L., & Hops, H. Training of marital skills: Some problems and concepts. In H. Leitenberg (Ed.), *Handbook of Behavior Modification.* New York: Appleton-Century-Crofts, 1976.

Patton, B. R., & Giffin, K. *Interpersonal Communication: Basic Text and Readings.* New York: Harper & Row, 1974.

Paul, G. L. Behavior modification research: Design and tactics. In C. M. Franks (Ed.), *Behavior Therapy: Appraisal and Status.* New York: McGraw-Hill, 1969.

Pemberton, D. A., & Benady, D. R. Consciously rejected children. *British Journal of Psychiatry,* 1973, 123, 575–578.

Perlow, A. D., & Mullins, S. C. Marital satisfaction as perceived by the medical student's spouse. *Journal of Medical Education,* 1976, 51, 726–734.

Perls, F. *The Gestalt Approach: Eye Witness to Therapy.* Ben Lomond, CA: Science and Behavior Books, 1973.

Perls, F., Hefferline, R. E., & Goodman, P. *Gestalt Therapy: Excitement and Growth in the Human Personality.* New York: Delta, 1965.

Perls, F. *Gestalt Therapy Verbatim.* Lafayette, CA: Real People Press, 1969.

Pew, M. L., & Pew, W. L. Adlerian marriage counseling. *Journal of Individual Psychology,* 1972, 28, 192–202.

Pfeil, E. Role expectations when entering into marriage. *Journal of Marriage and the Family,* 1968, 30, 161–165.

Phillips, C., & Toomin, L. *Staving Off Divorce: Techniques for Counseling the Troubled Couple.* Burbank, CA: California Family Study Center, 1975.

Phillips, E. L., & Wiener, D. N. *Short-term Psychotherapy and Structured Behavior Change.* New York: McGraw-Hill, 1966.

Pineo, P. C. Disenchantment in the later years of marriage. *Marriage and Family Living,* 1961, 23, 3–11.

Piven, F. F., & Cloward, R. A. *Regulating the Poor: The Functions of Public Welfare.* New York: Pantheon, 1971.

Pollard, W. E., & Mitchell, T. R. Decision theory analysis of social power. *Psychological Bulletin,* 1972, 78, 433–446.

Polster, E., & Polster, M. *Gestalt Therapy Integrated: Contours of Theory and Practice.* New York: Brunner/Mazel, 1973.

Pomeroy, W. Sexual myths of the 1970's. *Medical Aspects of Human Sexuality,* 1977, 11(1), 62–74.

Pondy, L. R. Organizational conflict: Concepts and models. *Administrative Science Quarterly,* 1967, 12, 296–320.

Pope, H., & Mueller, C. W. The intergenerational transmission of marital instability: Comparisons by race and sex. *Journal of Social Issues,* 1976, 32, 49–66.

Porter, A. M. W. Depressive illness in general practice: A demographic study and a controlled trial of imipramine. *British Medical Journal,* 1970, 28, 773–778.

Powell, L. C., Blakeney, P., Croft, H., & Pulliam, G. P. Rapid treatment approach to human sexual inadequacy. *American Journal of Obstetrics and Gynecology*, 1974, *119*(1), 89–97.

Powers, E. C. *An Attempt to Develop a Scale to Measure the Principle of Least Interest*. Unpublished manuscript, Department of Sociology, Ohio State University, 1964.

Price-Bonham, S. A comparision of weighted and unweighted decision-making scores. *Journal of Marriage and the Family*, 1976, *38*, 629–640.

Prochaska, J., & Prochaska, J. Twentieth century trends in marriage and marital therapy. In T. J. Paolino & B. S. McCrady (Eds.), *Marriage and Marital Therapy: Psychoanalytic, Behavioral and Systems Theory Perspectives*. New York: Brunner/Mazel, 1978.

Prugh, D. G., & Brody, B. Brief relationship therapy in the military setting. *American Journal of Orthopsychiatry*, 1946, *16*, 707–721.

Pruitt, D. G. Reciprocity and credit building in a laboratory dyad. *Journal of Personality and Social Psychology*, 1968, *8*, 143–147.

Pruitt, D. G., & Johnson, D. F. Mediation as an aid to face saving in negotiation. *Journal of Personality and Social Psychology*, 1970, *14*, 239–246.

Purcell, J. P. Illusion and reality: A closer look at the dynamics of cohabitation, marriage, and commitment. *Dissertation Abstracts International*, 1976, *37*, 1925.

Raft, D., Spencer, R. F., Toomey, T., & Brogan, D. Depression in medical outpatients: Use of the Zung scale. *Diseases of the Nervous System*, 1977, *38*, 999–1004.

Rahe, R. H. The pathway between subjects' recent life changes and their near future illness reports: Representative results and methodological issues. In B. S. Dohrenwend & B. P. Dohrenwend (Eds.), *Stressful Life Events: Their Nature and Effects*. New York: John Wiley and Sons, 1974.

Ramey, J. W. Intimate groups and networks: Frequent consequences of sexually open marriage. *The Family Coordinator*, 1975, *24*, 515–530.

Rappaport, J., Gross, T., & Lepper, C. Modeling, sensitivity training, and instruction: Implications for the training of college student volunteers and for outcome research. *Journal of Consulting and Clinical Psychology*, 1973, *40*, 99–107.

Raskin, D. E., & Klein, Z. E. Losing a symptom through keeping it: A review of paradoxical treatment techniques and rationale. *Archives of General Psychiatry*, 1976, *33*, 548–555.

Rausch, H. L., Barry, W. A., Hertel, R. K., & Swain, M. A. *Communication Conflict and Marriage*. San Francisco: Jossey-Bass, 1974.

Raush, M. Interaction sequences. *Journal of Personality and Social Psychology*, 1965, *2*, 487–499.

Raven, B. H., Centers, R., & Rodrigues, A. The bases of conjugal power. In R. E. Cromwell & D. H. Olson (Eds.), *Power in Families*. New York: John Wiley and Sons, 1975.

Rawlings, M. L. Development of interpersonal relationships in marriage through imputational and perceived interactional convergence. *Dissertation Abstracts International*, 1975, *35*(11-A), 7423.

Razani, J. Ejaculatory incompetence treated by deconditioning anxiety. *Journal of Behavior Therapy and Experimental Psychiatry*, 1972, *3*, 65–67.

Reckless, J., & Geiger, N. Impotence as a practical problem. In H. F. Dowling (Ed.), *Disease-a-Month*. Chicago: Year Book Medical Publishers, May 1975.

Rehm, L. P. Mood, pleasant events, and unpleasant events: Two pilot studies. *Journal of Consulting and Clinical Psychology*, 1978, *46*, 854–859.

Reid, W. J., & Shyne, A. W. *Brief and Extended Casework*. New York: Columbia University Press, 1969.

Reisinger, J. J. Effects of erotic stimulation and masturbation training upon situational orgasmic dysfunction. *Journal of Sex and Marital Therapy*, 1978, *4*, 177–185.

Renne, K. S. Correlates of dissatisfaction in marriage. *Journal of Marriage and the Family*, 1970, *32*, 54–67.

Renne, K. S. Health and marital experience in an urban population. *Journal of Marriage and the Family*, 1971, *33*, 338–350.

Resick, P. A., Welsh, B. K., Zitomer, E. A., Spiegel, D. K., Meidlinger, J. C., & Long, B. R.

Predictors of marital satisfaction, conflict and accord: A preliminary revision of the Marital Interaction Coding System, *Journal of Applied Behavior Analysis*, in press.

Reusch, J. The role of communication in therapeutic transactions. *Journal of Communication*, 1963, *13*, 132–139.

Rice, D. G., Gurman, A. S., & Razin, A. M. Therapist, sex, style and orientation. *Journal of Nervous and Mental Disease*, 1974, *159*, 413–421.

Rice, P. F. *The Adolescent: Development, Relationships, and Culture.* Boston: Allyn and Bacon, 1975.

Richardson, T. A. Hypnotherapy and frigidity. *American Journal of Clinical Hypnosis*, 1963, *5*, 194–199.

Riedel, D. C., Tischler, G. L., & Myers, J. K. *Patient Care Evaluation in Mental Health Programs.* Cambridge, MA: Ballinger Publishing Co., 1974.

Riskin, J., & Faunce, E. E. Family interaction scales. *Archives of General Psychiatry*, 1970, *22*, 504–537.

Risley, T. R. The social context of self control. In R. B. Stuart (Ed.), *Behavioral Self Management.* New York: Brunner/Mazel, 1977.

Robinson, C. H. *The Effects of Observational Learning on Sexual Behavior and Attitudes in Orgasmic Dysfunctional Women.* Unpublished doctoral dissertation, University of Hawaii, 1974.

Robinson, E. A., & Price, M. G. *Behavioral and Self-Report Correlates of Marital Satisfaction.* Paper presented at the Annual Meeting of the Association for Advancement of Behavior Therapy, December 1976.

Rochlin, G. *Man's Aggression: The Defense of the Self.* New York: Delta Books, 1973.

Roen, P. R. Impotence: A concise review. *New York Journal of Medicine*, 1965, *65*, 2576–2582.

Rogers, C. A process conception of psychotherapy. *American Psychologist*, 1958, *13*, 141–149.

Rogers, C. A theory of therapy, personality, and interpersonal relationships as developed in the client-centered framework. In S. Koch (Ed.), *Psychology: A Study of a Science. III. Formulations of the Person and the Social Context.* New York: McGraw-Hill, 1959.

Rogers, C. *On Becoming a Person.* Boston: Houghton Mifflin, 1961.

Rogers, C. R. The necessary and sufficient conditions of therapeutic personality change. *Journal of Consulting Psychology*, 1957, *21*, 95–103.

Rogers, L. S., Lipetz, M. E., Dworin, J., & Cohen, I. H. A multiple-correlation approach to factors relating to marital satisfaction. *Proceedings, 80th Annual Convention,* American Psychological Association, Washington, DC, 1972.

Rogers, M. F. Instrumental and infra-resources: The bases of power. *American Journal of Sociology*, 1974, *79*, 1418–1433.

Rokeach, M. A theory of organization and change within value–attitude systems. *Journal of Social Issues*, 1968, *24*, 13–33.

Rokeach, M. *The Nature of Human Values.* New York: Macmillan Co., 1973.

Rokeach, M., & Kliejunas, P. Behavior as a function of attitude-toward-object and attitude-toward-situation. *Journal of Personality and Social Psychology*, 1972, *22*, 194–201.

Rollins, B. C., & Bahr, S. J. A theory of power relationships in marriage. *Journal of Marriage and the Family*, 1976, *38*, 619–627.

Rollins, B. C., & Cannon, K. L. Marital satisfaction over the family life cycle: A re-evaluation. *Journal of Marriage and the Family*, 1974, *36*, 271–283.

Rollins, B. C., & Feldman, H. Marital satisfaction over the family cycle. *Journal of Marriage and the Family*, 1970, *32*, 20–27.

Rose, S. D. *Group Therapy: A Behavioral Approach.* Englewood Cliffs, NJ: Prentice-Hall, 1977.

Rosenberg, S., & Jones, R. A. A method for investigating and representing a person's implicit theory of personality: Theodore Dreiser's view of people. *Journal of Personality and Social Psychology*, 1972, *22*, 372–386.

Rosenberg, S., & Olshan, K. Evaluative and descriptive aspects of personality perception. *Journal of Personality and Social Psychology*, 1970, *16*, 619–626.

Rosenstock, F., & Kutner, B. Alienation and family crisis. *The Sociological Quarterly*, 1967, *8*, 397–405.

Ross, L. The intuitive psychologist and his shortcomings: Distortions in the attribution process. In L. Berkowitz (Ed.), *Advances in Experimental Social Psychology* (Vol. 10). New York: Academic Press, 1977.

Rossi, A. S. Transition to parenthood. *Journal of Marriage and the Family* 1968, *30*, 26–39.

Roth, M. Seeking common ground in contemporary psychiatry. *Proceedings of the Royal Society of Medicine*, 1969, *62*, 765–772.

Rotter, J. B. *Social Learning and Clinical Psychology.* Englewood Cliffs, NJ: Prentice-Hall, 1954.

Rotter, J. B. Some implications of a social learning theory for the practice of psychotherapy. In D. J. Levis (Ed.), *Learning Approaches to Therapeutic Behavior Change.* Chicago: Aldine, 1970.

Rubin, Z. *Lovers and Other Strangers: The Development of Intimacy in Encounters and Relationships.* Paper presented at the Annual Convention of the American Psychological Association, Honolulu, September 1972.

Rubin, Z. *Liking and Loving.* New York: Holt, Rinehart and Winston, 1973.

Russell, B. *Power.* London: Allen and Unwyn, 1938.

Rutledge, A. L. *Premarital Counseling.* Cambridge, MA: Schenkman, 1966.

Ryder, R. G. Husband–wife dyads versus married strangers. *Family Process,* 1968, *7*, 223–228.

Ryle, A., & Lipshitz, S. Recording change in marital therapy with the reconstruction grid. *British Journal of Medical Psychology,* 1975, *48*, 39–48.

Safilios-Rothschild, C. Patterns of familial power and influence. *Sociological Focus,* 1969, *2*, 7–19.

Sager, C. J. Sexual dysfunctions and marital discord. In H. S. Kaplan (Ed.), *The New Sex Therapy.* New York: Brunner/Mazel, 1974.

Sager, C. J. The role of sex therapy in marital therapy. *American Journal of Psychiatry,* 1976, *133*, 555–558.

Sahakian, W. S. *The History of Philosophy.* New York: Barnes and Noble, 1968.

Sampson, R. V. *Equality and Power.* London: Heinemann, 1965.

Sampson, R. V. *The Psychology of Power.* New York: Vintage Books, 1968.

Sarason, S. B., Levine, M. I., Goldenberg, I., Cherlin, D. S., & Benner, E. M. *Psychology in Community Settings: Clinical, Educational, Vocational, Social Aspects.* New York: John Wiley and Sons, 1966.

Sarbin, T. R. Role theory. In G. Lindzey (Ed.), *Handbook of Social Psychology.* Reading, MA: Addison-Wesley Publishing Co., 1954.

Satir, V. *Conjoint Family Therapy.* Palo Alto, CA: Science and Behavior Books, 1964.

Savicki, V. Outcomes of nonreciprocal self-disclosure strategies. *Journal of Personality and Social Psychology,* 1972, *23*, 271–276.

Scanzoni, J. A social system analysis of dissolved and existing marriages. *Journal of Marriage and the Family,* 1968, *30*, 452–461.

Scanzoni, J. H. *Opportunity and the Family.* New York: The Free Press, 1970.

Schaffer, L. F., & Shoben, E. J. Common aspects of psychotherapy. In B. G. Berenson & R. R. Carkhuff (Eds.), *Sources of Gain in Counseling and Psychotherapy.* New York: Holt, Rinehart and Winston, 1967.

Scheff, T. J. Toward a sociological model of consensus. *American Sociological Review,* 1967, *32*, 32–45.

Scheflen, A. E. Human communication: Behavioral programs and their integration and interaction. *Behavioral Science,* 1968, *13*, 44–55.

Scheflen, A. E. *How Behavior Means.* Garden City, NY: Anchor Books, 1974.

Scheidel, T. M. *Speech Communication and Human Interaction.* Glenview, IL: Scott, Foresman, 1972.

Schelling, T. C. *The Strategy of Conflict.* New York: Oxford University Press, 1963.

Schlein, S. *Training Dating Couples in Empathic and Open Communication: An Experimental Evaluation of a Potential Preventative Mental Health Program.* Unpublished doctoral dissertation, Pennsylvania State University, 1971.

Schlenker, B. R., Bonoma, T., Tedeschi, J. T., & Pivnick, W. P. Compliance to threats as a function of the wording of the threat and the exploitativeness of the threatener. *Sociometry*, 1970, *33*, 394–408.

Schless, A. P., Schwartz, L., Goetz, C., & Mendels, J. How depressives view the significance of life events. *British Journal of Psychiatry*, 1974, *125*, 406–410.

Schneid, H. *Marriage*. New York: Leon Amiel Publisher, 1973.

Schneiders, A. *Adolescents and the Challenge of Maturity*. Milwaukee, WI: Bruce Publishing Co., 1965.

Schneidman, B., & McGuire, L. Group therapy for nonorgasmic women: Two age levels. *Archives of Sexual Behavior*, 1976, *5*, 239–247.

Schofield, W. *Psychotherapy: The Purchase of Friendship*. Englewood Cliffs, NJ: Prentice-Hall, 1964.

Schuham, A. I. Power relations in emotionally disturbed and normal family triads. *Journal of Abnormal Psychology*, 1970, *75*, 30–37.

Schuham, A. I. Activity, talking time, and spontaneous agreement in disturbed and normal family interaction. *Journal of Abnormal Psychology*, 1972, *79*, 68–75.

Schulman, M. L. Idealization in engaged couples. *Journal of Marriage and the Family*, 1974, *36*, 139–147.

Scodel, A. Induced collaboration in some non-zero-sum games. *Journal of Conflict Resolution*, 1962, *6*, 335–340.

Scoresby, A. L. *The Marriage Dialogue*. Reading, MA: Addison-Wesley Publishing Co., 1977.

Scott, W. A., & Peterson, C. Adjustment, pollyannaism, and attraction to close relationships. *Journal of Consulting and Clinical Psychology*, 1975, *43*, 872–880.

Sedney, M. A. *Process of Sex-Role Development during Life Crises of Middle-aged Women*. Paper presented at the Annual Meeting of the American Psychological Association, San Francisco, August 1977.

Seeman, J. Counselor judgments of therapeutic process and outcome. In C. R. Rogers & R. F. Dymond (Eds.), *Psychotherapy and Personality Change*. Chicago: University of Chicago Press, 1954.

Semans, J. H. Premature ejaculation: A new approach. *Southern Medical Journal*, 1956, *49*, 353–358.

Serber, M., & Laws, R. *Tenderness*. San Luis Obispo, CA: Film produced by Behavioral Alternatives, 1974. (Available from Diana Serber-Corenman, Atascadero State Hospital, Atascadero, CA.)

Shannon, C. E., & Weaver, W. *The Mathematical Theory of Communication*. Urbana: University of Illinois Press, 1949.

Shazer, S. Brief hypnotherapy of two sexual dysfunctions: The crystal ball technique. *The American Journal of Clinical Hypnosis*, 1978, *20*, 203–208.

Shelling, T. C. *The Strategy of Conflict*. New York: Oxford University Press, 1963.

Shepard, H. A. Responses to situations of competition and conflict. In E. Boulding (Ed.), *Conflict Management in Organizations*. Ann Arbor, MI: Foundation for Research on Human Behavior, 1961.

Sherif, M., & Sherif, C. W. *An Outline of Social Psychology*. New York: Harper and Brothers, 1956.

Shibutani, T. *Society and Personality*. Englewood Cliffs, NJ: Prentice-Hall, 1961.

Shinn, M. Father absence and children's cognitive development. *Psychological Bulletin*, 1978, *85*, 295–324.

Shlien, J. M., Mosak, H. H., & Dreikurs, R. Effects of time limits: A comparison of client-centered and Adlerian psychotherapy. *American Psychologist,* 1960, *14*, 41.

Shlien, J. M., Mosak, H. H., & Dreikurs, R. Effect of time limits: A comparison of two psychotherapies. *Journal of Counseling Psychology*, 1962, *9*, 31–34.

Shoben, E. J. Psychotherapy as a problem in learning theory. *Psychological Bulletin*, 1949, *46*, 366–392.

Shoffner, S. M. Use of videotape learning packages: A marital enrichment field experiment with two delivery systems. *Dissertation Abstracts International*, 1977, *37*, 8001–8002.

Shomer, R. W., Davis, A. H., & Kelley, H. H. Threats and the development of coordination: Further studies of the Deutsch and Krauss trucking game. *Journal of Personality and Social Psychology*, 1966, 4, 119–126.

Shortell, J., Epstein, S., & Taylor, S. P. Instigation to aggression as a function of degree of defeat and the capacity for massive retalization. *Journal of Personality*, 1970, 38, 313–328.

Shostrum, E. L., & Kavanaugh, J. *Between Man and Woman*. Los Angeles: Nash, 1971.

Siegel, S., & Fouraker, L. E. *Bargaining and Group Decision Making*. New York: McGraw-Hill, 1960.

Siegman, A. W. Father absence during early childhood and antisocial behavior. *Journal of Abnormal Psychology*, 1966, 71, 71–74.

Sigal, J. J., Barrs, C. B., & Doubilet, A. L. Problems in measuring the success of family therapy in a common clinical setting: Impasse and solutions. *Family Process*, 1976, 15, 225–234.

Sigall, H., & Aronson, E. Opinion change and the gain–loss of interpersonal attraction. *Journal of Experimental Social Psychology*, 1967, 3, 178–188.

Silver, A. W., & Derr, J. A comparison of selected personality variables between parents of delinquent and non-delinquent adolscents. *Journal of Clinical Psychology*, 1966, 22, 49–50.

Simmel, G. *The Sociology of George Simmel*. New York: The Free Press, 1964.

Simon, H. A. A behavioral model of rational choice. *Quarterly Journal of Economics*, 1955, 69, 99–118.

Simpson, R. L. *Theories of Social Exchange*. Morristown, NJ: General Learning Press, 1972.

Sines, L. K. The relative contribution of four kinds of data to accuracy in personality assessment. *Journal of Consulting Psychology*, 1959, 23, 483–492.

Singh, S. B., Nigam, A., & Saxena, N. K. Study in the cases of marital disharmony. *Indian Journal of Clinical Psychology*, 1976, 3, 47–52.

Skinner, B. F. *Science and Human Behavior*. New York: Macmillan Co., 1953.

Skinner, B. F. *Beyond Freedom and Dignity*. New York: Alfred A. Knopf, 1971.

Skolnick, A. *The Intimate Environment: Exploring Marriage and the Family*. Boston, MA: Little, Brown and Co., 1973.

Slaney, R. B. Therapist and client perceptions of alternative roles for the facilitative conditions. *Journal of Consulting and Clinical Psychology*, 1978, 46, 1146–1147.

Sloan, L., & Latane, B. Sex and sociability in rats. *Journal of Experimental Social Psychology*, 1974, 10, 147–158.

Sloane, R., Cristal, A., Pepernick, M., & Staples, F. Role preparation and expectancy of improvement in psychotherapy. *Journal of Nervous and Mental Disease*, 1970, 150, 18–26.

Sloane, R. B., Staples, F. R., Cristol, A. H., Yorkston, N. J., & Whipple, K. *Psychotherapy Versus Behavior Therapy*. Cambridge, MA: Harvard University Press, 1975.

Sluzki, C. E., & Beavin, J. Symmetry and complementarily: An operational definition and a typology of dyads. In P. Watzlawick & J. H. Weakland (Eds.), *The Interactional View: Studies at the Mental Research Institute, Palo Alto, 1965-1974*. New York: W. W. Norton, 1977.

Sluzki, C. E., Beavin, J., Tarnopolsky, A., & Veron, E. Transactional disqualification: Research on the double bind. *Archives of General Psychiatry*, 1967, 16, 494–504.

Small, L. *The Briefer Psychotherapies*. New York: Brunner/Mazel, 1971.

Smith, C. G., & Tannenbaum, A. S. Organizational control structure: A comparative analysis. *Human Relations*, 1963, 16, 299–331.

Smith, J. R., & Smith, L. G. *Beyond Monogamy: Recent Studies of Sexual Alternatives in Marriage*. Baltimore: John Hopkins University Press, 1974.

Smith, T. E. Foundations of parental influence upon adolescents: An application of social power theory. *American Sociological Review*, 1970, 35, 860–872.

Smith, V. G., & Hammond, D. C. *Relationship Therapy*. San Francisco: Jossey-Bass, 1980.

Smith, W. P., & Anderson, A. J. Threats, communication, and bargaining. *Journal of Personality and Social Psychology*, 1975, 32, 76–82.

Snyder, C. R. Acceptance of personality interpretations as a function of assessment procedures. *Journal of Consulting and Clinical Psychology*, 1974, *42*, 150.

Snyder, C. R., & Larson, G. R. A further look at student acceptance of general personality interpretations. *Journal of Consulting and Clinical Psychology*, 1972, *38*, 384–388.

Snyder, M., Tanke, E. D., & Berscheid, E. Social perception and interpersonal behavior: On the self-fulfilling nature of social stereotypes. *Journal of Personality and Social Psychology*, 1977, *35*(9), 656–666.

Snyder, W. U. Clinical methods: Psychotherapy. In *Annual review of Psychology* (Vol. 1). Palo Alto, CA: Annual Reviews, 1950.

Sobotka, J. J. An evaluation of Afrodex in the management of male impotency: A double-blind cross over study. *Current Therapeutic Research*, 1969, *11*, 87–94.

Solomon, L. The influence of some types of power relationships and game strategies upon the development of interpersonal trust. *Journal of Abnormal and Social Psychology*, 1960, *61*, 223–230.

Solomon, M. A. The staging of family treatment: An approach to developing the therapeutic alliance. *Journal of Marriage and Family Counseling*, 1977, *3*, 59–66.

Sorenson, D. L. The relationship of perceptual incongruity and defensive style to marital discord. *Dissertation Abstracts International*, 1974, *35*, 3037–3038.

Spanier, G. B. Measuring dyadic adjustment: New scales for assessing the quality of marriage and similar dyads. *Journal of Marriage and the Family*, 1976, *38*, 15–28.

Spanier, G. B., Lewis, R. A., & Cole, C. L. Marital adjustment over the family life cycle: The issue of curvilinearity. *Journal of Marriage and the Family*, 1975, *37*, 263–275.

Spence, J. The personality scale of manifest anxiety. *Journal of Abnormal and Social Psychology*, 1953, *48*, 285–290.

Spitzer, R., Endicott, J., Fleiss, J., & Cohen, J. The psychiatric status schedule. *Archives of General Psychiatry*, 1970, *23*, 41–55.

Spitzer, R. L., Endicott, J., & Cohen, G. N. *Psychiatric Status Schedule: Informant Form.* New York: Biomedics Research, State Department of Mental Hygiene, 1966.

Sprenkle, D. H., & Olson, D. H. L. Circumplex model of marital systems: An empirical study of clinic and non-clinic couples. *Journal of Marriage and Family Counseling*, 1978, *4*, 59–74.

Sprey, J. Family power structure: A critical comment. *Journal of Marriage and the Family*, 1972, *34*, 235–238.

Sprey, J. Family power and process: Toward a conceptual integration. In R. E. Cromwell & D. H. Olson (Eds.), *Power in Families.* New York: John Wiley and Sons, 1975.

Stack, S. The effects of marital dissolution on suicide. *Journal of Marriage and the Family*, 1980, *42*, 83–92.

Stapert, J. C., & Clore, G. L. Attraction and disagreement-produced arousal. *Journal of Personality and Social Psychology*, 1969, *13*, 64–70.

Stapleton, R. E., Nacci, P., & Tedeschi, J. T. Interpersonal attraction and the reciprocation of benefits. *Journal of Personality and Social Psychology*, 1973, *28*, 199–205.

Stein, P. J. Singlehood: An alternative to marriage. *Family Coordinator*, 1975, *24*, 489–503.

Steinfeld, G. J. Decentering and family process: A marriage of cognitive therapies. *Journal of Marriage and Family Counseling*, 1978, *4*(3), 61–69.

Steinmetz, S. K., & Straus, M. A. I. General introduction: Social myth and social system in the study of intra-family violence. In S. K. Steinmetz & M. A. Straus (Eds.), *Violence in the Family.* New York: Dodd Mead, 1974.

Stern, R. S., & Marks, I. M. Contract therapy for obsessive–compulsive neurosis with marital discord. *British Journal of Psychiatry*, 1973, *123*, 681–684.

Sternberg, D. P., & Beier, E. G. *Changing Patterns of Conflict in Marriage: A Followup Study of 51 Newlywed Couples.* Paper presented at the Western Psychological Association Meetings, Portland, OR, April 1972.

Stevens, C. M. *Strategy and Collective Bargaining Negotiation.* New York: McGraw-Hill, 1963.

Stevens, J. O. *Awareness: Exploring, Experimenting, Experiencing.* Lafayette, CA: Real People Press, 1971.

Stevenson, I. Is the human personality more plastic in infancy and childhood? *American Journal of Psychiatry,* 1957, *114,* 152–161.

Stieper, D. R., & Wiener, D. N. *Dimensions of Psychotherapy: An Experimental and Clinical Approach.* Chicago: Aldine, 1965.

Stone, W. F. Patterns of conformity in couples varying in intimacy. *Journal of Personality and Social Psychology,* 1973, *27,* 413–418.

Storms, M. D. Videotape and the attribution process: Reversing the perspective of actors and observers. *Journal of Personality and Social Psychology,* 1973, *27,* 165–175.

Straker, M. A review of short-term psychotherapy. *Diseases of the Nervous System,* 1977, *38,* 813–816.

Straus, M. A. Measuring families. In H. T. Christensen (Ed.), *Handbook of Marriage and the Family.* Chicago: Rand McNally, 1964. (a)

Straus, M. A. Power and support structure of the family in relation to socialization. *Journal of Marriage and the Family,* 1964, *26,* 318–326.

Straus, M. A. Communication, creativity, and problem-solving ability of middle and working-class families in three societies. In W. W. Lambert & R. Weisbrod (Eds.), *Comparative Perspectives on Social Psychology.* Boston: Little, Brown and Co., 1971.

Straus, M., & Tallman, I. SINFAM: A technique for observational measurement and experimental study of families. In J. Aldous, T. Condon, R. Hill, M. Straus, & I. Tallman (Eds.), *Family Problem Solving.* Hinsdale, IL: Dryden Press, 1971.

Strodtbeck, F. L. The family as a three-person group. *American Sociological Review,* 1954, *19,* 23–29.

Strodtbeck, F. L. The family in action. *Child Study,* 1958, *34,* 14–18.

Strong, J. R. A marital conflict resolution model: Redefining conflict to achieve intimacy. *Journal of Marriage and Family Counseling,* 1975, *1,* 269–276.

Stroup, A. L. Family formation. In J. B. Turner (Ed.-in-chief), *Encyclopedia of Social Work,* Seventeenth Issue (Vol. 1). Washington, DC: National Association of Social Workers, 1977.

Strupp, H. H., Fox, R. E., & Lessler, K. *Patients View Their Psychotherapy.* Baltimore: The Johns Hopkins Press, 1969.

Stuart, F., Stuart, R. B., Maurice, W. L., & Szasz, G. *Sexual Adjustment Inventory.* Research Press, 2612 N. Mattis, Champaign, IL 61820. 1975.

Stuart, R. B. Decentration in the development of children's moral and causal judgment. *The Journal of Genetic Psychology,* 1967, *111,* 59–68.

Stuart, R. B. Operant–interpersonal treatment for marital discord. *Journal of Consulting and Clinical Psychology,* 1969, *33,* 675–682.

Stuart, R. B. Assessment and change of the communicational patterns of juvenile delinquents and their parents. In R. D. Rubin, H. Fensterheim, A. A. Lazarus, & C. M. Franks (Eds.), *Advances in Behavior Therapy.* New York: Academic Press, 1971. (a)

Stuart, R. B. Behavioral contracting with the families of delinquents. *Journal of Behavior Therapy and Experimental Psychiatry,* 1971, *2,* 1–11. (b)

Stuart, R. B. *Trick or Treatment.* Champaign, IL: Research Press, 1971. (c)

Stuart, R. B. Situational versus self-control. In R. D. Rubin, H. Fensterheim, J. D. Henderson, & L. P. Ullman (Eds.), *Advances in Behavior Therapy.* New York: Academic Press, 1972.

Stuart, R. B. *Premarital Counseling Inventory.* Champaign, IL: Research Press, 1973. (a)

Stuart, R. B. The role of social work education in innovative human services. In F. W. Clark, D. R. Evans, & L. A. Hamerlynck (Eds.), *Implementing Behavioral Programs for Schools and Clinics.* Champaign, IL: Research Press, 1973. (b)

Stuart, R. B. *Treatment Contract.* Champaign, IL: Research Press, 1975.

Stuart, R. B. Operant–interpersonal treatment for marital discord. In D. H. L. Olson (Ed.), *Treating Relationships.* Lake Mills, IA: Graphic Press, 1976.

Stuart, R. B. *Act Thin: Stay Thin.* New York: W. W. Norton, 1978.

Stuart, R. B. Ethical guidelines for behavior therapy. In S. Turner, K. Calhoun, & H. Adams (Eds.), *Handbook of Clinical Behavior Therapy.* New York: John Wiley and Sons, 1980. (a)

Stuart, R. B. *Getting Marriage Therapy Off on the Right Foot.* New York: BMA/Guilford, 1980. (b)

Stuart, R. B. *Learning To Maintain Marriage Therapy Gains.* New York: BMA/Guilford, 1980. (c)

Stuart, R. B. Weight loss and beyond: Are they taking it off and keeping it off? In P. O. Davidson & S. M. Davidson (Eds.), *Behavioral Medicine: Changing Health Lifestyles.* New York: Brunner/Mazel, 1980. (d)

Stuart, R. B. *Remarriage: Deciding to Do It and Making It Last.* New York: W. W. Norton, in press.

Stuart, R. B., & Braver, J. *Positive and Negative Exchanges between Spouses and Strangers.* Unpublished manuscript, University of Michigan, 1973.

Stuart, R. B., & Guire, K. Some correlates of the maintenance of weight lost through behavior modification. *International Journal of Obesity,* 1979, *3,* 87–96.

Stuart, R. B., & Lederer, W. J. *The Marriage Grid.* New York: W. W. Norton, in press.

Stuart, R. B., & Lott, L. A. Behavioral contracting with delinquents: A cautionary note. *Journal of Behavior Therapy and Experimental Psychiatry,* 1972, *3,* 161–169.

Stuart, R. B., & Roper, B. Behavior therapy for marital discord: A reconnaissance. In G. Gotesdam (Ed.), *Trends in Behavior Therapy.* New York: Academic Press, 1979.

Stuart, R. B., & Stuart, F. *Marital Precounseling Inventory.* Research Press, 2612 N. Mattis, Champaign, IL 61820. 1973.

Stuart, R. B., & Tripodi, T. Experimental evaluation of three time-constrained behavioral treatments for predelinquents and delinquents. In R. D. Rubin, J. P. Brade, & J. D. Henderson (Eds.), *Advances in Behavior Therapy* (Vol. 4). New York: Academic Press, 1973.

Stuart, R. B., Tripodi, T., Jayaratne, S., & Camburn, D. An experiment in social engineering in serving the families of delinquents. *Journal of Abnormal Child Psychology,* 1976, *4,* 243–261.

Stuckert, R. P. Role perception and marital satisfaction: A configurational approach. *Marriage and Family Living,* 1963, *25,* 415–419.

Styker, S. Role-taking accuracy and adjustment. *Sociometry,* 1957, *20,* 286–296.

Sullivan, M. W. *From Tension to Relaxation.* Menlo Park, CA: Granger Doyle, 1964.

Sumner, W. G. *Folkways.* Boston: Ginn, 1911.

Sundland, D., & Barker, E. N. The orientations of psychotherapists. *Journal of Consulting Psychology,* 1962, *26,* 201–212.

Szasz, T. S. *The Myth of Mental Illness.* New York: Harper and Row, 1964.

Tallman, I. The family as a small problem solving group. *Journal of Marriage and the Family,* 1970, *32,* 94–104.

Tanner, L. B. *Voices from Women's Liberation.* New York: New American Library, 1971.

Taylor, D. The development of interpersonal relationships: Social penetration processes. *Journal of Social Psychology,* 1968, *75,* 79–90.

Taylor, D. A., Altman, I., & Sorrentino, R. Interpersonal exchange as a function of reward/cost and situational factors: Expectancy confirmation–disconfirmation. *Proceedings, 76th Annual Convention,* American Psychological Association, Washington, DC, 1968.

Taylor, D. A., Altman, I., & Sorrentino, R. Interpersonal exchange as a function of rewards and costs and situational factors: Expectancy confirmation–disconfirmation. *Journal of Experimental Social Psychology,* 1969, *5,* 324–339.

Taylor, D. W., Berry, P. C., & Block, C. H. Does group participation when using brainstorming facilitate or inhibit creative thinking? *Administrative Science Quarterly,* 1958, *3,* 23–47.

Taylor, J. G. *The Behavioral Basis of Perception.* New Haven, CT: Yale University Press, 1962.

Taylor, J. W. Relationship of success and length in psychotherapy. *Journal of Consulting Psychology,* 1956, *20,* 332.

Tedeschi, J. T. (Ed.). *The Social Influence Processes.* Chicago, IL: Aldine, 1972.

Tedeschi, J. T., Schlenker, B. R., & Lindskold, S. The exercise of power and influence: The source of influence. In J. T. Tedeschi (Ed.), *The Social Influence Processes*. Chicago: Aldine, 1972.

Terman, L. A. *Psychological Factors in Marital Happiness*. New York: McGraw-Hill, 1938.

Tharp, R. G. Dimensions of marriage roles. *Marriage and Family Living*, 1963, 25, 389–404. (a)

Tharp, R. G. Psychological patterning in marriage. *Psychological Bulletin*, 1963, 60, 97–117. (b)

Thibaut, J. W., & Kelley, H. H. *The Social Psychology of Groups*. New York: John Wiley and Sons, 1959.

Thomas, E. J. *Marital Communication and Decision-Making: Analysis, Assessment and Change*. New York: The Free Press, 1977.

Thomas, W. I., & Thomas, D. S. *The Child in America*. New York; Alfred E. Knopf, 1928.

Thorndike, E. L. Animal intelligence: An experimental study of the associative processes in animals. *Psychological Review: Monograph Supplement*, 1898, 2, Whole No. 8.

Thorne, F. C. *Integrative Psychology*. Brandon, VT: Clinical Psychology Publishing Co., 1967.

Thorne, F. C. *Psychological Case Handling* (Vols. 1 & 2). Brandon, VT: Clinical Psychology Publishing Co., 1968.

Thornton, A. Children and marital stability. *Journal of Marriage and the Family*, 1977, 39, 531–540. (a)

Thornton, A. Decomposing the remarriage process. *Population Studies*, 1977, 31, 283–291. (b)

Tiger, L., & Shepher, J. *Women in the Kibbutz*. New York: Harcourt Brace, 1975.

Tinker, R. H. Dominance in marital interaction. *Proceedings, 81st Annual Convention*, American Psychological Association, Washington, DC, 1973.

Tolman, E. C. *Purpose Behavior in Animals and Man*. New York; Appleton, 1932.

Torrey, E. F. *The Mind Game: Witchdoctors and Psychiatrists*. New York: Emerson Hall Publishers, 1972.

Trotta, M. *Labor Arbitration: Principles, Practices, Issues*. New York: Simmons-Boardman, 1961.

Truax, C., & Wargo, D. Effects of vicarious therapy pretraining and alternate sessions on outcome of group psychotherapy with outpatients. *Journal of Consulting and Clinical Psychology*, 1969, 33, 509–521.

Truax, C. B. Effective ingredients in psychotherapy. *Journal of Counseling Psychology*, 1963, 10, 256–263.

Truax, C. B., & Carkhuff, R. R. *Toward Effective Counseling and Psychotherapy: Training and Practice*. Chicago: Aldine, 1967.

Truax, C. B., & Mitchell, K. M. Research on certain therapist interpersonal skills in relation to process outcome. In A. E. Bergin & S. L. Garfield (Eds.), *Handbook of Psychotherapy and Behavior Change*. New York: John Wiley and Sons, 1971.

Tsoi-Hoshmand, L. The limits of quid pro quo in couple therapy. *The Family Coordinator*, 1975, 24, 51–54.

Tsoi-Hoshmand, L. Marital therapy: An integrative behavioral-learning model. *Journal of Marriage and Family Counseling*, 1976, 2, 179–191.

Tubbs, S. L., & Moss, S. *Human communication: An Interpersonal Perspective*. New York: Random House, 1974.

Tuma, A. H., May, P. R. A., Yale, C., & Forsythe, A. B. Therapist experience, general clinical ability, and treatment outcome in schizophrenia. *Journal of Consulting and Clinical Psychology*, 1978, 46, 1120–1126.

Turk, J. L., & Bell, N. W. Measuring power in families. *Journal of Marriage and the Family*, 1972, 34, 215–222.

Turner, F. B. Common characteristics among people seeking professional marriage counseling. *Marriage and Family Living*, 1954, 16, 143–144.

Turner, J. L., Foa, E. B., & Foa, U. G. Interpersonal reinforcers: Classification, interrelationship, and some differential properties. *Journal of Personality and Social Psychology*, 1971, 19, 168–180.

Turner, R. H. *Family Interaction*. New York: John Wiley and Sons, 1970.

Tuthill, J. F. Impotence. *The Lancet*, 1955, 1, 124–128.

Udry, J. R. *The Social Context of Marriage* (3rd ed.). Philadelphia: J. B. Lippincott Co., 1974.

Udry, J. R., Nelson, H. A., & Nelson, R. O. An empirical investigation of some widely held beliefs about marital interaction. *Marriage and Family Living*, 1961, *23*, 388–390.

Ulrich, R. E., Stachnik, T. J., & Stainton, W. R. Student acceptance of generalized personality interpretations. *Psychological Reports*, 1963, *13*, 831–834.

U.S. Bureau of the Census. *1970 Census of the Population, Volume II:4C. Marital Status*. Washington, DC: U.S. Government Printing Office, 1970.

U.S. Bureau of the Census. *Number, Timing and Duration of Marriages and Divorces in the United States: June 1975*. Current Populations Reports, Series P-20, No. 297, 1976.

U.S. Department of Commerce. *We, the American Young Marrieds*. Washington, DC: Superintendent of Documents, 1973.

U.S. Department of Commerce. *Social Indicators 1976: Selected Data on Trends and Conditions in the United States*. Washington, DC: U.S. Superintendent of Documents, 1977.

U.S. Department of Commerce. *Population Profile of the United States: 1977*. Current Population Reports, Series P-20, No. 423, 1978.

U.S. Public Health Service. *A Concurrent Validational Study of the NCHS General Well-Being Schedule*. Hyattsville, MD: USDHEW Publication No. (HRA) 78-1347, 1977.

Vaihinger, H. *The Philosophy of As-If* (trans. by C. K. Ogden). New York: Scribners, 1924.

Valle, S. K., & Marinelli, R. P. Training in human relations skills as a preferred mode of treatment for married couples. *Journal of Marriage and Family Counseling*, 1975, *1*, 359–365.

van der Veen, F. *Content Dimensions of the Family Concept*. Paper presented at the meeting of the American Psychological Association, Washington, DC, 1971.

Veevers, J. E. The moral careers of voluntary childless wives: Notes on the defense of a variant world view. *The Family Coordinator*, 1975, *24*, 473–488.

Venema, H. B. Marriage enrichment: A comparison of the behavioral exchange negotiation and communication models. *Dissertation Abstracts International*, 1976, *36*, 4184–4185.

Veroff, J., & Feld, S. *Marriage and Work in America: A Study of Motives and Roles*. New York: Van Nostrand Reinhold Co., 1970.

Vincent, C. E. Barriers to the development of marital health as a health field. *Journal of Marriage and Family Counseling*, 1977, *3*(3), 3–11.

Vincent, J. P., Weiss, R. L., & Birchler, G. R. A behavioral analysis of problem solving in distressed and nondistressed married and stranger dyads. *Behavior Therapy*, 1975, *6*, 475–487.

Von Bertalanffy, L. An outline of general systems theory. *British Journal of Philosophy of Science*, 1950, *1*, 134–165.

Von Bertalanffy, L. *General Systems Theory*. New York: George Braziller, 1968.

Wallace, D., & Rothaus, P. Communication, group loyalty, and trust in the PD game. *Journal of Conflict Resolution*, 1969, *13*, 370–380.

Wallach, M. S., & Strupp, H. H. Dimensions of psychotherapists' activities. *Journal of Consulting Psychology*, 1964, *28*, 120–125.

Waller, W. *The Family: A Dynamic Interpretation*. New York: Cordon Co., 1938.

Wallerstein, J. S., & Kelly, J. B. The effects of parental divorce: Experiences of the child in later latency. *American Journal of Orthopsychiatry*, 1976, *46*, 256–269.

Walster, E., & Walster, G. W. *A New Look at Love*. Reading, MA: Addison-Wesley Publishing Co., 1978.

Warren, N., & Rice, L. Structuring and stabilizing of psychotherapy for low-prognosis clients. *Journal of Consulting and Clinical Psychology*, 1972, *39*, 173–181.

Waskow, I. E., & Parloff, M. B. *Psychotherapy Change Measures: Report of the Clinical Branch Outcome Measures Project*. Rockville, MD: DHEW Publication No. (ADM) 74-120, 1975.

Wattie, B. Evaluating short-term casework in a family agency. *Social Casework*, 1973, *54*, 608–616.

Watzlawick, P. *An Anthology of Human Communication*. Palo Alto, CA: Science and Behavior Books, 1964.

Watzlawick, P. The psychotherapeutic technique of "reframing." In J. L. Claghorn (Ed.), *Successful Psychotherapy*. New York: Brunner/Mazel, 1976.

Watzlawick, P. The utopia syndrome. In P. Watzlawick & J. H. Weakland (Eds.), *The Interactional View: Studies at the Mental Research Institute, Palo Alto, 1965-1974*. New York: W. W. Norton, 1977.

Watzlawick, P., & Beavin, J. Some formal aspects of communication. In P. Watzlawick & J. H. Weakland (Eds.), *The Interactional View: Studies at the Mental Research Institute, Palo Alto, 1965-1974*. New York: W. W. Norton, 1974.

Watzlawick, P., & Weakland, J. H. (Eds.). *The Interactional View: Studies at the Mental Research Institute, Palo Alto, 1965-1974*. New York: W. W. Norton, 1977.

Watzlawick, P., Beavin, J. H., & Jackson, D. D. *Pragmatics of Human Communication: A Study of Interactional Patterns, Pathologies, and Paradoxes*. New York: W. W. Norton, 1967.

Watzlawick, P., Beavin, J., Sikorski, L., & Mecia, B. Protection and scapegoating in pathological families. *Family Process*, 1970, *9*, 27-39.

Watzlawick, P., Weakland, J. H., & Fisch, R. *Change: Principles of Problem Formation and Problem Resolution*. New York: W. W. Norton, 1974.

Weakland, J. H., Fisch, R., Watzlawick, P., & Bodin, A. M. Brief therapy: Focused problem resolution. *Family Process*, 1974, *13*, 141-168. (Also in P. Watzlawick & J. H. Weakland [Eds.], *The Interactional View: Studies at the Mental Research Institute, Palo Alto, 1965-1974*. New York: W. W. Norton, 1977.)

Weed, L. L. Medical records that guide and teach. *New England Journal of Medicine*, 1968, *278*, 593-600, 652-657.

Wegner, D. M., & Vallacher, R. R. *Implicit Psychology: An Introduction to Social Cognition*. New York: Oxford University Press, 1977.

Weick, K. E. Task acceptance dilemmas: A site for research on cognition. In S. Feldman (Ed.), *Cognitive Consistency*. New York: Academic Press, 1966.

Weick, K. E. Group processes, family processes, and problem solving. In J. Aldous, T. Condon, R. Hill, M. Strauss, & I. Tallman (Eds.), *Family Problem Solving: A Symposium on Theoretical Methodological, and Substantive Concerns*. Hinsdale, IL: Dryden Press, 1971.

Weil, M. Extramarital relationships: A reappraisal. *Journal of Clinical Psychology*, 1975, *3*, 723-725.

Weiner, B. *Theories of Motivation*. Chicago: Markham, 1972.

Weiss, R. L., & Isaac, J. *Behavior vs. Cognitive Measures as Predictors of Marital Satisfaction*. Paper presented at the Western Psychological Association Meeting, Los Angeles, April 1976.

Weiss, R. L., & Margolin, G. Assessment of marital conflict and accord. In A. R. Ciminero, K. S. Calhoun, & H. E. Adams (Eds.), *Handbook of Behavioral Assessment*. New York: John Wiley and Sons, 1977.

Weiss, R. L., Hops, H., & Patterson, G. R. A framework for conceptualizing marital conflict: A technology for altering it, some data for evaluating it. In L. A. Hamerlynck, L. C. Handy, & E. J. Mash (Eds.), *Behavior Change: Methodology, Concepts and Practice*. Champaign, IL: Research Press, 1973.

Weiss, R. L., Birchler, G. R., & Vincent, J. P. Contractual models for negotiation training in marital dyads. *Journal of Marriage and the Family*, 1974, *36*, 321-330.

Weissman, M. M., & Myers, J. K. Rates and risks of depressive symptoms in a United States urban community. *Acta Psychiatrica Scandinavia*, 1978, *57*, 219-231.

Weitzman, L. J. To love, honor, and obey? Traditional legal marriage and alternative family forms. *The Family Coordinator*, 1975, *24*, 531-548.

Wells, J. G. A critical look at personal marriage contracts. *The Family Coordinator*, 1976, *25*, 33-37.

Wener, A. E., & Rehm, L. P. Depressive affect: A test of behavioral hypotheses. *Journal of Abnormal Psychology*, 1975, *84*, 221-227.

Werner, C., & Latane, B. Responsiveness and communication medium in dyadic interaction. *Bulletin of the Psychonomic Society*, 1976, *8*, 569-571.

Wertheim, E. The science and typology of family systems. II. Further theoretical and practice considerations. *Family Process*, 1975, *14*, 285-310.

White, R. W. *The Abnormal Personality*. New York: The Roland Press, 1956.

Wieman, R. J., Shoulders, D. I., & Farr, J. H. Reciprocal reinforcement in marital therapy. *Journal of Behavior Therapy and Experimental Psychiatry*, 1974, *5*, 291-295.

Wiener, H. *The Human Use of Human Beings: Cybernetics and Society*. New York: Doubleday Paperback, 1954.

Wile, D. B. Personality styles and therapy styles. *Psychotherapy: Theory, Research and Practice*, 1976, *13*, 303-307.

Wile, D. B. Ideological conflicts between clients and psychotherapists. *American Journal of Psychotherapy*, 1977, *31*, 437-449.

Wilkening, E. A., & Bharadwaj, L. K. Dimensions of aspirations, work roles and decision-making of farm husbands and wives in Wisconsin. *Journal of Marriage and the Family*, 1967, *29*, 703-711.

Wilkins, W. Expectancy of therapeutic gain: An empirical and conceptual critique. *Journal of Consulting and Clinical Psychology*, 1973, *40*, 69-77.

Williams, L. K., Hoffman, R., & Mann, F. An investigation of the control graph: Influence in a staff organization. *Social Forces*, 1959, *37*, 189-195.

Williams, R. *American Society: A Sociological Interpretation*. New York: Alfred A. Knopf, 1951.

Williams, R. M. Values. In E. Sills (Ed.), *International Encyclopedia of the Social Sciences*. New York: Macmillan Co., 1968.

Willis, R. H. Conformity, independence, and anticonformity. *Human Relations*, 1965, *18*, 373-388.

Wills, T. A., Weiss, R. L., & Patterson, G. R. *A Behavioral Analysis of the Determinants of Marital Satisfaction*. Paper presented at the Annual Meeting of the Western Psychological Association, Portland, OR, April 1972.

Wills, T. A., Weiss, R. L., & Patterson, G. R. A behavioral analysis of the determinants of marital satisfaction. *Journal of Consulting and Clinical Psychology*, 1974, *42*, 802-811.

Wilson, W. Cooperation and the cooperativeness of the other player. *Journal of Conflict Resolution*, 1969, *13*, 110-117.

Wilson, W., & Insko, C. Recency effects in face-to-face interaction. *Journal of Personality and Social Psychology*, 1968, *9*, 21-23.

Wincze, J. P., & Caird, W. K. *The Effects of Systematic Desensitization and Video Desensitization in the Treatment of Essential Sexual Dysfunction in Women*. Paper presented at convention of the Association for the Advancement of Behavior Therapy, Miami, 1973.

Wincze, J. P., & Caird, W. K. The effects of systematic desensitization and video desensitization in the treatment of essential sexual dysfunction in women. *Behavior Therapy*, 1976, *7*, 335-342.

Winter, W. D., Ferreira, A. J., & Bowers, N. Decision-making in married and unrelated couples. *Family Process*, 1973, *12*, 83-94.

Wolberg, L. R. Methodology in short-term therapy. *American Journal of Psychiatry*, 1965, *122*, 135-140.

Wolberg, L. R. Methodology in short-term psychotherapy. In H. H. Barten (Ed.), *Brief Therapies*. New York: Behavioral Publications, 1971.

Wolf, H. F. *Philosophy for the Common Man*. New York: Philosophical Library, 1951.

Wolgast, E. H. Do husbands or wives make the purchasing decisions? *Journal of Marketing*, 1958, *23*, 151-158.

Wolpe, J. *Psychotherapy by Reciprocal Inhibition*. Palo Alto, CA: Stanford University Press, 1958.

Woodworth, R. S., & Schlosberg, H. *Experimental Psychology.* New York: Holt, 1954.

Worchel, P., & Schuster, S. D. Attraction as a function of drive state. *Journal of Experimental Research in Personality,* 1966, *1,* 277–281.

Wright, G. C., & Stetson, D. M. The impact of no-fault divorce law reform on divorce in American states. *Journal of Marriage and the Family,* 1978, *40,* 575–580.

Wrong, D. H. Some problems in defining social power. *American Journal of Sociology,* 1968, *73,* 673–681.

Yalom, D. D., & Lieberman, M. A. A study of encounter group casualties. *Archives of General Psychiatry,* 1971, *25*(1), 16–30.

Yalom, I. *Theory and Practice of Group Psychotherapy.* New York: Basic Books, 1970.

Young, R. E., Becker, A. L., & Pike, K. L. *Rhetoric: Discovery and Change.* New York: Harcourt, Brace and World, 1970.

Yulis, S. Generalization of therapeutic gain in the treatment of premature ejaculation. *Behavior Therapy,* 1976, *7,* 355–358.

Zeiss, A. M., Rosen, G. M., & Zeiss, R. A. Orgasm during intercourse: A treatment strategy for women. *Journal of Consulting and Clinical Psychology,* 1977, *45*(5), 891–895.

Zeiss, R. A. Self-directed treatment for premature ejaculation: Preliminary case reports. *Journal of Behavior Therapy and Experimental Psychiatry,* 1977, *8,* 87–91.

Zeiss, R. A., & Zeiss, A. M. *Prolong Your Pleasure.* New York: Pocket Books, 1978.

Zeiss, R. A., Christensen, A., & Levine, A. G. Treatment for premature ejaculation through male-only groups. *Journal of Sex and Marital Therapy,* 1978, *4,* 139–143.

Zilbergeld, B. Group treatment of sexual dysfunction in men without partners. *Journal of Sex and Marital Therapy,* 1975, *1,* 204–214.

Zilbergeld, B. *Male Sexuality.* Boston: Little, Brown and Co., 1978.

Zimbardo, P. G. The cognitive control of motivation. *Transactions of the New York Academy of Sciences,* 1966, *28,* 902–922.

Zimbardo, P. G. *The Cognitive Control of Motivation.* Glenview, IL: Scott, Foresman, 1969.

Zubin, J. Discussion of symposium on newer approaches to personality assessment. *Journal of Personality Assessment,* 1972, *36,* 427–434.

Zuk, G. H. The go-between process in family therapy. *Family Process,* 1966, *5,* 163–178.

Zuk, G. H. Family therapy. *Archives of General Psychiatry,* 1967, *16,* 71–79.

Zuk, G. H. *Process and Practice in Family Therapy.* Haverford, PA: Psychiatry and Behavior Science Books, 1975.

Zuk, G. H. Family therapy: Clinical hodgepodge or clinical science? *Journal of Marriage and Family Counseling,* 1976, *2,* 299–303.

Zuk, G. H. Values and family therapy. *Psychotherapy: Theory, Research and Practice,* 1978, *15,* 48–55.

Zung, W. W. K. A self-rating depression scale. *Archives of General Psychiatry,* 1965, *12,* 63–70.

AUTHOR INDEX

Boldface page numbers indicate material in tables and figures.

S U B J E C T   I N D E X

Boldface page numbers indicate material in tables and figures.

U.S. Public Health Service, 106, **131**
Utility, subjective expected, 257
Utopia syndrome, 54

Vaginal dilation, 148, 149, 348, 349
Vaginal orgasm, 351
Vaginismus, treatment of, 311, 315, 317, 347–351
Validation (*see also* Goals of therapy, values/
        philosophy in)
    in communication, 235
    consensual, 70
    convergent, 64
Values
    and action, 22
    clarification of, 93
    and culture, 286
    and religion, 100, 101
    and science, 62
    and therapeutic practice, 22–25

Venn diagrams, 293
Veterans Administration, 140
Vibrators and sexuality, 334, 352
Videotapes
    for communication exercises, 96
    for desensitization, 344
    for psychotherapy, 161
    for sex education, 355, 356
Vital marriage, 100

Widows, **9**, **10**, **12**
Willingness-to-Change Questionnaire, 90, **124**
Win–lose trap, 292

Yohimbine, 333
Young's rectal dilators, 350

Zero-sum games, 292
Zung Self-Rating Depression Scale, 106